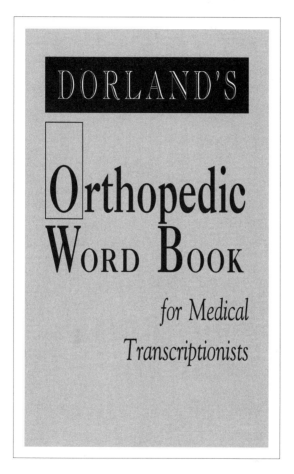

DORLAND'S

Orthopedic Word Book

for Medical Transcriptionists

DORLAND'S

Orthopedic WORD BOOK

for Medical Transcriptionists

Series Editor
SHARON B. RHODES, CMT, RHIT

Edited & Reviewed by:
Arlaine Walsh, CMT

W.B. SAUNDERS COMPANY
A Harcourt Health Sciences Company

Philadelphia London New York St. Louis Sydney Toronto

W.B. Saunders Company
A Harcourt Health Sciences Company

The Curtis Center
Independence Square West
Philadelphia, Pennsylvania 19106

Library of Congress Cataloging-in-Publication Data

Dorland's orthopedic word book for medical transcriptionists / Sharon Rhodes,
Arlaine Walsh, editors.—1st ed.

p. cm.

ISBN 0-7216-9390-3

1. Orthopedics—Terminology. 2. Medical transcription—Terminology. I. Title:
   Orthopedic word book for medical transcriptionist. II. Rhodes, Sharon
   B. III. Walsh, Arlaine.

RD723.D668 2002

616.7′01′4—dc21   2001034185

Dorland's Orthopedic Word Book for
Medical Transcriptionists   ISBN 0-7216-9390-3

Printed in the United States of America.

Last digit is the print number: 9 8 7 6 5 4 3 2 1

PREFACE

I am proud to present the *Dorland's Orthopedic Word Book for Medical Transcriptionists* — one of the ongoing series of word books being compiled for the professional medical transcriptionist. For over one hundred years, W.B. Saunders has published the *Dorland's Illustrated Medical Dictionary*. With the advent of medical transcription, it became the dictionary of choice for medical transcriptionists.

When I was approached in the fall of 1999 to help develop a new series of word books for W.B. Saunders, I have to admit the thought absolutely overwhelmed me. The *Dorland's Illustrated Medical Dictionary* was one of my first book purchases when I began my transcription career over thirty years ago. To be invited to participate in this project is an honor I could never have imagined for myself!

Transcriptionists need and will continue to need trusted up-to-date resources to help them research difficult terms quickly. In developing the *Dorland's Orthopedic Word Book for Medical Transcriptionists*, I had access to the entire *Dorland's* terminology database for the book's foundation. In addition to this immense database, a context editor, Arlaine Walsh, CMT, a recognized leader in the field of medical transcription, was selected to review the material from the database, to contribute new and unique terms, and to remove outdated and obsolete ones. With Arlaine's extensive research and diligent work, I believe this to be the most up-to-date word book for the field of orthopedics.

In developing the orthopedic word book, I wanted the size to be manageable so the book would be easy to handle, provide a durable long-lasting binding, and use a type font large enough to read while providing extensive terminology.

Anatomical plates were added as well as identification of anatomical landmarks. Additionally, a list of the most frequently prescribed drugs has been included.

Although I have tried to produce the most thorough word book for orthopedics available to medical transcriptionists, it is difficult to include every term as the field of medicine is constantly evolving. As you discover new terms, please feel free to share them with me for inclusion in the next edition of the *Dorland's Orthopedic Word Book for Medical Transcriptionists.*

I may be reached at the following e-mail address: Sharon@TheRhodes.com.

SHARON B. RHODES, CMT, RHIT
Brentwood, Tennessee

A
A band
A disk

AAA bone

AAI
activating adjusting instrument

AAROM
active ankle joint complex range of motion

AB/AD
abductor/adductor
AB/AD ratio

A band

ABAQUS modeling program

abarthrosis

abarticular

abarticulation

Abbe operation

Abbott
A. brace
A. gouge
A. knee approach
A. method
A. splint
A.-Carpenter posterior approach
A.-Fisher-Lucas hip arthrodesis
A.-Gill epiphyseal plate exposure
A.-Gill epiphysiodesis
A.-Gill osteotomy
A.-Lucas arthrodesis
A.-Lucas shoulder operation

ABC
aneurysmal bone cyst

ABD
abduction

abduct

abduction (ABD)
a. contracture
hip a.
humerothoracic a.

abductor
a. digiti quinti (ADQ)
a. hallucis
hyperdynamic a. hallucis

Abernethy fascia

ABI
ankle-brachial index

ablation
cartilage a.

abscess
arthrifluent a.
bone a.
Brodie a.
button a.
growth-plate a.
horseshoe a.
intraosseous a.
midpalmar a.
paraspinal a.
paravertebral a.
Pott a.
psoas a.
retrosternal a.
spinal a.
subaponeurotic a.
subfascial a.
subgaleal a.
subperiosteal a.
subphrenic a.
syphilitic a.
thecal a.

absorptiometry
dual-energy x-ray a. (DEXA)
peripheral dual-energy x-ray a. (pDEXA)

absorption
bone a.
bony a.
shock a.
Weber-Vasey traction-a.

1

abut

abutment
    ulnocarpal a.

abutted

abutting

AC
    acromioclavicular
        AC arthroplasty
        AC articulation
        AC injury classification
        AC joint
        AC joint separation
        AC ligament
        AC separation

ACA
    American Chiropractic Association

acampsia

acantha

acanthoma

acceleration/deceleration injury

accelerator
    linear a. (LINAC)

Access Ostase blood test

access
    eccentric a. of ankle rotation

accessiflexor

accessoria
    ossa carpalia a.

accessorius
    talus a.

accessory
    a. atlantoaxial ligament
    a. bone
    a. collateral ligament
    a. communicating tendon
    a. digit
    a. lateral collateral ligament

accessory *(continued)*
    a. motion
    a. movement technique
    a. navicular cast
    a. ossicle
    a. ossification center of calcaneus
    a. phalanx
    a. sesamoid

accommodation
    a. curve
    a. reflex

accommodative
    a. brace
    a. orthosis

Accu-Back back support

Accuflate tourniquet

Accu-Flo
    A. polyethylene bur hole cover
    A. silicone rubber bur hole cover
    A. ultrafiltration system

Acculength arthroplasty measuring system

Accu-Line
    A. dual pivot
    A. femoral resector
    A. guide
    A. knee instrumentation
    A. tibial resector

AccuPressure heel cup

ACDF
    anterior cervical diskectomy and fusion

Ace
    A. bandage reduction
    A. Unifix fixation
    A.-Colles fracture frame
    A.-Fisher fixation

acetabula *(plural of* acetabulum)

acetabular
    a. allograft
    a. angle of Sharp
    a. augmentation graft
    a. component
    a. cup arthroplasty
    a. cup peg drill guide
    a. cup template
    a. endoprosthesis
    a. extensile approach
    a. gauge
    a. labrum
    a. osteolysis
    a. posterior wall fracture
    a. prosthesis
    a. prosthetic interface
    a. prosthetic liner
    a. protrusio deformity
    a. reamer
    a. rim fracture
    a. seating hole
    a. spacer
    a. trial set

acetabulectomy

acetabuli
    ligamentum transversum a.

acetabuloplasty
    Albee a.
    Pemberton a.
    shelf a.

acetabulum *pl.* acetabula
    deep-shelled a.
    dysplastic a.
    floor of the a.
    intrapelvic protrusio aceta-
        buli
    malunited a.
    protrusio acetabuli
    transverse ligament of a.
    true a.
    weightbearing dome of a.

ACF
    anterior cervical fusion

achilleocalcaneal
    a. plantar system

achilleocalcaneal *(continued)*
    a. vascular network

Achilles
    A. bulge sign
    bursa of A. tendon
    A. heel pad
    A. jerk
    A. peritendinitis
    A. squeeze test
    A. tendinitis
    A. tendon (AT)
    A. tendon advancement
    A. tendon lengthening
    A. tendon reflex
    A. tendon repair
    A. tendon rupture (ATR)
    A. tenotomy

Achillis
    tendo A.

achillobursitis

achillodynia
    Albert a.

achillorrhaphy

achillotenotomy

Achillotrain active Achilles ten-
    don support

achondroplasia

achondroplastic dwarfism

Ackerman criteria for osteomy-
    elitis

ACL
    anterior cruciate ligament
        Cincinnati ACL brace
        ACL drill
        ACL drill guide
        ACL graft
        ACL graft knife
        Pinn ACL guide system
        ACL reconstruction
        ACL repair

Acland
    A. clamp

Acland *(continued)*
    A. clamp-applying forceps
    A. clamp approximator

aclasis
    diaphyseal a.
    tarsoepiphyseal a.

ACLR
    anterior capsulolabral reconstruction

acorn
    Midas Rex a.
    a. reamer

acoustic myography

ACP
    anterior cervical plate

Acra-Cut wire pass drill

Acrel ganglion

ACRM
    American College of Rehabilitative Medicine

acrocontracture

acrodysesthesia

acrokinesia

AcroMed
    A. screw
    A. VSP fixation system
    A. VSP plate

acromial
    a. angle
    a. spur
    a. spur index (ASI)

acromiale
    os a.

acromioclavicular (AC)
    a. arthroplasty
    a. articulation
    a. injury classification
    a. joint
    a. joint separation
    a. ligament
    a. separation

acromioclaviculare
    ligamentum a.

acromiocoracoid ligament

acromiohumeral
    a. interval (AHI)

acromion
    nonunion of a.

acromionectomy
    Armstrong a.

acromioplasty
    anterior a.
    arthroscopic a.
    decompressive a.
    McLaughlin a.
    McShane-Leinberry-Fenlin a.
    Neer a.
    Rockwood anterior a.

acromioscapular

acromyotonia

acromyotonus

acro-osteolysis

acro-osteosclerosis

acropachy

acropachyderma
    a. with pachyperiostitis

acropectorovertebral dysplasia

acrostealgia

acrylic
    a. bone cement
    a. cap splint
    a. orthotic device
    a. template splint

Acryl-X

ACS
    anterior compartment syndrome

ACSM
    American College of Sports Medicine

Acthar

actinic keratosis

actinomycosis

activating adjusting instrument
  (AAI)

activation
  latency of a.
  order of a.

active
  a. ankle joint complex
    range of motion (AAROM)
  a. integral range of motion
    (AIROM)
  a. knee extension (AKE)
  a. motion testing (AMT)
  a. and passive range of mo-
    tion
  a. range of movement
  a. range of motion exer-
    cises
  a. release technique (ART)

active-assisted
  a.-a. range of motion
  a.-a. range of motion exer-
    cise

active-assistive

Activella

activity
  biphasic endplate a.
  cingulate gyrus a.
  a. configuration
  a's of daily living (ADL)
  diversional a.
  endplate a.
  functional a.
  increased insertional a.
  insertion a.
  A. Losses Assessment
    (ALA)
  monophasic endplate a.
  opsonic a.
  a.-pattern analysis
  pivoting and cutting a.
  push-pull a.

activity *(continued)*
  sudomotor a.
  volitional a.

actual leg length test

actuator
  NYU-Hosmer electric elbow
    and prehension a.

ACU-derm wound dressing

AcuDriver osteotome

ACU-dyne antiseptic

Acufex
  A. ankle distractor
  A. arthroscopic instrumen-
    tation
  A. curet
  A. distractor pin
  A. double-lumen arthro-
    scopic cannula
  A. gouge
  A. grasper
  A. MosaicPlasty compre-
    hensive system
  A. osteotome
  A. TAG rod
  A. tibial guide

Acuflex

AcuMatch (femoral hip prosthe-
  sis)
  A. A Series
  A. L Series
  A. M Series

Adair Dighton syndrome

Adair screw compressor

adamantinoma

Adams
  A. forward-bending test
  A. hip operation
  A. position test
  A. procedure
  A. saw
  A. scoliosis test
  A. splint

Adams *(continued)*
    A. transmalleolar arthrodesis
    A. view

adapter *(variant of* adaptor*)*

Adapteur multi-functional drill guide

Adaptic
    A. dressing

adaptive equipment

adaptor *(spelled also* adapter*)*
    Christmas tree a.
    chuck a.
    Collet screwdriver a.
    French a.
    Grace plate 4-hole a.
    Hudson chuck a.
    Jacobs chuck a.
    Lloyd a.
    Mayfield a.
    SACH foot a.

ADD
    adduction

adduction (ADD) *(sometimes dictated* "a-d-duction"*)*
    a. contracture
    Edgarton-Grand thumb a.
    flexion-a.
    a. fracture
    a. osteotomy
    a. traction technique

adductocavus
    metatarsus a.

adductor
    a. aponeurosis
    a. hallucis longus
    a. hallucis tendon
    a. longus muscle rupture
    a. magnus
    a. magnus a. flap
    a. pollicis brevis tendon
    a. pollicis muscle
    a. tendon and lateral capsule release

adductor *(continued)*
    a. tenotomy and obturator neurectomy (ATON)

adductovarus
    metatarsus a. (MTA)
    true metatarsus a. (TMA)

adductus
    congenital metatarsus a.
    dynamic metatarsus a.
    forefoot a.
    metatarsus a. (MTA)
    metatarsus primus a. (MPA)
    midfoot a.
    pes equinovarus a.
    true metatarsus a. (TMA)

adenine arabinoside (ara-A)

adenosine thallium scan

adhesion
    filmy a.
    intraarticular a.
    subacromial bursal a.
    subdeltoid bursal a.

adhesive
    APR cement fixation a.
    Aron Alpha a.
    Biobrane a.
    a. capsulitis
    Coe-pak a.
    Coverlet a.
    cyanoacrylate a.
    fibrin glue a.
    Histoacryl glue a.
    hydroxyapatite a.
    Implast a.
    ligand a.
    LLPS hydroxyapatite a.
    methyl methacrylate a.
    Orthomite II a.
    Palacos cement a.
    Surfit a.
    Zimmer low viscosity a.

adipofascial flap

adiposis dolorosa

A disk

ADJ
adjustable dynamic joint

Adjusta-Wrist
A. hinge
A. splint

ADK
Automated Disposable Keratome

Adkins
A. spinal arthrodesis
A. spinal fusion

ADL
activities of daily living

Adlone Injection

ADM
abductor digiti minimi

adolescent
a. idiopathic scoliosis (AIS)
a. kyphosis
a. scoliosis

adrenocorticotropic hormone
(ACTH)

ADQ
abductor digiti quinti

adrenergic vagal function

adrenoleukodystrophy (ADL)

ADROM
ankle dorsiflexion range of
motion

Adson
A. bur
A. cerebellar retractor
A. drill guide
A. drill guide forceps
A. hemilaminectomy retractor
A. hypophyseal forceps
A. laminectomy chisel
A. maneuver

Adson (continued)
A. maneuver test
A. periosteal elevator
A. rongeur
A. saw guide
A. sign
A. spiral drill
A. suction tube
A. test
A. twist drill
A.-Rogers perforating drill

ADT
anterior drawer test

advancement
Achilles tendon a.
Atasoy V-Y a.
calcaneonavicular liga-
ment–tibialis posterior
tendon a.
Chandler patellar a.
en bloc a.
a. flap
heel cord a. (HCA)
Johnson pronator a.
Lloyd-Roberts-Swann tro-
chanteric a.
Maquet a.
Murphy heel cord a.
patellar a.
plantar calcaneonavicular
ligament–tibialis poste-
rior tendon a.
profundus a.
trochanteric a.
vastus medialis a. (VMA)
Wagner profundus a.
Wagner trochanteric a.

adventitia

adventitial

adventitious

A-E, AE
above-elbow
A-E amputation

AEP
auditory evoked potential

AER
    abduction-external rotation

Aeroaid

Aeroplast dressing

Aesculap
    A. bipolar cautery
    A. clamp
    A. drill
    A. forceps
    A. head holder
    A. saw
    A.-PM noncemented femoral prosthesis

affection
    patellar a.

AFI total hip replacement prosthesis

Aflexa

AFO
    ankle-foot orthosis
        articulated AFO
        AFO brace sock
        Type C-50, C-90 AFO

Aftate

afterpotential
    negative a.
    positive a.

AGC
    anatomically graduated component
        AGC Biomet total knee system
        AGC femoral prosthesis
        AGC knee prosthesis
        AGC tibial prosthesis

AGE
    angle of greatest extension

Agee
    A. carpal tunnel release system

Agee (continued)
    A. force-couple splint reduction
    A. 4-pin fixation device
    A. WristJack external fixator
    A. WristJack fracture reduction system

agenesis
    Bayne classification of radial a.
    caudal-spinal a.
    radial a.
    sacral a.

agenetic fracture

agent
    antiosteoclastic a.
    chondroprotective a.
    chymopapain blocking a.
    nociceptor a.
    phlogistic a.
    uricosuric a.

AGF
    angle of greatest flexion

Aggressor device

Agliette
    A. measurement
    A. supracondylar osteotomy

Agnew splint

Ahern trochanteric débridement

AHI
    acromiohumeral interval
    Arthritis Helplessness Index

AHO
    acute hematogenesis osteomyelitis

AHSC
    Arizona Health Science Center
        AHSC elbow prosthesis

AHSC *(continued)*
  AHSC-Volz elbow prosthesis
  AHSC-Volz hinge

A-hydroCort

AIIS
  anterior inferior iliac spine
  AIIS avulsion fracture

Aiken osteotomy

AIM
  Ace intramedullary
  AIM CPM (continuous passive motion)
  AIM femoral nail system

aimer
  Arthrotek femoral a.
  tibial a.

AIMS
  Arthritis Impact Measurement Scale

Ainslie acrylic splint

Aircast
  A. Air-Stirrup brace
  A. ankle brace
  A. Cryo/Cuff
  A. Stirrup
  A. Swivel-Strap
  A. Swivel-Strap brace

Airex
  A. balance pad
  A. mat

Airfoam splint

AirGEL ankle brace

Air-Limb

AirLITE support pad

AIROM
  active integral range of motion

Air-Soft splint

AirStance pylon

Air-Stirrup ankle brace

AIS
  Abbreviated Injury Scale
  adolescent idiopathic scoliosis

AITA modular trauma system

Aitken
  A. classification of epiphyseal fracture
  A. femoral deficiency
  A. hip class

AJ
  ankle jerk

AJC
  ankle joint complex

A-K, AK
  above-knee
  A-K amputation

AKA
  above-knee-amputation

AKE
  active knee extension
  AKE test

Akin
  A. bunionectomy
  chevron-A. double osteotomy
  distal A. phalangeal osteotomy
  A. operation
  A. proximal phalangeal osteotomy

ALA
  Activity Losses Assessment

ala *pl.* alae
  sacral a.

Alanson
  A. amputation
  A. amputation technique

Albee
  A. acetabuloplasty
  A. hip arthrodesis

Albee *(continued)*
    A. olive-shaped bur
    A. operation
    A. osteotome
    A.-Delbet operation

Albers-Schönberg marble bone

Albert
    A. achillodynia
    A. operation

Albinus muscle

Albright
    A. dystrophy
    A. osteodystrophy
    A. syndrome
    A.-McCune-Sternberg syndrome

Alexander
    A. chisel
    A. costal periosteotome
    A. periosteal elevator
    A. technique
    A.-Farabeuf periosteotome

Alexian Brothers overhead frame

Alginate dressing

algodystrophy syndrome

aligner
    Charnley femoral inlay a.
    femoral a.
    patellar a.
    tibial a.

alignment
    extramedullary a.

Aliplast pad

ALL
    anterior longitudinal ligament

Allen
    A. arthroscopic elbow positioner
    A. arthroscopic knee positioner

Allen *(continued)*
    A. arthroscopic wrist positioner
    A. head screwdriver
    A. maneuver
    A. open reduction of calcaneal fracture
    A. shoulder arthroscopy
    A. sign
    A. test
    A. wrench
    A.-Brown prosthesis
    A.-Ferguson Galveston pelvic fixation
    A.-Kocher clamp

Allevyn wound dressing

Allgower suture technique

alligator grasping forceps

Allis
    A. clamp
    A. maneuver
    A. sign
    A. test
    A. tissue forceps

AllMed PF

AlloAnchor RC

allodynia

Allofix cortical bone pin

allogenic bone graft

allogenous bone graft

allograft
    acetabular a.
    bone a.
    bone-tendon-bone a.
    femoral cortical ring a.
    femoral diaphyseal a.
    MTE a.
    osteochondral a.

AlloGrip bone vise

AlloMatrix injectable putty

Allo-Pro hip system

alloy
>cobalt-based a.
>cobalt-chromium a.
>Elgiloy metal a.
>stainless steel a.
>Ti-6A1-4V a.
>Ti-Nidium a.
>titanium a.
>Vitallium a.
>Wood a.

Allplast

Allport retractor

Alouette
>A. amputation
>A. operation

Alpha-BSM

ALPS
>anterior locking plate system
>>Amset ALPS

ALPSA
>anterior labrum periosteum shoulder arthroscopic lesion
>>ALPSA lesion

ALRI
>anterolateral rotary instability
>>ALRI test

Alsberg
>A. angle
>A. triangle

Alta
>A. cancellous screw
>A. CFX reconstruction rod
>A. cortical screw
>A. cross-locking screw
>A. lag screw
>A. modular trauma system
>A. screw
>A. tibial-humeral rod
>A. tibial nail
>A. transverse screw

altitudinal anopsia

Alumafoam splint

Alvar
>A. bolt
>A. condylar bolt

Alznner orthosis

amalgam

AMBI
>AMBI compression hip screw
>AMBI fixation
>AMBI hip screw

Ambulator shoes

AMD
>arthroscopic microdiskectomy
>articular motion device

AME bone growth stimulator

Amfit
>A. custom orthosis
>A. digitizer
>A. orthosis

Amici
>A. disk
>line of A.
>striae of A.

AML trial hip component

Amoss sign

amphiarthrodial disk

amphiarthrosis

Amplatz anchor system

amputation
>above-elbow (A-E) a.
>above-knee (A-K) a.
>Alanson a.
>Alouette a.
>aperiosteal a.
>Béclard a.
>below-elbow (B-E) a.

amputation *(continued)*
  below-knee (B-K) a.
  Berger interscapular a.
  Bier a.
  border ray a.
  Bunge a.
  Burgess below-knee a.
  button toe a.
  Callander a.
  Carden a.
  central a.
  chop a.
  Chopart hindfoot a.
  cineplastic a.
  circular a.
  circular supracondylar a.
  closed a.
  closed-flap a.
  coat-sleeve a.
  a. in contiguity
  a. in continuity
  corporectomy a.
  cutaneous a.
  Dieffenbach a.
  disarticular a.
  double-flap a.
  Dupuytren a.
  eccentric a.
  elliptic a.
  fishmouth a.
  forefoot digital a.
  forequarter a.
  Gordon-Taylor hindquarter a.
  Gritti a.
  Gritti-Stokes a.
  guillotine a.
  Hancock a.
  hand a.
  Hey a.
  hindquarter a.
  interilioabdominal a.
  interinnominoabdominal a.
  interpelviabdominal a.
  interscapulothoracic a.
  Jaboulay a.
  kineplastic a.
  Kirk a.
  Langenbeck a.

amputation *(continued)*
  Larrey a.
  Le Fort a.
  linear a.
  Lisfranc a.
  MacKenzie a.
  McKittrick transmetatarsal a.
  Maisonneuve a.
  major a.
  Malgaigne a.
  mediotarsal a.
  minor a.
  mixed a.
  modified Boyd a. of ankle and distal tibial physis
  musculocutaneous a.
  oblique a.
  open a.
  osteoplastic a.
  oval a.
  periosteoplastic a.
  phalangophalangeal a.
  Pirogoff a.
  ray a.
  racket a.
  rectangular a.
  Ricard a.
  spontaneous a.
  Stokes a.
  subastragalar a.
  subperiosteal a.
  Syme a.
  Teale a.
  transfemoral a.
  a. by transfixion
  transmetatarsal a.
  transtibial a.
  traumatic a.
  Tripier a.
  Vladimiroff-Mikulicz a.
  Wagner modification of Syme a.
  Wagner two-stage Syme a.

amputee

AMREX
  AMREX muscle stimulator

AMREX *(continued)*
 AMREX therapeutic ultra-
  sound

AMS
 antimigration system

Amspacher
 A.-Messenbaugh closing
  wedge osteotomy
 A.-Messenbaugh technique

Amstutz
 A. cemented hip prosthesis
 A. femoral component
 A. resurfacing technique
 A. total hip replacement
 A.-Wilson osteotomy

AMT
 active motion testing

amyotrophy
 Aran-Duchenne a.
 neuralgic a.

aerobe

ANA
 antinuclear antibody

anabolic steroid

anaerobic
 a. cellulitis
 a. infection
 a. osteomyelitis

analgesia
 patient-controlled a. (PCA)

analysis
 activity-pattern a.
 bioelectrical impedance a.
  (BIA)
 bradykinetic a.
 EMED gait a.
 Fourier a.
 gait a.
 Kaplan-Meier a.
 lateral flexion dynamic vis-
  ual a.
 Mann-Whitney a.
 occipital fiber a.
 trapezius fiber a.

Anametric
 A. total knee prosthesis
 A. total knee system

anapophysis

anastomosis
 fishmouth a.
 flexor tendon a.
 Martin-Gruber a.

anatomically graduated component (AGC)

anatomic porous replacement
 (APR)

anchor
 Anchorlok soft tissue su-
  ture a. system
 AxyaWeld bone a.
 BioRoc a.
 BioSphere a.
 E-Z Roc a.
 Fastlin threaded a.
 Isola spinal implant sys-
  tem a.
 Mitek a.
 PaBa a.
 Panalok absorbable a.
 ROC a.

anconeal

anconeus

anconoid

Anderson
 A. fixation apparatus
 A. medial-lateral grind test
 A. modification of Berndt-
  Harty classification
 A. screw placement tech-
  nique
 A. splint
 A. tibial pseudarthrosis
  classification
 A.-D'Alonzo odontoid frac-
  ture classification
 A.-Fowler anterior calca-
  neal osteotomy

Anderson *(continued)*
    A.-Fowler calcaneal displacement osteotomy
    A.-Green growth prediction
    A.-Hutchins unstable tibial shaft fracture
    A.-Neivert osteotome

Andersson hip status system

Andrews
    A. anterior instability test
    A. iliotibial band reconstruction
    A. iliotibial band tenodesis
    A. lateral tenodesis

AnergiX.RA

anergy

aneroid gauge

AnervaX.RA

anesthesia
    ankle block a.
    Bier block a.
    digital block a.
    graded spinal a.
    intrathecal a.
    peripheral nerve block a.
    regional a.
    ring block a.
    spinal a.
    supraclavicular brachial block a.
    toe-block a.

aneurysmal bone cyst (ABC)

Angell-James dissector

Anghelescu sign

angiography
    digital subtraction a.

angiokeratoma

angiomatosis
    skeletal-extraskeletal a.

angle
    acetabular a.
    acetabular a. of Sharp

angle *(continued)*
    acromial a.
    Alsberg a.
    anatomic intermetatarsal a.
    antegonial a.
    anteroposterior talocalcaneal a. (APTC)
    articular facet a.
    Baumann a.
    Beatson combined ankle a.
    bimalleolar a.
    Böhler calcaneal a.
    Böhler lumbosacral a.
    Bowman a.
    C a.
    calcaneal inclination a.
    calcaneoplantar a.
    calcaneotibial a.
    capital epiphyseal a.
    capitolunate a.
    center edge a. of Wiberg
    central collodiaphyseal a. (CCD)
    cervicothoracic pedicle a.
    Citelli a.
    Clarke arch a.
    Cobb lumbar a.
    Cobb scoliosis a.
    Codman a.
    condylar a.
    a. of congruence
    costal a.
    costolumbar a.
    costophrenic a.
    costosternal a.
    costovertebral a. (CVA)
    a. of declination
    distal articular set a.
    distal metatarsal articular a.
    a. of divergence
    dorsoplantar talometatarsal a.
    dorsoplantar talonavicular a.
    Drennan metaphyseal-epiphyseal a.
    elevation a.
    Engel a.

angle *(continued)*
   Euler a.
   eulerian a.
   external a. of border of
     tibia
   external a. of scapula
   facet a.
   femorotibial a. (FTA)
   Ferguson sacral base a.
   flexion a.
   Fowler-Philip a.
   Glissane crucial a.
   gonial a.
   a. of greatest extension
     (AGE)
   a. of greatest flexion (AGF)
   hallux dorsiflexion a.
   hallux valgus a.
   hallux valgus interphalan-
     geus a.
   Hibbs metatarsocalcane-
     al a.
   Hilgenreiner a.
   hip joint a. (HJA)
   humeral-ulnar a.
   a. of inclination
   a. of incongruity
   increased carrying a.
   infrasternal a. of thorax
   intermetatarsal a.
   internal a. of tibia
   intrascaphoid a.
   Kite a.
   Konstram a.
   kyphotic a.
   lateral plantar metatarsal a.
   lateral talocalcaneal a.
   lateral tarsometatarsal a.
   Laurin a.
   Lisfranc articular set a.
   lumbosacral joint a.
   mandibular a.
   a. of Mary
   Meary metarsotalar a.
   medial a. of humerus
   medial a. of scapula
   medial a. of tibia
   mediolateral radiocarpal a.
   Merchant congruence a.

angle *(continued)*
   metaphyseal-diaphyseal a.
   metaphyseal-epiphyseal a.
   metatarsocalcaneal a.
   metatarsotalar a.
   metatarsus adductus a.
   metatarsus primus a.
   Mikulicz a.
   negative congruence a.
   occipitocervical a.
   Pauwels a.
   pedicle axis a.
   pelvic a.
   pelvivertebral a.
   physeal a.
   proximal articular set a.
     (PASA)
   Q (quadriceps) a.
   resting forefoot supina-
     tion a.
   sacral base a.
   sacrofemoral a.
   sacrohorizontal a.
   sacrovertebral a.
   sagittal pedicle a.
   scapholunate a.
   Sharp acetabular a.
   Southwick lateral slip a.
   sternoclavicular a.
   subscapular a.
   talar axis–first metatarsal
     base a. (TAMBA)
   talar-tilt a.
   talocalcaneal a.
   talocrural a.
   talometatarsal a.
   talonavicular a.
   tarsometatarsal a.
   a. of thoracic inclination
   tibiofemoral a.
   tibiotalar a.
   TMA-thigh a.
   toe-out a.
   tuber a.
   tuber-joint a.
   ulnar humeral a.
   valgus a.
   varus MTP (metatarsophal-
     angeal) a.

angle *(continued)*
> Wiberg center edge a.
> Wiberg fracture a.
> Wiltse a.

angled
> a. arthroscope
> a. awl
> a. blade fixation plate
> a.-down forceps
> a. jaw rongeur
> a. Scoville curet
> a.-up forceps

angulated fracture

angulation
> anterior a.

angulatory malunion

angulus
> a. acromialis
> a. acromii
> a. costae
> a. inferior scapulae
> a. infrasternalis
> a. lateralis scapulae
> a. lateralis tibiae
> a. medialis scapulae
> a. medialis tibiae
> a. superior scapulae

anhydrotic

anisodactylous

anisodactyly

anisomelia

anisosthenic

anisotropic disk

ankle
> a. arthrodesis
> a. arthroplasty
> a.-brachial index (ABI)
> Buechel-Pappas total a.
> a. clonus
> a. contracture orthosis
> C stance a.
> a. disarticulation
> a. equinus
> a. eversion

ankle *(continued)*
> a. jerk
> a. joint complex (AJC)
> medial ligament of a.
> neuropathic a.
> a. orthosis
> a. stabilizer
> tailor's a.
> transmalleolar a.

ankylose

ankylosing
> a. spondylitis

ankylosis
> bony a.
> extraarticular a.
> extracapsular a.
> false a.
> fibrous a.
> ligamentous a.
> intracapsular a.
> shoulder a.
> spurious a.
> true a.
> vertebral a.

anlage
> fibular a.
> ulnar a.

annular *(spelled also anular)*
> congenital a. band
> a. fiber
> a. fibrosis
> a. groove
> a. ligament
> a. periradial recess

annulotomy

annulus *(spelled also anulus)*

anomalous
> a. insertion

anonychia

anopsia
> altitudinal a.

anserine bursitis

anserinus
> pes a.

Anspach
   A. cementome
   A. power drill
   A. reamer

antalgic gait

antebrachial
   a. cutaneous nerve
   a. fascia
   a. fascial graft

antecubital fossa

antegonial angle

antegrade method

antenatal dislocation

anterior
   a. acromioplasty
   a. angulation
   a. ankle impingement
   a. atlantooccipital membrane
   a. atlantoodontoid interval
   a. axillary approach
   a. calcaneal osteotomy
   a. calcaneal process fracture
   a. capsulolabral reconstruction (ACLR)
   a. cervical body fusion
   a. cervical diskectomy and fusion (ACDF)
   a. cervicothoracic junction surgery
   a. collateral ligament
   a. column osteosynthesis
   a. compartment syndrome
   a. cord impingement
   a. corpectomy
   a. cruciate instability with pivot shift
   a. cruciate ligament (ACL)
   a. distraction instrumentation
   a. drawer sign
   a. drawer test
   a. epineurotomy
   a. glenoid labrum
   a. horn meniscal tear

anterior *(continued)*
   a. humeral line
   a. iliofemoral technique
   a. inferior iliac spine (AIIS)
   a. innominate
   a. labrum periosteum shoulder arthroscopic lesion (ALPSA)
   a. tibiofibular joint
   a. tibiofibular ligament
   a. transthoracic approach
   a. Zielke instrumentation

anterior-inferior
   a.-i. compression
   a.-i. fusion with SSI
   a.-i. glide
   a.-i. listhesis
   a.-i. movement

anterius
   ligamentum capitis fibulae a.
   ligamentum longitudinale a.
   ligamentum meniscofemorale a.
   ligamentum sacrococcygeum a.
   ligamentum talofibulare a.
   ligamentum tibiofibulare a.

anterocentral portal

anterodistal

anteroinferior
   a. spondylolisthesis

anterolateral
   a.-anteromedial rotary instability
   a. femorotibial ligament tenodesis
   a. raphe
   a. rotary instability (ALRI)

anterolisthesis

anteromedial
   a.-posteromedial rotary instability

anteroposterior (AP)
   a. talocalcaneal angle (APTC)

anteroproximal

anterosuperior

antetorsion
    femoral a.

anteversion
    femoral a.

antibody
    AE1 a.
    AE3 a.
    antihistocompatibility a.
    antinuclear a. (ANA)

anticavitation drill

antifungal

antiglide plate

antimigration system (AMS)

antipodagric

antirheumatic

antispastic

antitonic

anular

anulus (*spelled also* annulus)
    a. fibrosus
    a. fibrosus disci interverte-
        bralis

AO
    ankle orthosis
    Arbeitsgemeinschaft für os-
        teosynthesefragen
            AO-Denis-Weber classi-
                fication of ankle frac-
                ture
            AO group shoulder ar-
                throdesis
    atlantooccipital
        AO blade plate
        AO brace
        AO cancellous screw
        AO classification
        AO classification of an-
            kle fracture

AO (*continued*)
    AO compression appa-
        ratus
    AO condylar blade
        plate
    AO contoured T plate
    AO contouring appa-
        ratus
    AO cortex screw
    AO drill bit
    AO dynamic compres-
        sion plate
    AO external fixation
    AO femoral distractor
    AO fixateur interne
    AO group shoulder ar-
        throdesis
    AO lag screw
    AO minifragment set
    narrow AO dynamic
        compression plate
    AO notched instrumen-
        tation
    AO plate bender
    AO pseudoisochro-
        matic color plate test
    AO reconstruction
        plate
    AO reduction forceps
    AO screw fixation
    AO semitubular plate
    AO slotted medullary
        nail
    AO spinal internal fixa-
        tion
    AO spongiosa screw
    T-shaped AO plate

AOA
    AOA cervical immobiliza-
        tion brace
    AOA halo cervical traction

AO-ASIF (*also* AO/ASIF)
    AO-ASIF compression plate
    AO-ASIF fiaxteur interne
    AO-ASIF orthopedic im-
        plant

AO-ASIF *(continued)*
 AO-ASIF screw

AOFAS
 American Orthopaedic
 Foot and Ankle Society

AOL
 anterior oblique ligament

AP
 action potential
 anterior and posterior
 anteroposterior

A-P cutter

aparthrosis

APD
 automated percutaneous
 diskectomy

Apert
 A. disease
 A. syndrome

apertura
 a. pelvica inferior
 a. pelvica superior
 a. pelvis inferior
 a. pelvis superior

aperture
 spinal a.

apex *pl.* apices
 a. capitis fibulae
 a. dorsal angulation
 a. of head of fibula
 a. of head of patella
 a. ossis sacralis
 a. ossis sacri
 a. patellae
 a. vertebra

APLD
 automated percutaneous
 lumbar diskectomy

Apley
 A. compression test
 A. distraction test
 A. scratch test

Apley *(continued)*
 A. sign
 A. test
 A. traction

Apligraf

Apofix cervical instrumentation

Apollo
 A. DXA bone densitometry
 system
 A. hip system
 A. knee system

aponeurosis *pl.* aponeuroses
 abdominal a.
 adductor a.
 a. of biceps muscle of arm
 bicipital a.
 a. bicipitalis
 clavicoracoaxillary a.
 crural a.
 digital a.
 external intercostal a.
 falciform a. of rectus abdominis muscle
 femoral a.
 a. glutealis
 a. of insertion
 internal intercostal a.
 meniscal a.
 a. musculi bicipitis brachii
 a. palmaris
 a. plantaris
 Sibson a.
 subscapular a.
 supraspinous a.
 temporal a.
 vertebral a.

aponeurotic

aponeurotomy

apophyseal
 a. fracture
 a. joint

apophysis *pl.* apophyses
 a. anularis
 iliac a.

apophysis *(continued)*
   medial epicondylar a.
   odontoid a.
   a. ossium
   slipped vertebral a.
   spinal process a.
   vertebral ring a.

apophysitis
   calcaneal a.
   iliac a.

apparatus
   Anderson fixation a.
   AO compression a.
   Axer compression a.
   Buck traction a.
   Calandruccio triangular
     compression a.
   Cameron fracture a.
   Charnley a.
   coracoclavicular a.
   DeWald spinal a.
   Deyerle fixation a.
   electric bone stimulation a.
   external skeletal fixation a.
   four-bar external fixation a.
   halo vest a.
   Hodgen a.
   Ilizarov a.
   internal fixation a.
   Kirschner a.
   Kronner external fixation a.
   Küntscher traction a.
   a. ligamentosus colli
   McLaughlin osteosynthes-
     is a.
   Müller compression a.
   Nauth traction a.
   optoelectric meauring a.
   Parham-Martin fracture a.
   Quengel a.
   Redi-Trac traction a.
   Rezaian external fixation a.
   Sayre a.
   subneural a.
   Sutter-CPM knee a.
   Taylor a.
   Vidal-Adrey modified Hoff-
     man external fixation a.

apparatus *(continued)*
   Volkov-Oganesian external
     fixation a.
   Wagner external fixation a.
   Wagner-Schanz screw a.
   Zickel supracondylar fixa-
     tion a.

appliance
   Jobst a.

apposition
   axonal a.
   facet a.

appositional growth

approach
   Abbott-Carpenter poster-
     ior a.
   acetabular extensile a.
   acetabular knee a.
   anterior axillary a.
   anterior transthoracic a.
   anterolateral a.
   anteromedial retropharan-
     geal a.
   Bailey-Badgley anterior cer-
     vical a.
   Banks-Laufman a.
   Berger-Bookwalter poster-
     ior a.
   bilateral ilioinguinal a.
   bilateral sacroiliac a.
   Bosworth a.
   Boyd-Sisk a.
   Brackett-Osgood knee a.
   Brackett-Osgood poster-
     ior a.
   Brodsky-Tullos-Gartsman a.
   Bruner a.
   Bruser lateral a.
   Bryan-Morrey elbow a.
   Campbell posterior should-
     er a.
   Carnesale acetabular exten-
     sile a.
   Carnesale hip a.
   Cloward cervical disk a.
   Colonna-Ralston ankle a.
   Coonse-Adams knee a.

approach *(continued)*
- Cubbins shoulder a.
- Darrach-McLaughlin a.
- deltoid-splitting shoulder a.
- deltopectoral a.
- dorsalward a.
- dorsolateral a.
- dorsomedial a.
- dorsoplantar a.
- dorsoradial a.
- dorsorostral a.
- dorsoulnar a.
- DuVries a.
- extrabursal a.
- extraperitoneal a.
- extrapharyngeal a.
- Fowler-Philip a.
- Gatellier-Chastang a.
- Gatellier-Chastang ankle a.
- Gatellier-Chastang posterolateral a.
- Guleke-Stookey a.
- Hardinge femoral a.
- Harmon cervical a.
- Harris anterolateral a.
- Hirschhorn compression a.
- Hoffmann a.
- Hoppenfeld-Deboer a.
- iliofemoral a.
- ilioinguinal a.
- intraforaminal a.
- ipsilateral a.
- Kocher-Gibson posterolateral a.
- Kocher-Langenbeck a.
- Koenig-Schaefer medial a.
- lateral Ollier a.
- lateral parapatellar a.
- Lazepen-Gamidov anteromedial a.
- Leslie-Ryan anterior axillary a.
- Letournel-Joudet a.
- Ludloff medial a.
- McAfee a.
- McConnell extensile a.
- McFarland-Osborne lateral a.

approach *(continued)*
- McWhorter posterior shoulder a.
- Mears-Rubash a.
- medial parapatellar capsular a.
- midlateral a.
- Minkoff-Jaffe-Menendez posterior a.
- Mize-Bucholz-Grogan a.
- Molesworth-Campbell elbow a.
- Moore posterior a.
- Moore-Southern a.
- Ollier arthrodesis a.
- Osborne posterior a.
- patella turndown a.
- Perry extensile anterior a.
- Pfannenstiel transverse a.
- Pogrun lateral a.
- posterior costrotransversectomy a.
- posterior occipitocervical a.
- posterior transolecranon a.
- proprioceptive neuromuscular facilitation a.
- Putti posterior a.
- Reinert acetabular extensile a.
- Roos a.
- saber-cut a.
- Senegas hip a.
- Smith-Petersen-Cave-Van Gorder anterolateral a.
- Somerville anterior a.
- Southwick-Robinson anterior cervical a.
- subclavicular a.
- thoracolumbar retroperitoneal a.
- transbrachioradialis a.
- transcalcaneal a.
- transolecranon a.
- transtrochanteric a.
- triradiate transtrochanteric a.
- volarward a.
- Wadsworth elbow a.

approach *(continued)*
    Wagner a.
    Wagoner posterior a.
    Watson-Jones a.
    Wiltberger anterior cervical a.
    Wiltse a.
    Wiltse-Spencer paraspinal a.
    Yee posterior shoulder a.
    Z-plasty a.

appropulsive gait

approximator
    Acland clamp a.
    Bruni-Wayne clamp a.
    Buncke-Schulz a.
    clamp a.
    double-clamp a.
    Henderson clamp a.
    hook a.
    Ikuta clamp a.
    Iwashi clamp a.
    Kleinert-Kutz clamp a.
    Lalonde tendon a.
    Lemmon sternal a.
    sternal a.
    Van Beek nerve a.

APR
    anatomic porous replacement

apraxia

apraxic gait

apron
    quadriceps a.

APTC
    anteroposterior talocalcaneal angle

AquaMED dry hydrotherapy

Aquaphor gauze dressing

Aqua/Whirl bath

Arafiles elbow arthrodesis

Aran-Duchenne amyotrophy

arc
    reflex a.

arcade of Frohse

arch
    anterior a. of atlas
    axillary a.
    costal a.
    crural a.
    femoral a., superficial
    fibrous a. of soleus muscle
    a. of foot
    a. height
    inguinal a.
    Langer axillary a.
    lateral a.
    longitudinal a.
    longitudinal a., lateral
    longitudinal a., medial
    longitudinal a. of foot
    medial a.
    metatarsal a.
    neural a. of vertebra
    palmar a.
    popliteal a.
    posterior a. of atlas
    pubic a.
    a. of ribs
    subpubic a.
    supraorbital a. of frontal bone
    tendinous a. of lumbodorsal fascia
    tendinous a. of soleus muscle
    transverse a. of foot
    a. of vertebra
    vertebral a.

"arch and slouch" position

Archimedean drill

arcuate-popliteal complex

arcuatum
    ligamentum popliteum a.

arcus
    a. atlantis
    a. iliopectineus
    a. inguinalis

arcus *(continued)*
　a. palmaris profundis
　a. palmaris superficialis
　a. parietoccipitalis
　a. pedis longitudinalis
　a. pedis transversalis
　a. pedis transversus distalis
　a. pedis transversus proximalis
　a. plantaris
　a. plantaris profundus
　a. pubicus
　a. pubis
　a. tendineus
　a. tendineus fasciae pelvis
　a. tendineus musculi solei
　a. vertebrae
　a. vertebralis
　a. volaris profundus
　a. volaris superficialis

area
　arch peak a.
　a. intercondylaris anterior tibiae
　a. intercondylaris posterior tibiae
　Cohnheim a's
　dorsolumbar a.
　odontoid-axial a.
　puboischial a.
　trapezial a.

areflexia

arm
　mini C-a.
　XiScan mini C-a.
　Yasargil Leyla retractor a.

armboard
　Flexisplint flexed a.

Armistead
　A. technique
　A. ulnar lengthening operation

Armstrong
　A. acromionectomy
　A. plate

Army osteotome

Army-Navy retractor

Arnold
　bigeminate ligaments of A.
　deep bifurcate ligaments of A.
　A. lumbar brace
　trigeminate ligaments of A.
　A.-Chiari malformation
　A.-Chiari syndrome

Aronson-Prager technique

arrest
　epiphyseal a.
　greater trochanteric apophyseal a.
　growth a.

ART
　active release technique

arteritis
　brachiocephalic a.
　a. brachiocephalica
　Takayasu a.

artery
　first dorsal metatarsal a. (FDMA)
　genicular a.

Arth-Aid

arthralgia
　subtalar a.

arthrectomy

arthrempyesis

Arthrex
　A. coring reamer
　A. sheathed interference screw
　A. zebra pin

arthritic

arthritis *pl.* arthritides
　acute hematogenous a.
　acute rheumatic a.
　acute suppurative a.

arthritis *(continued)*
    Bekhterev (Bechterew) a.
    Brucella a.
    calcaneocuboid joint a.
    Charcot a.
    cricoarytenoid a.
    crystal-induced a.
    a. deformans
    degenerative a.
    enteropathic a.
    erosive a.
    exudative a.
    Fries score for rheumato-
      id a.
    fungal a.
    gonococcal septic a.
    gouty a.
    A. Helplessness Index (AHI)
    hemophiliac a.
    hypotrophic a.
    A. Impact Measurement
      Scale (AIMS)
    infectious a.
    Jaccoud a.
    juvenile rheumatoid a.
    Marie-Strümpell a.
    migratory a.
    mutilans rheumatoid a.
    mycobacterial a.
    oligoarticular a.
    pantalocrural a.
    patellofemoral a.
    pauciarticular a.
    pisotriquetral a.
    polyarticular a.
    postmenopausal a.
    psoriatic a.
    pyogenic a.
    radiocarpal a.
    rheumatoid a.
    Rome criteria for rheuma-
      toid a.
    septic a.
    seronegative rheumatoid a.
    seropositive rheumatoid a.
    silicone a.
    staphylococcal a.
    Steinbrocker classification
      of rheumatoid a.

arthritis *(continued)*
    suppurative a.
    tibiotalar a.
    Tom Smith a.
    traumatic a.
    tuberculous a.
    viral-associated a.

ArthroCare
    A. wand

arthrocele

arthrocentesis

arthrochalasis

arthrochondritis

arthroclasia

arthroclisis

arthrodesed digit

arthrodesis
    Abbott-Fisher-Lucas hip a.
    Adams transmalleolar a.
    Adkins spinal a.
    Albee hip a.
    AO group shoulder a.
    Arafiles elbow a.
    atlantoaxial a.
    Baciu-Filibiu dowel ankle a.
    Baciu-Filibiu transmalleo-
      lar a.
    Badgley a.
    Barr-Record ankle a.
    Barrasso-Wile-Gage a.
    Batchelor-Brown extra-ar-
      ticular subtalar a.
    Benyi modification of Lam-
      brinudi triple a.
    Blair-Morris-Bunn-Hand
      ankle a.
    Bosworth femoroischial a.
    Brett a.
    Brewster triple a.
    Brittain ischiofemoral a.
    Brockman-Nissen a.
    Brooks atlantoaxial a.
    calcaneocuboid (CC) a.
    calcaneopelvic a.
    calcaneotibial a.

arthrodesis *(continued)*
  Campbell-Akbarnia a.
  Campbell-Rinehard-Kalenak
    anterior a.
  Carceau-Brahms ankle a.
  cervical a.
  Chapchal knee a.
  Charcot hip a.
  Chamley ankle a.
  Charnley-Houston should-
    er a.
  Chuinard-Petersen ankle a.
  Cloward cervical a.
  Compere-Thompson a.
  coracoclavicular a.
  cuneiform joint a.
  Dennyson-Fulford subta-
    lar a.
  distal fibulotalar a.
  distraction bone block a.
  Dunn-Brittain triple a.
  Elmslie triple a.
  Enneking knee a.
  Enneking resection-a.
  extraarticular a.
  failed triple a.
  fibulotalar a.
  first cuneiform joint a.
  first cuneiform–navicular
    joint a.
  first metatarsal–first cunei-
    form a.
  Gallie ankle a.
  Gallie atlantoaxial a.
  Gant hip a.
  Garceau-Brahms a.
  Ghormley a.
  Gill-Stein a.
  glenohumeral a.
  Glissane a.
  Goldner spinal a.
  Graham ankle a.
  Grice-Green extra-articular
    subtalar a.
  Guttmann subtalar a.
  Haddad-Riordan a.
  hallux interphalangeal
    joint a.
  Harris-Beath a.

arthrodesis *(continued)*
  Heiple a.
  Hibbs a.
  hindfoot a.
  Hoke triple a.
  Horwitz-Adams a.
  Ilizarov ankle a.
  Johannson-Barrington a.
  joint a.
  Kickaldy-Willis a.
  knee a.
  Lambrinudi a.
  Lambrinudi triple a.
  Lapidus a.
  Lipscomb modified Mc-
    Keever a.
  Lisfranc a.
  lunotriquetral a.
  McKeever metatarsophal-
    angeal a.
  Mann modified Mc-
    Keever a.
  Marcus-Balourdas-Heiple
    transmalleolar a.
  metatarsocuneiform a.
  midcarpal a.
  Millender-Nalebuff a.
  Moberg a.
  modified Lapidus a.
  Müller a.
  Nalebuff a.
  Naughton-Dunn triple a.
  naviculocuneiform joint a.
  panastragaloid a.
  pantalar a.
  para-articular a.
  Pontenza a.
  Pridie ankle a.
  Putti knee a.
  radiocarpal a.
  resection a.
  Richards a.
  Ryerson triple a.
  scaphocapitolunate
    (SCL) a.
  scaphotrapeziotrapezoid a.
  scapulothoracic a.
  Scoffert triple a.

arthrodesis *(continued)*
 Siffert-Forster-Nachamie a.
 Soren a.
 spinal a.
 Steindler elbow a.
 Stewart-Harley transmalleolar ankle a.
 Stone a.
 subtalar a.
 talonavicular a.
 tarsometatarsal truncated-
  wedge a.
 tibiocalcaneal a.
 tibiotalar a.
 tibiotalocalcaneal a.
 triple a.
 triquetrum-lunate a.
 triscaphe a.
 truncated tarsometatarsal a.
 Uematsu shoulder a.
 ulnocarpal a.
 Watson-Jones a.
 Whitecloud-LaRocca cervical a.
 Wilson-Johansson-Barring-
  ton cone a.

arthrodiastasis

arthrodynia

arthrodysplasia

arthroempyesis

arthroereisis
 subtalar a.

Arthro-Flo arthroscopic irrigation system

arthrogenic gait

arthrogryposis
 a. multiplex congenita
 neurogenic a.

arthrokatadysis

arthrokleisis

arthrolith

arthrology

Arthro-Lok system

arthrolysis

arthromeningitis

arthrometer
 Medmetric knee ligament a.

arthrometric knee laxity measurement

arthroncus

arthroneuralgia

arthronosus

arthropathic

arthropathology

arthropathy
 Charcot a.
 chondrocalcific a.
 crystal a.
 cuff-tear a.
 finger joint a.
 hemophilic a.
 inflammatory a.
 Jaccoud a.
 joint a.
 neuropathic a.
 psoriatic a.
 pyrophosphate a.
 sacroiliac joint a.
 seronegative a.

arthrophyte

arthroplasty
 ablative a.
 acetabular cup a.
 acromioclavicular a.
 Ashworth hand a.
 Aufranc cup a.
 Aufranc-Turner a.
 Austin Moore a.
 autogenous interpositional
  shoulder a.
 Bechtol a.

arthroplasty *(continued)*
  bipolar hip a.
  Bowers radial a.
  Bryan a.
  Campbell interpositional a.
  capitellocondylar total elbow a.
  capsular interposition a.
  carpometacarpal a.
  Carroll and Taber a.
  cementless total hip a.
  Charcot a.
  Charnley low-friction hip a.
  Charnley total hip a.
  Clayton forefoot a.
  Colonna trochanteric a.
  condylar implant a.
  convex condylar-implant a.
  Coonrad-Morrey total elbow a.
  Cracchiolo forefoot a.
  Cracchiolo-Sculco implant a.
  Cubbins a.
  Dewar-Barrington a.
  distraction a.
  duToit-Roux a.
  DuVries a.
  Eaton implant a.
  Eaton volar plate a.
  Eden-Hybbinette a.
  elbow a.
  ELP stem for hip a.
  Ewald capitellocondylar total elbow a.
  Ewald elbow a.
  Ewald-Walker kinematic knee a.
  Ewald-Walker knee a.
  extensor brevis a.
  Girdlestone resection a.
  Gristina-Webb total shoulder a.
  Gunston a.
  Harrington total hip a.
  hemijoint a.
  hemiresection interposition a.

arthroplasty *(continued)*
  hip a.
  Hungerford-Krackow-Kenna knee a.
  ICLH double cup a.
  Inglis triaxial total elbow a.
  Jaccoud a.
  Keller resection a.
  knee a.
  Kocher-McFarland hip a.
  Koenig metatarsophalangeal joint a.
  Kutes a.
  McAtee-Tharias-Blazina a.
  McKee-Farrar total hip a.
  Mann-DuVries a.
  Mark II Sorrells hip a.
  Mayo resection a.
  Memford-Gurd a.
  metacarpophalangeal joint a.
  Meuli a.
  Millender a.
  modified Keller resection a.
  mold acetabular a.
  monospherical total shoulder a.
  Morrey-Bryan total elbow a.
  Mould a.
  Müller hip a.
  NEB (New England Baptist) hip a.
  Niebauer trapeziometacarpal a.
  noncemented total hip a.
  Press-Fit condylar knee a.
  Putti-Platt a.
  Regnauld modification of Keller a.
  resection a.
  sacroiliac joint a.
  Sauvé-Kapandji a.
  Schlein elbow a.
  Silastic lunate a.
  silicone rubber a.
  silicone wrist a.
  Smith-Petersen cup a.

arthroplasty *(continued)*
    Steffee thumb a.
    tendon interposition a.
    Thompson a.
    total articular replacement a. (TARA)
    total elbow a.
    total hip a.
    total joint a.
    total knee a.
    total shoulder a.
    total wrist a.
    triaxial total elbow a.
    Tupper a.
    ulnar hemiresection interposition a.
    unicompartmental knee a.
    Vainio a.
    Vitallium cup a.
    volar plate a.
    Volz total wrist a.
    Wilson-McKeever a.

Arthropor
    A. acetabular cup
    A. cup pad
    A. cup prosthesis
    A. oblong cup for acetabular defect

ArthroProbe

arthropyosis

arthroscope
    Dyonics a.
    Eagle straight-ahead a.
    fiberoptic a.
    Panoview a.
    Sapphire View a.
    Storz oblique a.
    Stryker viewing a.
    Wolf a.

arthroscopically-assisted anterior cruciate ligament reconstruction

arthroscopy
    Allen shoulder a.
    a. basket forceps
    diagnostic a.

arthroscopy *(continued)*
    diagnostic a. and débridement
    diagnostic and operative a. (DOA)
    Gillquist a.
    a. grasping forceps
    lateral hip a.
    midcarpal a.
    radiocarpal a.
    second-look a.

arthrosis
    crystal-induced a.
    Eaton CMC (carpometacarpal) a. *(stages I–IV)*
    Enneking knee a.
    subtalar a.
    uncovertebral a.

arthrosynovitis

Arthrotek
    A. calibrated cylinder
    A. femoral aimer
    A. Ellipticut instrumentation

arthrotome

arthrotomy
    Magnuson-Stack shoulder a.
    medial parapatellar a.
    parapatellar a.
    subtalar a.

arthroxesis

ArthroWand
    CAPS A.

articular
    a. cartilage autografting
    a. facet angle
    a. ligamentous system

articulated
    a. external fixator
    a. tension device

articulatio
    a. acromioclavicularis

articulatio *(continued)*
   a. atlantoaxialis lateralis
   a. atlantoaxialis mediana
   a. atlantoepistrophica
   a. atlantooccipitalis
   a. calcaneocuboidea
   a. capitis costae
   a. capitis humeri
   articulationes capitulorum
      costarum
   articulationes carpi
   articulationes carpometa-
      carpales
   a. carpometacarpalis polli-
      cis
   articulationes carpometa-
      carpeae
   a. carpometacarpea pollicis
   a. cartilaginea
   articulationes cinguli mem-
      bri inferioris
   articulationes cinguli mem-
      bri superioris
   articulationes cinguli pec-
      toralis
   articulationes cinguli pel-
      vici
   a. cochlearis
   articulationes columnae
      vertebralis
   a. complexa
   a. composita
   a. condylaris
   a. condylaris inversa
   articulationes costochon-
      drales
   a. costotransversaria
   articulationes costoverte-
      brales
   a. cotylica
   a. coxae
   a. coxofemoralis
   a. crurotalaris
   a. cubitalis
   a. cubiti
   a. cuneocuboidea
   a. cuneonavicularis
   a. ellipsoidea
   a. fibrosa

articulatio *(continued)*
   a. genualis
   a. genus
   a. glenohumeralis
   a. humeri
   a. humeroradialis
   a. humeroulnaris
   a. iliofemoralis
   articulationes intercarpales
   articulationes intercarpeae
   articulationes interchon-
      drales
   articulationes intercunei-
      formes
   articulationes intermetacar-
      pales
   articulationes intermetacar-
      peae
   articulationes intermetatar-
      sales
   articulationes intermetatar-
      seae
   articulationes interphalan-
      geae manus
   articulationes interphalan-
      geales manus
   articulationes interphalan-
      geae pedis
   articulationes interphalan-
      geales pedis
   articulationes intertarsales
   a. lumbosacralis
   articulationes manus
   a. mediocarpalis
   a. mediocarpea
   articulationes membri in-
      ferioris liberi
   articulationes membri su-
      perioris liberi
   articulationes metacarpo-
      phalangeae
   articulationes metacarpo-
      phalangeales
   articulationes metatarso-
      phalangeae
   articulationes metatarso-
      phalangeales
   a. ossis pisiformis
   a. ovoidalis

articulatio *(continued)*
    articulationes pedis
    a. plana
    a. radiocarpalis
    a. radiocarpea
    a. radioulnaris
    a. radioulnaris distalis
    a. radioulnaris proximalis
    a. sacrococcygea
    a. sacroiliaca
    a. sellaris
    a. simplex
    a. spheroidea
    a. sternoclavicularis
    articulationes sternocosta-
      les
    a. subtalaris
    a. synovialis
    a. talocalcanea
    a. talocalcaneonavicularis
    a. talocruralis
    a. talonavicularis
    a. tarsi transversa
    a. tarsi transversa Choparti
    articulationes tarsometa-
      tarsales
    articulationes tarsometa-
      tarseae
    a. tibiofibularis
    a. trochoidea
    articulationes vertebrales
    articulationes zygapophy-
      siales
articulation
    acromioclavicular a.
    atlantoaxial a.
    atlantooccipital a.
    bicondylar a.
    brachiocarpal a.
    brachioradial a.
    brachioulnar a.
    calcaneocuboid a.
    capitular a.
    carpometacarpal a.
    carporadial a.
    chondrosternal a.
    Chopart a.

articulation *(continued)*
    collateral ligament of MCP
      a's
    collateral ligament of MTP
      a's
    condylar a.
    coracoclavicular a.
    costocentral a.
    costovertebral a.
    coxofemoral a. of Buisson
    crurotalar a.
    cubital a.
    cubitoradial a.
    cuneocuboid a.
    cuneonavicular a.
    glenohumeral a.
    humeroradial a.
    humeroulnar a.
    iliofemoral a.
    iliosacral a.
    intercarpal a.
    intercuneiform a.
    intermetacarpal a.
    intermetatarsal a's
    interphalangeal a.
    intertarsal a.
    lumbosacral a.
    metacarpocarpal a.
    metacarpophalangeal a.
    metatarsocuneiform a.
    metatarsophalangeal a.
    occipitoatlantal a.
    occipitocervical a.
    palmar ligaments of inter-
      phalangeal a's
    patellofemoral a.
    phalangeal a's
    a. of pisiform bone
    pisocuneiform a.
    proximal interphalangeal
      (PIP) a.
    proximal radioulnar a.
    radiocapitellar a.
    radiocarpal a.
    radioscaphoid a.
    radioulnar a.
    sacrococcygeal a.
    sacroiliac a.

articulation *(continued)*
    scapuloclavicular a.
    spheroidal a.
    sternoclavicular a.
    sternocostal a's
    subtalar a.
    talocalcaneonavicular a.
    talocrural a.
    talonavicular a.
    tarsometatarsal a's
    tibiofibular a.
    ulnolunate a.
    ulnotriquetral a.
    Vermont spinal fixator a.
    zygapophyseal a's

artifact
    stimulus a.

Artisan cement system

assessment
    Activity Losses A. (ALA)
    BFM arm impairment a.
    ergonomic a.
    functional a.
    Jebsen a. of hand function
    Moire topographic scolios-
      is a.
    Musculoskeletal
      Function A.
    Tinetti gait a.

ARUM Colles fixation pin

Asch
    A. forceps
    A. splint

Ashhurst
    A. leg splint
    A.-Bromer ankle fracture

ASI
    acromial spur index

ASIF
    Association for the Study
      of Internal Fixation
        ASIF chisel
        ASIF right-angle blade
          plate

ASIF *(continued)*
    ASIF screw
    ASIF screw pin

ASIn
    anterosuperior internal il-
      ium movement

Asnis
    A. cannulated cancellous
      screw
    A. 3 cannulated screw sys-
      tem
    A. pin
    A. pinning
    A. technique

Aspen cervical collar

Aspinwall transverse ligament
    test

ASSI Lalonde dynamic compres-
    sion bone clamp

astasia-abasia gait

astragalus
    aviator's a.

asyndesis

asynergia

AT
    Achilles tendon

Atasoy
    A. triangular advancement
      flap
    A. V-Y advancement

atavicus
    metatarsus primus a.

atavistic tarsometatarsal joint

ataxia
    Bruns a.
    equilibratory a.
    Friedreich a.
    hereditary spinocerebel-
      lar a.
    locomotor a.

ataxic gait

Aten olecranon screw

Atkin epiphyseal fracture

Atkinson endoprosthesis

Atlanta
A. brace orthosis
A.–Scottish Rite abduction
orthosis

atlantal
a. transverse ligament

atlantis
arcus a.
ligamentum cruciforme a.
ligamentum transversum a.

atlantoaxial
a. arthrodesis
a. fracture-dislocation
a. luxation
a. rotary displacement
a. rotary subluxation

atlantooccipital (AO)

atlantoodontoid
a. interspace
a. joint

Atlas
A. modular humeral pros-
thesis
A. orthogonal percussion
instrument

atlas (C1)
cruciform ligament of a.
a. fracture
transverse ligament of a.

atlas-axis
a.-a. complex
a.-a. movement

ATON
adductor tenotomy and ob-
turator neurectomy

atonia

atony

ATR
Achilles tendon repair

ATR *(continued)*
Achilles tendon rupture

atrophia
a. musculorum lipomatosa

atrophy
arthritic a.
bone a.
disuse a.
a. of disuse
Erb a.
facioscapulohumeral mus-
cular a.
Hoffmann a.
interstitial a.
ischemic muscular a.
juvenile muscular a.
Landouzy-Dejerine a.
leaping a.
muscular a.
myopathic a.
posttraumatic a. of bone
pseudohypertrophic mus-
cular a.
rheumatic a.
infantile spinal muscular a.
Werdnig-Hoffmann spinal
muscular a.
Sudeck a.
thenar a.
Zimmerlin a.

attachment plaques

Attenborough total knee prosthesis

attentuation of tendon

attritional perforation

Aufranc
A. awl
A. cobra hip prosthesis
A. cobra retractor
A. concentric hip mold
A. cup arthroplasty
A. gouge
A. modification of Smith-Pe-
tersen cup
A. osteotome

Aufranc *(continued)*
    A. periosteal elevator
    A. reamer
    A.-Turner cemented hip
        prosthesis
    A.-Turner femoral compo-
        nent
    A.-Turner hip cup

Aufricht glabellar rasp

auger

AuRA

auranofin

aurothiomalate
    a. disodium
    sodium a.

Aussies-Isseis unstable scoliosis

Austin
    bicorrectional A. osteot-
        omy
    A. bunionectomy
    A. chevron osteotomy fu-
        sion
    A. osteotomy

Austin Moore
    A. M. arthroplasty
    A. M. extractor
    A. M. hemiarthroplasty
    A. M. pin
    A. M. prosthesis
    A. M. reamer

autochthonous graft

autocinesis

autocompression plate

autogene
    Soudre a.

autogenous
    a. bone graft
    a. fibular graft
    a. interpositional shoulder
        arthroplasty
    a. patellar ligament graft
    a. semitendinosus-gracilis
        graft

autograft
    bone-patellar a.
    free revascularized a.
    patellar bone-tendon-
        bone a.
    Russell fibular head a.

autografting
    articular cartilage a.

AuTolo Cure Process

Automated
    A. Disposable Keratome
        (ADK)
    A. OsteoGram 2000

automated
    a. percutaneous diskec-
        tomy (APD)
    a. percutaneous lumbar
        diskectomy (APLD)

Autophor
    A. ceramic total hip pros-
        thesis
    A. femoral prosthesis

autoreinforced polyglycolide
    rod

autotome drill

Auvard clamp

avascular
    a. fragment
    a. necrosis (AVN)
    a. necrosis of bone
    a. necrosis of the femoral
        head (AVNFH)
    a. sequestrum

aviator's astragalus

A-V Impulse system foot pump
    DVT prophylaxis device

AVN
    avascular necrosis

AVNFH
    avascular necrosis of the
        femoral head

avulsion
  a. chip fracture
  digitorum brevis a.
  a. fracture

awl
  angled a.
  Aufranc a.
  Carter Rowe a.
  DePuy a.
  Ender a.
  Ferran a.
  Küntscher a.
  Mark II Kodros radiolucent a.
  reaming a.
  Rush pin reamer a.
  Stedman a.
  Swanson scaphoid a.
  T-handled a.
  Zelicof orthopedic a.
  Zuelzer a.

Axel wire twister

Axer
  A. compression apparatus
  A. compression device
  A. lateral opening wedge osteotomy
  A.-Clark procedure

axial
  a. calcaneal projection
  a. calcaneal view
  a. compression of the foot
  a. compression test
  a. fixation
  a. loading injury
  a. load test
  a. manual traction test

axial *(continued)*
  a. multiplanar gradient refocused magnetic resonance image
  a. plane angular deformity biomechanics
  a. sesamoid projection

Axiom modular knee system

axis *pl.* axes
  bimalleolar-foot a.
  femoral shaft a.
  flexion-extension a.
  hypothalamoneurohypophyseal a. (HNA)
  interepicondylar a.
  ligamentum apicis dentis a.
  proximal reference a.
  tooth of a.
  transcondylar a. (TCA)
  transepicondylar a.
  transmalleolar a. (TMA)
  weightbearing a.
  X a.
  Y a.
  Z a.

axonal apposition

AxyaWeld
  A. bone anchor
  A. J-tip suture welding system

Ayers needle holder

Ayres tactile discrimination test

azotemic osteodystrophy

aztreonam

Baastrup
  B. disease
  B. syndrome

Babinski
  plantar B. response
  B. reflex
  B. sign
  B. test
  B.-Frohlich syndrome

BacFix system

Baciu
  B.-Filibiu dowel ankle ar-
    throdesis
  B.-Filibiu transmalleolar ar-
    throdesis

back
  b. brace
  flat b.
  functional b.
  hollow b.
  hump b.
  hunch b.
  b. knee
  poker b.
  b. range of motion (BROM)
  saddle b.

Backbar device

backcutting osteotome

backfire fracture

Backhaus
  B. towel clamp
  B. towel forceps
  B.-Jones towel clamp

Bacon bone rongeur

Badgley
  B. arthrodesis
  B. laminectomy retractor
  B. plate
  B. resection of iliac wing

Bado classification

Baer
  B. bone rongeur

Baer *(continued)*
  B. bone-cutting forceps

Bagby angled compression
  plate

Bahler hinge

Bailey
  B. conductor
  B.-Badgley anterior cervical
    approach
  B.-Badgley cervical spine
    fusion
  B.-Badgley technique
  B.-Cowley clamp
  B.-Dubow nail
  B.-Dubow osteotomy
  B.-Dubow rod
  B.-Gibbon rib contractor
  B.-Gigli saw guide
  B.-Morse clamp

BAK
  BAK cage
  BAK interbody fusion sys-
    tem

BAK/C cervical interbody fusion system

BAK/Proximity interbody fusion
  implant

Baker
  B. cyst
  B. patellar advancement
    operation
  B. translocation operation
  B.-Hill osteotomy

Balacescu closing wedge osteotomy

Baldan fracture splint

Balfour
  B. clamp
  B. self-retaining retractor

Balkan
  B. femoral splint
  B. frame

ball
- b. bur
- b. extractor
- chondrin b.
- Gertie b.
- Gymnic b.
- Jurgan pin b.
- Silastic b.
- Thera-Band exercise b.
- b.-tipped Kuntscher guide

Ballantine
- B. clamp
- B. hemilaminectomy retractor

Ballenger
- B. knife
- B. periosteotome
- B.-Hajek chisel

ballottable

ballottement
- b. of patella
- b. test

Bamberger-Marie disease

band
- A b.
- AO tension b.
- aponeurotic b.
- congenital annular b.
- H b.
- I b.
- iliopatellar b.
- iliotibial b. (ITB)
- M b.
- Maissiat b.
- Parham b.
- Simonart b.
- periosteal b.
- Z b.

bandage
- Barton b.
- Comperm tubular elastic b.
- Conco elastic b.
- Desault wrist b.
- Elastoplast b.
- Esmarch b.

bandage *(continued)*
- Gibney b.
- Helenca b.
- Heliodorus b.
- Hueter b.
- Kerlix b.
- Kling b.
- Orthoflex elastic plaster b.
- Ortho-Trac adhesive skin traction b.
- plaster b.
- Redigrip pressure b.
- Silesian b.
- stockinette b.
- TubeGauz b.
- Tubigrip b.
- Velpeau b.
- Webril b.

Bandi procedure

Bane
- B. bone rongeur
- B.-Hartmann bone rongeur

Bankart
- B. fracture
- B. lesion
- B. operation
- B. reconstruction
- B. shoulder dislocation
- B. shoulder repair
- B. shoulder repair set
- B.-Putti-Platt operation

Banks
- B. bone graft
- B.-Laufman approach

Bannon-Klein implant

bantenadesis

bar
- calcaneonavicular b.
- Denis Browne b.
- Fillauer b.
- Gerster traction b.
- Leyla b.
- Livingston intramedullary b.
- lumbrical b.
- opponens b.

bar *(continued)*
    spondylitic b.
    spondylotic b.
    stabilizing b.
    Stephen spreader b.
    unsegmented vertebral b.
    valgus b.
    Zielke derotator b.

Bárány-Nylen maneuver

Barrasso-Wile-Gage arthrodesis

barbotage

Bardeleben bone-holding forceps

Bard-Parker
    B.-P. blade
    B.-P. handle
    B.-P. knife
    B.-P. scalpel

Barker operation

Barkow
    internal interosseous ligaments of B.
    B. ligament
    plantar external ligaments of B.

Barlow
    B. maneuver
    B. sign
    B. test

Barnes curve

Barouk
    B. button space for hallux valgus deformity
    B. cannulated bone screw
    B. microscrew with shortening osteotomy

Barr
    B. anterior transfer
    B. bolt
    B. pin
    B. tendon transfer operation
    B.-Record ankle arthrodesis

Barraquer needle holder

Barre test

barrier
    Capset (calcium sulfate) bone graft b.

Barsky operation

Barthel index

Bartlett nail fold

Barton
    B. fracture
    B. operation

Bart-Pumphrey syndrome

basement membrane

basilar
    b. artery migraine
    b. crescentic osteotomy
    b. femoral neck fracture
    b. metatarsal osteotomy

Basile hip screw

basioccipital

basis
    b. metacarpalis
    b. metatarsalis
    b. ossis metacarpalis
    b. ossis metacarpi
    b. ossis metatarsalis
    b. ossis metatarsi
    b. ossis sacri
    b. patellae
    b. phalangis digitorum manus
    b. phalangis digitorum pedis
    b. scapulae

basivertebral

basket
    Acufex meniscal b.
    b. forceps
    b. rongeur
    Schutte shovel nose b.

basocervical fracture

Bassett
    B. electrical stimulation
        system
    B. sign

Batchelor
    B. plate
    B.-Brown extra-articular
        subtalar arthrodesis

Batch-Spittler-McFaddin knee
    disarticulation

Bateman hemiarthroplasty

bath
    Aqua/Whirl b.
    contrast b.
    galvanic b.
    paraffin b.
    whirlpool b.

Battle sign

Batzdorf cervical wire passer

Bauer
    B.-Jackson classification
    B.-Tondra-Trusler opera-
        tion
    B.-Tondra-Trusler tech-
        nique

Bauerfeind
    B. ankle brace
    B. Malleolic ankle orthosis
    B. Comprifix knee brace

Baumann angle

Baumrucker clamp irrigator

Bavarian splint

Baxter-D'Astous procedure

Baylor metatarsal splint

Bayne classification of radial
    agenesis

BBC
    biceps brachialis, coraco-
        brachialis
        BBC muscle

B-E, BE
    below-elbow
        B-E amputation

beach chair position

beaked cervicomedullary junc-
    tion

beaklike
    b. osteophyte
    b. osteophyte formation

Beall-Webel-Bailey technique

Beasley-Babcock forceps

Beath
    B. bone intermedullary peg
    B. needle
    B. pin

Beatson combined ankle angle

Beaty
    B. lateral orthosis
    B. lateral release

Beaufort seating orthosis

Beau line

Beaver blade handle

Bechterew (*variant of*
    Bekhterev)

Bechtol
    B. acetabular component
    B. arthroplasty
    B. hip prosthesis
    B. screw

Beck
    B. disease
    B.-Steffee total ankle pros-
        thesis

Becker
    B. muscular dystrophy
    B. orthopedic spinal sys-
        tem (BOSS)
    B. tendon repair
    B. variant of Duchenne dys-
        trophy

Beckman retractor

Béclard amputation

Becton open reduction

bed
    BioDyne b.
    Borg-Warner b.
    Carrom orthopedic b.
    Chick-Foster orthopedic b.
    CircOlectric b.
    Clinitron air b.
    DMI orthopedic b.
    Hausted orthopedic b.
    Hill-Rom orthopedic b.
    Joerns orthopedic b.
    orthopedic b.
    Roho b.
    Stryker b.

Beeson cast spreader

Behçet syndrome

Bekhterev (*spelled also* Bechterew)
    B. arthritis
    B. disease
    B. spondylitis
    B. test
    B.-Mendel reflex

Bell
    B. nerve
    B.-Dally cervical dislocation
    B.-Tawse open reduction technique

Bellemore-Barrett closing wedge osteotomy

Bellini ligament

Belos compression plate

bender
    AO plate b.
    Bunnell knuckle b.
    DePuy rod b.
    Luque rod b.
    plate b.
    rod b.

Bendixen-Kirschner traction

BeneFin clinical shark cartilage

Bennett
    B. comminuted fracture
    B. dislocation
    B. lesion

Benyi modification of Lambrinudi triple arthrodesis

Berens
    B. muscle clamp
    B. muscle clamp forceps

Berg balance test

Berger
    B. capsulodesis
    B. disease
    B. interscapular amputation
    B. operation
    B.-Bookwalter posterior approach

Bergman mallet

Bergstrom needle

Berke clamp

Berliner percussion hammer

Berman
    B.-Gartland metatarsal osteotomy
    B.-Moorehead metal locator

Bermuda spica cast

Berndt
    B. hip ruler
    B.-Hardy classification of transchondral fracture

Bernhard clamp

Berstein cast table

Bertin
    B. hip retractor
    B. ligament

Bertolotti syndrome

Besnier rheumatism

Bethesda bone

Bethune
B. clamp
B. periosteal elevator
B.-Coryllos rib shears

Beurrier connector

bevel-point Rush pin

Beyer
B. rongeur
B.-Stille rongeur
B.-Stille bone rongeur

BFM arm impairment assessment

BIA
bioelectrical impedance analysis

BIAS total hip system

BICAP cautery

bicentric prosthesis

biceps
b. brachialis, coracobrachialis (BBC)
b. brachialis muscle
b. brachii muscle
b. brachii tendon
b. femoris
b. femoris muscle
b. femoris tendon
b. groove
b. internal lesion
b. jerk
b. jerk reflex test
b. reflex
b. tendinitis

Bichat ligament

bicipital
b. groove

Bickel
B. intramedullary nail
B. intramedullary rod
B.-Moe procedure

bicondylar
b. knee prosthesis
b. T-shaped fracture

Bielschowsky-Janský disease

Bier
B. amputation
B. block
B. block anesthesia
B. operation

bifid
b. graft
b. thumb deformity

bifida
spina b.

biframed distraction technique

Bigelow
B. ligament
B. septum

Bilhaut-Cloquet procedure

Bilos
B. extractor
B. pin extractor

bimalleolar

Bi-Metric hip prosthesis

Biobrane adhesive

Bioclusive
B. select transparent film dressing
B. transparent film dressing

bioconcave vertebra

BioCuff

Biodex
B. isokinetic dynamometer

BioDyne bed

bioelectrical impedance analysis (BIA)

biofeedback
B. 5DX

biofeedback *(continued)*
  electromyographic b.

BioFit Press-Fit acetabular prosthesis

Biofix
  B. absorbable rods and screws
  B. system pin

Bioflex magnetic brace

Bio-Gel decubitus pillow

Bioglass

Biolox Aluminia

biomaterial
  Zenotech b.

biomechanics
  axial plane angular deformity b.

BioMed TENS unit

Biomet
  B. acetabular cup
  B. cement-removal hand chisel
  B. custom implant
  B. fracture brace
  B. MARS acetabular component
  B. Maxim knee system
  B. metal-on-metal articulation hip system

Biometric prosthesis

Bio-Moore endoprosthesis

Bionix absorbable cannulated screw

Bio-Oss synthetic bone

BioPolyMeric graft

biopsy
  Fosnaugh nail b.

BioRCI bioabsorbable screw

BioRoc anchor

BioScrew

BioSorbFX SR plate and screw

BioSphere anchor

BioStinger

BioStop G

Biotex implant metal

Biothotic foot orthosis

bipartite fracture

bipivotal hinge knee brace

Bircher
  B. bone-holding clamp
  B. meniscus knife

Birkett hernia

Bishop bone clamp

bit
  drill b.
  Howmedica microfixation system drill b.

B-K, BK
  below-knee
    B-K amputation

Blackburne-Peel ratio

Black Max mid-size knee component

blade
  Bard-Parker b.
  Gigli saw b.
  Hebra b.
  Müller compression b.
  b. plate
  b. plate fixation
  Smillie-Beaver b.

Blair
  B. talar body fusion blade plate
  B. tibiotalar arthrodesis blade plate
  B.-Morris-Bunn-Hand ankle arthrodesis

Blalock clamp

Bledsoe cast brace

blister
    b. of bone
    fracture b.

block
    axillary b.
    Bier b.
    bone b. procedure
    brachial plexus b.
    conduction b.
    depolarization b.
    digital nerve b.
    facet joint b.
    field b.
    Gill posterior bone b.
    hand b.
    Hara infiltration b.
    interscalene b.
    median nerve b.
    metacarpal b.
    Mikhail bone b.
    musculocutaneous nerve b.
    nerve b.
    nerve root b.
    peripheral nerve b.
    recurrent median nerve b.
    scalene b.
    sciatic leg b.
    sphenopalatine ganglion b.
    spinal cord b.
    stellate sympathetic gan-
        glion b.
    ulnar nerve b.

blocker's exostosis

Bloom splint

Blount
    B. brace
    B. disease
    B. displacement osteotomy
    B. epiphysiodesis
    B. knee retractor
    B. osteotome
    B. splint

Blount (continued)
    B. stapling
    B.-Schmidt Milwaukee
        brace

blow-in fracture

blow-out fracture

Blumensaat line

Blumenthal bone rongeur

Blundell-Jones hip osteotomy

Bobath method

Bobechko spreader

Bodner retractor

body
    artificial vertebral b.
    cartilaginous loose b.
    fibrous loose b.
    Kelvin b.
    newtonian b.
    oryzoid b's
    osteocartilaginous b.
    osteocartilaginous loose b.
    pedunculated loose b.
    rice b.
    Schmorl b.
    talar b.
    vertebral b.

BodyIce cold pack

Böhler (spelled also Boehler)
    B. brace
    B. calcaneal angle
    B. calcaneal view
    B. clamp
    B. fracture frame
    B. lumbosacral angle
    B. pin
    B. skintight cast
    B. stirrup
    B. tong traction
    B.-Braun frame
    B.-Braun splint
    B.-Knowles hip pin
    B.-Steinman pin holder

Bohlman
- B. anterior cervical verte-brectomy
- B. cervical fusion tech-nique
- B. pin
- B. triple wire technique

Boies forceps

Boldrey brace

Bollinger knee brace

bolt
- Alvar b.
- Alvar condylar b.
- Barr b.
- cannulated b.
- DePuy b.
- Fenton tibial b.
- Herzenberg b.
- hexhead b.
- Hubbard-Nylok b.
- No-Lok b.
- Recon proximal drill gui-de b.
- transfixion b.
- Webb-Andreesen condy-lar b.

Bombelli
- B.-Mathys-Morscher hip prosthesis
- B.-Morscher femoral com-ponent

bone
- AAA b.
- b. absorption
- accessory b.
- acromial b.
- Albers-Schönberg marble b.
- b. allograft
- antigen-extracted alloge-neic b.
- astragaloid b.
- astragaloscaphoid b.
- b. autogenous graft
- Bethesda b.
- Bio-Oss synthetic b.
- b.-biting forceps

bone *(continued)*
- bleeding b.
- blister of b.
- b. block procedure
- bridging b.
- b. bur
- cadaver b.
- calcaneocuboid b.
- Calcitite b.
- b. canaliculi
- cancellous b.
- capitate b.
- carpal b.
- chalky b.
- b. chip graft
- coccygeal b.
- collar b.
- compact b.
- cortical b.
- corticocancellous b.
- cribriform b.
- cuboid b.
- cuneiform b.
- b. curet
- b.-cutting forceps
- b. cyst fracture
- demineralized b.
- eburnated b.
- endochondral b.
- b. femoral plug
- b. flap fixation plate
- b. forceps
- fragmental b.
- hamate b.
- heterotopic b.
- b.-holding forceps
- hydroxyapatite b.
- hyoid b.
- innominate b.
- Interpore b.
- ischial b.
- ivory b.
- Kiel b.
- lamellar b.
- lamellated b.
- lenticular b. of hand
- lunate b.
- lunocapitate b.
- marble b.

bone *(continued)*
- b. marrow graft
- metacarpal b.
- metatarsal b.
- morcellated b.
- morcellized b.
- b. morphogenic protein
- navicular b.
- nonlamellated b.
- occipital b.
- odontoid b.
- omovertebral b.
- osteonal lamellar b.
- osteopenic b.
- osteoporotic b.
- pagetoid b.
- b. peg epiphysiodesis
- Pirie b.
- pisiform b.
- pyramidal b.
- radial b.
- b. reamer
- replacement b.
- b. replacement material
- resurrection b.
- rudimentary b.
- sacral b.
- scaphoid b.
- b. scintigraphy
- segmentally demineralized b.
- semilunar b.
- sesamoid b.
- b.-splitting forceps
- spongy b.
- subchondral b.
- supracollicular spike of cortical b.
- talonavicular b.
- tarsal b.
- b.-tendon-b. allograft
- thoracic b's
- tip of sacral b.
- trabeculae of b.
- trapezium b.
- trapezoid b.
- trapezoid b. of Henle
- trapezoid b. of Lyser
- b. trephine

bone *(continued)*
- triquetral b.
- b. trough
- ulnar b.
- uncinate b.
- b. union
- wormian b.
- woven b.
- xiphoid b.

Bone Care International

bone cement
- acrylic b. c.
- CMW b. c.
- DePuy 1 b. c.
- Endurance b. c.
- Implast b. c.
- low-viscosity b. c.
- Osteobond copolymer b. c.
- Palacos b. c.
- Palacos radiopaque b. c.
- PMMA (polymethyl methacrylate) b. c.
- polymerized b. c.
- polymethyl methacrylate (PMMA) b. c.
- Simplex P b. c.
- Surgical Simplex P b. c.
- Zimmer b. c.
- Zimmer low-viscosity b. c.

Bone Collector device

Bonefos

bone graft
- advancement b. g.
- allogenic b. g.
- allogenous b. g.
- Banks b. g.
- bicortical iliac b. g.
- cadaver b. g.
- cancellous b. g.
- cancellous morselized b. g.
- Chuinard autogenous b. g.
- Codivilla b. g.
- cortical b. g.
- corticocancellous b. g.
- b. g. extrusion
- Gillies b. g.
- hemicylindrical b. g.

bone graft *(continued)*
    iliac crest b. g.
    McFarland b. g.
    McMaster b. g.
    Matti-Russe b. g.
    medullary b. g.
    morcellized b. g.
    Nicoll cancellous b. g.
    onlay b. g.
    osteoperiosteal b. g.
    particulate cancellous b. g.
    pedicle b. g.
    Russe b. g.
    Ryerson b. g.
    b. g. shoe horn
    sliding wedge local b. g.
    Soto-Hall b. g.
    split calvarial b. g.
    Weiland iliac crest b. g.
    Wolfe-Kawamoto b. g.

Boneloc cement

Bone Mulch screw

BonePlast

BoneSource hydroxyapatite cement

Bonfiglio
    B. bone replacement material
    B. modification

Bonner position

Bonney
    B. clamp
    B.-Kessel dorsiflexionary tilt-up osteotomy

bony
    b. ankylosis
    b. eburnation
    b. exostosis
    b. osteophyte
    b. purchase
    b. slurry
    b. slurry leakage

boot
    Cryo/Cuff b.
    De Lorme b.

boot *(continued)*
    derotation b.
    Gibney b.
    Markell brace b.
    pneumatic compression b.
    Profore b.
    sequential pneumatic compression b.
    Unna b.
    Unna paste b.
    Venodyne b.
    "Western b." in open fracture

Boplant Surgibone

Borchardt olive-shaped bur

Borchgrevin traction

Borden-Spence-Herman osteotomy

border
    cryptotic medial b.
    lateral acromial b.
    medial b.
    scapulovertebral b.
    vertebral b.

Borg-Warner bed

Borge clamp

Borggreve
    B. limb rotation
    B. method
    B.-Hall technique

Bornholm disease

BOSS
    Becker orthopedic spinal system

Boston
    B. brace thoracolumbosacral orthosis
    B. bivalve cast
    B. Classification System
    B. LINAC
    B. scoliosis brace
    B. soft body jacket

Bosworth
    B. approach

Bosworth *(continued)*
    B. coracoclavicular screw
    B. femoroischial arthrode-
        sis
    B. femoroischial transplant
    B. spine plate
    B. tendo calcaneus repair

Bouchard nodes

bouche de tapir

Bouge needle

Bourgery ligament

Bourneville disease

Bousquet external hypermobil-
    ity test

boutonnière
    b. deformity
    b. hand dislocation

Bovie
    B. cauterization
    B. electrocautery device
    B. knife

Bowen osteotome

Bowman
    B. angle
    B. disks

Bowditch law

Boyd
    B. hip disarticulation
    modified B. amputation of
        ankle and distal tibial
        physis
    B.-Sisk approach

Boyes
    B. muscle clamp
    B. test

Bozzini light conductor

brace
    abduction b.
    accommodative b.
    Aircast Air-Stirrup b.

brace *(continued)*
    Aircast ankle b.
    Aircast Swivel-Strap b.
    AirGEL ankle b.
    Air-Stirrup ankle b.
    ankle b.
    AO b.
    Arnold lumbar b.
    back b.
    Bauerfeind ankle b.
    Bauerfeind Comprifix
        knee b.
    Bioflex magnetic b.
    Biomet fracture b.
    bipivotal hinge knee b.
    Bledsoe cast b.
    Blount b.
    Blount-Schmidt Milwau-
        kee b.
    Böhler b.
    Boldrey b.
    Bollinger knee b.
    Boston scoliosis b.
    calcaneal b.
    caliper b.
    Callender derotational b.
    Cam Walker leg b.
    Capener b.
    Carpal Lok wrist b.
    CASH b.
    Castiglia ankle b.
    Centec Propoint knee b.
    cervical b.
    chairback b.
    Charleston scoliosis b.
    Charnley b.
    Chopart b.
    Cincinnati ACL b.
    collar b.
    contraflexion b.
    DACO b.
    DarcoGel ankle b.
    Dennyson cervical b.
    DePuy fracture b.
    derotation b.
    DonJoy ALP b.
    DonJoy Gold Point knee b.
    Duncan shoulder b.
    dynamic abduction b.

brace *(continued)*
- Exotec b.
- Fisher b.
- Flexor-hinge hand splint b.
- FLOAM ankle stirrup b.
- Florida back b.
- Florida contraflexion b.
- Florida hyperextension b.
- fracture b.
- Futuro wrist b.
- Galveston metacarpal b.
- Genutrain knee b.
- Goldthwait b.
- Guilford cervical b.
- halo b.
- Hennessy knee b.
- Hessing b.
- hinge b.
- hip b.
- Hoke lumbar b.
- Hudson TLSO b.
- Hudson-Jones knee cap b.
- hyperextension b.
- Ilfeld b.
- J-35 hyperextension b.
- J-45 contraflexion b.
- J-55 postfusion b.
- J-59 Florida b.
- Jewett contraflexion b.
- Jewett postfusion b.
- Jewett-Benjamin cervical b.
- Jones b.
- Kleinert postoperative traction b.
- Klenzak spring b.
- knee b.
- knee cage b.
- Knight b.
- knock-knee b.
- Korn Cage knee b.
- kyphosis b.
- LeCocq b.
- leg b.
- Lenox Hill derotational knee b.
- Lenox Hill Spectralite knee b.
- Lerman hinge b.
- Lorenz b.

brace *(continued)*
- Lovitt-Uhler modification of Jewett postfusion b.
- lumbar b.
- MacAusland lumbar b.
- McKee b.
- Medipedic multicentric knee b.
- Miami fracture b.
- Miami TLSO scoliosis b.
- Milwaukee b.
- Nakamura b.
- neck b.
- Neoprene hinged knee b.
- Nextep knee b.
- Newington b.
- Omni knee b.
- Oppenheim b.
- Orthomedics b.
- Ortho-Mold spinal b.
- Orthoplast fracture b.
- Os-5/Plus 2 knee b.
- OsteoArthritic knee b.
- Palumbo dynamic patellar b.
- Palumbo knee b.
- Patten-Bottom-Perthes b.
- Rolyan tibial fracture b.
- ROM knee b.
- Sarmiento fracture b.
- SAS II b.
- Sawa shoulder b.
- Schanz collar b.
- scoliosis b.
- Scottish Rite b.
- Seton hip b.
- shoulder b.
- Smedberg b.
- SOMI b.
- spinal b.
- Spinal Technology bivalve TLSO b.
- Stille b.
- Stromgren ankle b.
- Taylor back b.
- Teufel cervical b.
- Teurlings wrist b.
- Thermoskin b.

brace *(continued)*
    Thomas cervical collar b.
    TLSO b.
    Tomasini b.
    Townsend b.
    Tracker knee b.
    Tri-angle shoulder abduction b.
    turnbuckle ankle b.
    Ultrabrace b.
    unilateral calcaneal b. (UCB)
    Varney acromioclavicular b.
    Victorian b.
    Watco b.
    weightbearing b.
    Wilke boot b.
    wrist b.
    Yale b.
    Zimmer reamer b.
    Zinco CAM Walker b.

brachial
    b. plexus

brachialis

brachiocephalic vein

brachioradialis
    b. flap

brachymetatarsia

Brackett
    B. osteotomy
    B.-Osgood knee approach
    B.-Osgood posterior approach
    B.-Osgood-Putti-Abbott technique

Bradford frame

Brady leg splint

bradykinin

bradymetatarsalgia

Brady-Bishop-Tullos decompression

Bragard test

Brant aluminum splint

Brantigan
    B. cage
    B.-Voshell procedure

brassiere
    Jobst b.

Braun-Yasargil right-angle clip

Breck pin cutter

bregmatomastoid suture

Brett
    B. arthrodesis
    B.-Campbell tibial osteotomy

brevis
    coxa b.
    extensor carpi radialis b.
    extensor digitorum b.
    extensor hallucis b.
    extensor pollicis b.
    flexor carpi quinti b.
    flexor digiti quinti b.
    flexor digitorum b.
    flexor hallucis b.
    flexor pollicis b.
    peroneus b.
    radialis b.
    b. release

Brewster triple arthrodesis

Brickner position

bridge
    autograft b.
    b. graft
    b. of meniscus
    osseus b.
    tarsal b.

Bridge hip system

bridging
    b. bone
    b. callus
    heterotrophic ossification b.

Brigham prosthesis

brim
   pelvic b.
   quadrilateral b.

brisement
   b. forcé

Brissaud scoliosis

Bristow
   B. operation
   B. periosteal elevator
   B. procedure
   B.-Helfet procedure
   B.-May procedure

Brittain
   B. chisel
   B. ischiofemoral arthrode-
      sis

broach
   cemented b.
   cementless b.
   Charnley femoral b.
   ELP b.
   femoral prosthesis b.
   Harris b.
   Koenig metatarsal b.
   Mittlemeir b.
   orthopaedic b.
   Swanson metatarsal b.
   Zimmer femoral canal b.

Broberg-Morrey fracture

Broca
   pilaster of B.

Brockman-Nissen arthrodesis

Brodie
   B. abscess
   B. bursa
   B. disease
   B. knee
   B. ligament

Brodsky-Tullos-Gartsman approach

BROM
   back range of motion

bromhidrosis (*spelled also*
   bromidrosis)
   plantar b.

Brooker
   B. intramedullary nail
   B.-James tendon transfer
   B.-Wills nail

Brooks
   B. atlantoaxial arthrodesis
   B.-Gallie cervical fusion
   B.-Gallie cervical operation
   B.-Jones tendon transfer
   B.-Seddon pectoralis major
      tendon transfer
   B.-Seddon transfer tech-
      nique

Brophy periosteal elevator

Brown
   B. knee joint reconstruc-
      tion
   B.-Adson forceps
   B.-Cushing forceps
   B.-Mueller T-fastener set

Browne splint

Brown-Séquard
   B.-S. lesion
   B.-S. syndrome

Brucella arthritis

brucellosis
   spinal b.

Bruck disease

Brücke lines

Brudzinski
   B. test
   B.-Kernig test

Bruening
   B. chisel
   B.-Citelli rongeur

Bruger
   cul-de-sac of B.

Brun bone curet

Bruner approach

Bruni-Wayne clamp approximator

Brunn plaster shears

Brunnstrom method

Bruns ataxia

Brunswick-Mack rotating drill

Bruser lateral approach

Bryan
   B. arthroplasty
   B.-Morrey elbow approach

Bryant
   B. line
   B. sign
   B. traction

BTM hip system

buccinator
   b. muscle
   b. myomucosal flap

Buchanan disease

Buch-Gramcko gouge

Buchholz
   B. acetabular cup
   B. prosthesis

Buck
   B. bone curet
   B. convoluted traction device
   B. extension
   B. extension splint
   B. fascia
   B. method
   B. operation
   B. periosteal elevator
   B. traction apparatus
   B. traction splint

bucket-handle
   b.-h. fracture
   b.-h. plica
   b.-h. tear of meniscus

Buckley chisel

Bucky diaphragm

Budin hammer toe splint

Buechel-Pappas total ankle

Buerger
   B. disease
   B. test
   B.-Allen exercise

Buford complex

buildup (*noun*)

build up (*verb*)

bulbocavernosus reflex

bulla *pl.*, bullae

Bulldog clamp-applying forceps

bumper fracture

Buncke
   B. technique
   B.-Schulz approximator
   B.-Schulz clamp approximator

bundle
   medial neurovascular b.
   muscle b.
   posterolateral b.
   transverse b. of palmar aponeurosis
   Weissmann b.

Bunge amputation

bunion
   dorsal b.
   Estersohn osteotomy for tailor's b.
   tailor's b.

bunionectomy
   Akin b.

bunionectomy *(continued)*
    Austin b.
    chevron b.
    DuVries-Mann modified
      Z b.
    Hauser b.
    Joplin b.
    Kelikian modified Z b.
    Keller b.
    Lapidus b.
    McBride b.
    modified McBride b.
    osteotomy/b.
    Reverdin b.
    Reverdin-Laird b.
    Reverdin-McBride b.
    Silver b.
    Stone b.
    tailor's b.
    tricorrectional b.
    Wu b.

bunionette
    b.–hallux valgus–splayfoot

Bunnell
    B. atraumatic technique
    B. crisscross suture
    B. dissecting probe
    B. finger extension splint
    B. gutter splint
    B. knuckle bender
    B. modification of Steindler
      flexorplasty
    B. opponensplasty
    B. posterior tibial tendon
      transfer operation
    B. pull-out wire
    B. tendon repair
    B. tendon stripper
    B. tendon transfer
    B. tendon transfer tech-
      nique
    B. wire pull-out suture
    B.-Littler test

bupivacaine

bur *(spelled also* burr)
    Adson b.

bur *(continued)*
    Albee olive-shaped b.
    ball b.
    bone b.
    Borchardt olive-shaped b.
    Burwell b.
    Caparosa b.
    carbide b.
    coarse carbide cone b.
    crosscut b.
    decortication b.
    D'Errico enlarging drill b.
    Doyen cylindrical b.
    Dyonics arthroplasty b.
    enlarging b.
    finish b.
    Hall b.
    high-speed b.
    high-torque b.
    Midas Rex b.
    Ossotome b.
    paronychia b.
    pear b.
    Rotablator rotating b.
    Stille b.
    Zimmer rotary b.

Burford-Finochietto rib
  spreader

Burgess below-knee amputation

Burkhalter
    B. modification of Stiles-
      Bunnell technique
    B. transfer technique
    B.-Reyes method for pha-
      langeal fracture

Burnham finger splint

Burns
    B. test
    B.-Haney incision

burr *(variant of* bur)

bursa *pl.* bursae
    b. of Achilles
    b. of Achilles tendon
    acromial b.
    adventitious b.
    anconeal b.

bursa *(continued)*

anconeal b. of triceps muscle

b. anserina

anserine b.

anterior genual b.

bicipital b.

bicipitofibular b.

bicipitoradial b.

b. bicipitoradialis

Brodie b.

calcaneal b.

b. of calcaneal tendon

Calori b.

common peroneal b.

coracobrachial b.

coracoid b.

b. cubitalis interossea

cubitoradial b.

deep infrapatellar b.

deep lateral retroepicondyloid b.

deep patellar b.

deep postcalcaneal b.

deltoid b.

external inferior genual b.

external infracondyloid b.

external postgenual b.

fibular b.

b. of flexor carpi radialis muscle

gastrocnemiosemimembranous b.

genual b.

gluteal b.

gluteal intermuscular bursae

gluteofascial bursae

gluteofemoral bursae

bursae gluteofemorales

gluteotuberosal b.

humeral b.

b. iliaca subtendinea

b. iliopectinea

iliopectineal b.

b. of iliopsoas muscle

iliopubic vesicular b.

inferior b. of biceps femoris muscle

bursa *(continued)*

inferior subtendinous b. of biceps femoris muscle

infragenual b.

infrapatellar b.

b. infrapatellaris profunda

b. infrapatellaris subcutanea

bursae intermusculares musculorum gluteorum

internal superior genual bursae

internal supracondyloid b.

interosseous cubital b.

intertubercular b.

b. intratendinea olecrani

intratendinous supra-anconeal b.

ischiadic b.

b. ischiadica musculi glutei maximi

b. ischiadica musculi obturatorii interni

ischial b. of gluteus maximus muscle

ischial b. of obturator internus muscle

ischiogluteal b.

lateral b. of gastrocnemius muscle

lateral subtendinous b. of gastrocnemius muscle

b. of latissimus dorsi muscle

medial b. of gastrocnemius muscle

medial subtendinous b. of gastrocnemius muscle

medial supracondyloid b.

middle patellar b.

middle prepatellar b.

Monro b.

b. mucosa

b. mucosa submuscularis

mucous b.

multilocular b.

b. musculi bicipitis femoris inferior

bursa *(continued)*
  b. musculi bicipitis femoris superior
  b. musculi coracobrachialis
  b. musculi extensoris carpi radialis brevis
  b. musculi gastrocnemii lateralis
  b. musculi gastrocnemii medialis
  b. musculi infraspinati
  b. musculi latissimi dorsi
  b. musculi obturatoris interni
  b. musculi piriformis
  b. musculi poplitei
  b. musculi sartorii propria
  b. musculi semimembranosi
  b. musculi subscapularis
  b. musculi teretis majoris
  olecranon b.
  b. of olecranon
  b. of piriform muscle
  pisiform b.
  popliteal b.
  b. of popliteal muscle
  postcalcaneal b.
  posterior genual b.
  bursae praepatellares
  b. praepatellaris subcutanea
  b. praepatellaris subfascialis
  b. praepatellaris subtendinea
  prepatellar bursae
  bursae prepatellares
  b. prepatellaris profunda
  b. prepatellaris subaponeurotica
  b. prepatellaris subcutanea
  b. prepatellaris subfascialis
  b. prepatellaris subtendinea
  prespinous patellar b.
  pretibial b.
  bursae propriae musculi sartorii

bursa *(continued)*
  pyriform b.
  b. of quadratus femoris muscle
  retrocalcaneal b.
  retrocondyloid b.
  sciatic b. of gluteus maximus muscle
  sciatic b. of obturator internus muscle
  b. sciatica musculi glutei maximi
  b. sciatica musculi obturatorii interni
  semimembranosogastrocnemial b.
  semimembranous b.
  semitendinous b.
  subachilleal b.
  subacromial b.
  b. subacromialis
  subcalcaneal b.
  subclavian b.
  subcoracoid b.
  subcrural b.
  b. subcutanea
  b. subcutanea acromialis
  b. subcutanea calcanea
  b. subcutanea infrapatellaris
  b. subcutanea malleoli lateralis
  b. subcutanea malleoli medialis
  b. subcutanea olecrani
  b. subcutanea prepatellaris
  b. subcutanea tuberositatis tibiae
  subcutaneous b.
  subcutaneous acromial b.
  subcutaneous calcaneal b.
  subcutaneous infrapatellar b.
  subcutaneous b. of lateral malleolus
  subcutaneous b. of medial malleolus
  subcutaneous b. of olecranon

bursa *(continued)*
   subcutaneous patellar b.
   subcutaneous prepatel-
     lar b.
   subcutaneous synovial b.
   subcutaneous trochanter-
     ic b.
   subcutaneous b. of tuber-
     osity of tibia
   subdeltoid b.
   b. subdeltoidea
   b. subfascialis
   b. subfascialis prepatellaris
   subfascial prepatellar b.
   subfascial synovial b.
   subiliac b.
   subligamentous b.
   b. submuscularis
   submuscular synovial b.
   subpatellar b.
   b. subtendinea
   b. subtendinea iliaca
   b. subtendinea musculi bi-
     cipitis femoris inferior
   b. subtendinea musculi
     gastrocnemii lateralis
   b. subtendinea musculi
     gastrocnemii medialis
   b. subtendinea musculi in-
     fraspinati
   b. subtendinea musculi la-
     tissimi dorsi
   b. subtendinea musculi ob-
     turatorii interni
   bursae subtendineae mus-
     culi sartorii
   b. subtendinea musculi
     subscapularis
   b. subtendinea musculi ter-
     etis majoris
   b. subtendinea musculi ti-
     bialis anterioris
   b. subtendinea musculi ti-
     bialis posterioris
   b. subtendinea musculi tra-
     pezii
   b. subtendinea musculi tri-
     cipitis brachii
   b. subtendinea olecrani

bursa *(continued)*
   b. subtendinea prepatel-
     laris
   subtendinous b.
   subtendinous b. of anterior
     tibial muscle
   subtendinous iliac b.
   subtendinous b. of infraspi-
     natus muscle
   subtendinous b. of internal
     obturator muscle
   subtendinous b. of lateral
     head of gastrocnemius
     muscle
   subtendinous b. of latissi-
     mus dorsi muscle
   subtendinous b. of medial
     head of gastrocnemius
     muscle
   subtendinous b. of obtura-
     tor internus muscle
   subtendinous b. of poste-
     rior tibial muscle
   subtendinous prepatellar b.
   subtendinous bursae of
     sartorius muscle
   subtendinous b. of sub-
     scapularis muscle
   subtendinous synovial b.
   subtendinous b. of teres
     major muscle
   subtendinous b. of trape-
     zius muscle
   subtendinous b. of triceps
     muscle of arm
   superficial inferior infrapa-
     tellar b.
   superficial b. of knee
   superficial b. of olecranon
   superior b. of biceps fe-
     moris muscle
   supernumerary b.
   supragenual b.
   suprapatellar b.
   b. suprapatellaris
   synovial b.
   synovial b. of trochlea
   b. synovialis
   b. synovialis subcutanea

bursa *(continued)*
    b. synovialis subfascialis
    b. synovialis submuscularis
    b. synovialis subtendinea
    b. tendinis Achillis
    b. tendinis calcanei
    b. of tendon of Achilles
    trochanteric b. of gluteus
        maximus muscle
    trochanteric bursae of glu-
        teus medius muscle
    trochanteric b. of gluteus
        minimus muscle
    b. trochanterica musculi
        glutei maximi
    bursae trochantericae mus-
        culi glutei medii
    b. trochanterica musculi
        glutei minimi
    b. trochanterica subcuta-
        nea
    trochlear synovial b.
    tuberoischiadic b.
    ulnoradial b.
    Voshell b.

bursal
    b. cyst
    b. débridement
    b. inflammation
    b. sac
    b. tissue

bursitis
    Achilles b.
    adhesive b.
    anserine b.
    calcific b.
    chronic retrocalcaneal b.
    cubital b.
    iliopsoas b.
    infracalcaneal b.
    infrapatellar b.
    intermetatarsophalan-
        geal b.
    ischiogluteal b.
    medial gastrocnemius b.
    olecranon b.
    patellar b.

bursitis *(continued)*
    popliteal b.
    postcalcaneal b.
    prepatellar b.
    pyogenic b.
    radiohumeral b.
    retrocalcaneal b.
    scapulohumeral b.
    semimembranous b.
    septic b.
    subacromial b.
    subdeltoid b.
    subgluteal b.
    subscapularis b.
    superficial calcaneal b.
    tarsal navicular b.
    Tornwaldt b.
    trochanteric b.
    tuberculous trochanteric b.

bursocentesis

bursography

bursolith

bursopathy

bursotomy

burst
    b. fracture
    b.-type laceration

bursting dislocation

Burton sign

Burwell bur

Busenkell posterior hip retrac-
    tor

Busquet disease

Butcher saw

butterfly
    b. fracture
    b. fracture fragment

buttonhole
    b. deformity
    b. fracture
    b. rupture

buttress
    OMNI pretibial b.
    b. thread screw

Byars mandibular prosthesis

bypass
    extended tibial in situ b.

bypass *(continued)*
    femorodistal b.
    popliteus b.

BWM
    Bad Wildungen Metz
        BWM spine system

C
  C angle
  C clamp
  C stance ankle

C1
  atlas
    cruciform ligament of
      C1
    C1 fracture
    transverse ligament of
      C1

C1–C3 cruciate pulley

cable
  antirotation c.
  Dall-Miles c.
  Dwyer scoliosis c.
  Gallie fusion using c.
  Songer c.
  titanium c.
  c.-twister orthosis

Cabot
  C. leg splint
  C. posterior splint

cadaveric knee

cadence of gait

Cadenza girdle

Caffey disease

cage
  BAK c.
  Brantigan c.
  fusion c.
  Harms c.
  Ray threaded fusion c.
    (TFC)

Calandruccio
  C. impaction screw-plate
  C. triangular compression
    apparatus

calcaneal
  c. apophysitis
  c. L osteotomy
  c. tenodesis

calcanean

calcanectomy

calcanei (*plural of* calcaneus)

calcaneocavovarus
  c. deformity

calcaneocavus
  talipes c.

calcaneoclavicular ligament

calcaneocuboid (CC)
  c. arthrodesis
  c. subluxation

calcaneocuboideum
  ligamentum c.

calcaneofibulare
  ligamentum c.

calcaneofibular ligament (CFL)

calcaneonavicular
  c. bar resection
  c. ligament–tibialis poste-
    rior tendon advancement

calcaneopelvic arthrodesis

calcaneoplantar angle

calcaneoscaphoid

calcaneotibial
  c. angle
  c. arthrodesis

calcaneotibiale
  ligamentum c.

calcaneovalgus

calcaneus *pl.* calcanei
  displaced intraarticular c.
  c. secondarius
  talipes c.
  White-Kraynick tendo c.

calcar
  c. femorale
  c. pedis
  c. reamer

calcar *(continued)*
    c. trimmer with Zimmer-Hudson shank

calcificans
    chondrodystrophia c.

calcification
    flocculent foci of c.
    heterotropic c.
    paraarticular c.

calcified osteoid

calcinosis
    c. circumscripta
    c. intervertebralis
    tumoral c.

Calcitite
    C. bone
    C. graft

calcium
    c. alginate
    c. alginate dressing
    c. glubionate
    c. hydroxyapatite
    c. pyrophosphate dihydrate (CPPD)
    c. pyrophosphate dihydrate deposition

Caldani ligament

Caldwell
    C. hanging cast
    C.-Durham flatfoot technique
    C.-Durham tendon operation

calibrator
    screw depth c.

caliper
    Harpenden c.
    Thomas walking c.
    Townley femur c.
    Vernier c.

Callander amputation

Calleja exercises

Callender
    C. derotational brace
    C. technique hip prosthesis

callosal lesion

callus
    bone c.
    bridging c.
    ensheathing c.
    external c.
    florid c.
    fracture c.
    internal c.
    medullary c.
    myelogenous c.
    pinch c.
    shearing c.

Calman-Nicolle finger prosthesis

Calori bursa

Caltagirone chisel

Calvé-Perthes disease

calx

CAM, Cam
    controlled ankle motion

camera
    DyoCam 550 arthroscopic video c.

Cameron
    C. fracture apparatus
    C.-Haight periosteal elevator

Camitz tendon transfer

Cam Lok knee joint

Campbell
    C. ankle procedure
    C. cannulated screw
    C. interpositional arthroplasty
    C. ligament
    C. periosteal elevator
    C. posterior shoulder approach

Campbell *(continued)*
    C. rongeur
    C. tibial osteotomy
    C. traction splint
    C.-Akbarnia arthrodesis
    C.-Goldthwaite procedure
    C.-Rinehard-Kalenak anterior arthrodesis

Camper
    C. chiasma
    C. fascia

camptocormia

camptodactyly

camptomelia

camptomelic
    c. dwarfism

camptospasm

Camurati-Engelmann disease

Cam Walker brace

Canadian crutch

Canakis beaded hip pin

canal
    adductor c.
    Alcock c.
    calciferous c's
    c. of Frohse
    central c. of modiolus
    crural c.
    crural c. of Henle
    Guyon c.
    haversian c.
    humeral c.
    Hunter c.
    hydrops c.
    intersacral c.
    intramedullary c.
    obturator c.
    obturator c. of pubic bone
    pisohamate c.
    Richet tibio-astragalocalcaneal c.

canal *(continued)*
    spinal c.
    subsartorial c.
    talar c.
    tarsal c.
    Volkmann c.

Canale
    C. osteotomy
    C.-Kelly talar neck fracture

canaliculus *pl.* canaliculi
    bone canaliculi
    haversian c.

canalis
    c. adductorius
    c. carpi
    c. femoralis
    c. nutricius
    c. nutriens
    c. obturatorius
    c. sacralis
    c. spinalis
    c. subsartorialis
    c. vertebralis

Canavan-van Bogaert-Bertrand disease

cancellous
    c. bone
    c. morcellized bone graft
    c. versus cortical bone

cane
    adjustable c.
    English c.
    offset c.
    quadrapod c.
    single-point c.
    small-base quad c.
    tripod c.

cannula
    Acufex double-lumen arthroscopic c.
    Dyonics c.
    Eriksson muscle biopsy c.
    McCain TMJ c.
    microirrigating c.
    self-sealing c.
    Teflon c.

cannula *(continued)*
    zone-specific c.

Cantelli sign

cap
    acetabular c.
    Cloward drill guide c.
    knee c.
    Silipos mesh c.
    Zang metatarsal c.
    Zimmer tibial nail c.

Caparosa
    C. bur
    C. reamer

capeline bandage

Capello
    C. slim-line abduction pillow
    C. technique

Capener
    C. brace
    C. coil splint
    C. finger splint
    C. lateral rachiotomy

CAPIS
    CAPIS bone plate system
    CAPIS screw

capital
    c. epiphyseal angle
    c. femoral epiphysis
    c. fragment
    c. ligament

capitate
    c. bone
    c.-lunate joint

capitellar fracture

capitellocondylar
    c. total elbow arthroplasty
    c. unconstrained elbow
        prosthesis

capitellum
    Hahn-Steinthal fracture
        of c.
    Kocher-Lorenz fracture of c.

capitolunate angle

capitular epiphysis

capitulum
    c. costae
    c. fibulae
    c. humeri
    c. of humerus
    c. radii
    c. radiale humeri fracture
    c. ulnae

Capner
    C. gouge
    C. splint

caprolactam suture

CAPS ArthroWand

Capset (calcium sulfate) bone
    graft barrier

capsula
    c. articularis
    c. articularis acromioclavi-
        cularis
    c. articularis articulationis
        tarsi transversae
    c. articularis articula-
        tionum vertebrarum
    c. articularis atlantoaxialis
        lateralis
    c. articularis atlantoepistro-
        phica
    c. articularis atlantooccipi-
        talis
    c. articularis calcaneocu-
        boidea
    c. articularis capitis costae
    capsulae articulares carpo-
        metacarpeae
    c. articularis carpometacar-
        pea pollicis
    c. articularis costotransver-
        saria
    c. articularis coxae
    c. articularis cubiti
    capsulae articulares digito-
        rum manus

capsula *(continued)*
    capsulae articulares digitorum pedis
    c. articularis genus
    c. articularis humeri
    capsulae articulares intermetacarpeae
    capsulae articulares intermetatarseae
    capsulae articulares interphalangearum manus
    capsulae articulares interphalangearum pedis
    c. articularis manus
    capsulae articulares metacarpophalangeae
    capsulae articulares metatarsophalangeae
    c. articularis ossis pisiformis
    c. articularis radioulnaris distalis
    c. articularis sternoclavicularis
    c. articularis sternocostalis
    c. articularis talocalcanea
    c. articularis talocruralis
    c. articularis talonavicularis
    capsulae articulares tarsometatarseae
    c. articularis tibiofibularis

capsule
    anterior c.
    anteromedial c.
    articular c.
    cartilage c.
    elbow c.
    facet c.
    Gerota c.
    joint c.
    Kadian c.
    meniscofemoral c.
    meniscotibial c.
    metatarsophalangeal joint c.
    synovial c.
    talonavicular c.

capsule *(continued)*
    trapeziometacarpal c.

capsulectomy
    subtalar c.

capsulitis
    adhesive c.
    glenohumeral adhesive c.

capsulodesis
    Berger c.

capsulorrhaphy
    pants-over-vest c.
    Roux-duToit staple c.

capsulotomy
    stereotaxic anterior c.

caput
    c. breve musculi bicipitis brachii
    c. breve musculi bicipitis femoris
    c. costae
    c. distortum
    c. femoris
    c. fibulae
    c. fibulare
    c. humerale
    c. humerale musculi flexoris carpi ulnaris
    c. humerale musculi flexoris digitorum sublimis
    c. humerale musculi pronatoris teretis
    c. humeri
    c. humeroulnare musculi flexoris digitorum superficialis
    c. laterale musculi gastrocnemii
    c. laterale musculi tricipitis brachii
    c. longum musculi bicipitis brachii
    c. longum musculi bicipitis femoris
    c. longum musculi tricipitis brachii

caput *(continued)*
    c. mediale musculi gastroc-
        nemii
    c. mediale musculi tricipitis
        brachii
    c. metacarpale
    c. metatarsale
    c. musculi
    c. obliquum musculi adduc-
        toris hallucis
    c. obliquum musculi adduc-
        toris pollicis
    c. ossis metacarpalis
    c. ossis metacarpi
    c. ossis metatarsalis
    c. ossis metatarsi
    c. phalangis manus
    c. phalangis pedis
    c. planum
    c. radiale
    c. radiale musculi flexoris
        digitorum superficialis
    c. radii
    c. rectum musculi recti fe-
        moris
    c. reflexum musculi recti fe-
        moris
    c. talare
    c. tali
    c. transversum musculi ad-
        ductoris hallucis
    c. transversum musculi ad-
        ductoris pollicis
    c. ulnae
    c. ulnare musculi flexoris
        carpi ulnaris
    c. ulnare musculi pronato-
        ris teretis

carbide bur

carbon-tungsten rasp

Carborundum grinding wheel

Carceau-Brahms ankle arthrod-
    esis

Cardan screwdriver

Carden amputation

carious

Carleton spots

C-arm fluoroscope

Carnesale
    C. acetabular extensile ap-
        proach
    C. hip approach
    C. technique

carpal
    c.-intercarpal joint
    c.-metacarpal joint

Carpal Lok wrist brace

carpectomy
    Omer-Capen c.

carpometacarpal

carpophalangeal joint

carporadial articulation

carpus
    complex instability of c.

Carrell-Girard screw

carrier
    Cave-Rowe ligature c.

Carroll
    C.-Bennett retractor
    C.-Bunnell drill
    C.-Legg osteotome
    C.-Legg periosteal elevator
    C.-Smith-Petersen osteo-
        tome

Carrom orthopedic bed

CarTCell (liquefied cartilage ex-
    tract)
    C. NF (non-frozen)

Carter
    C. splint
    C. Rowe awl

Carticel autologous cultured
    chondrocytes

Carticin

cartilage
    c. ablation

cartilage *(continued)*
  athrodial c.
  articular c.
  BeneFin clinical shark c.
  calcified c.
  cellular c.
  circumferential c.
  connecting c.
  costal c.
  cryopreserved c.
  c.-derived inhibitor (CDI)
  diarthrodial c.
  eburnation of c.
  elastic c.
  ensiform c.
  epiphyseal c.
  falciform c's
  floating c.
  glenoid c.
  interarticular c.
  interosseous c.
  intervertebral c.
  investing c.
  knee c.
  mucronate c.
  obducent c.
  ossifying c.
  patellofemoral c.
  physeal c.
  precursory c.
  quadrangular c.
  reticular c.
  semilunar c. of knee joint
  sigmoid c's
  slipping rib c.
  sternal c.
  stratified c.
  torn knee c.
  triquetral c.
  triquetrous c.
  triradial c.
  triticeous c.
  Weitbrecht c.
  xiphoid c.
  Y c.

cartilagines *(plural of* cartilago)

cartilaginiform

cartilaginoid

cartilaginous

cartilago *pl.* cartilagines
  c. articularis
  c. ensiformis
  c. epiphysialis
  cartilagines falcatae

cartilagotropic

cartwheel fracture

CASH brace

CASP
  contoured anterior spinal
  plate

Caspar anterior instrumentation

Caspari
  C. arthroscopic portal
  C. repair

cast
  accessory navicular c.
  Bermuda spica c.
  bivalved cylinder c.
  Böhler skintight c.
  Boston bivalve c.
  Caldwell hanging c.
  Cotrel scoliosis c.
  Dehne c.
  c. with dorsal toe plate ex-
  tension
  flexion body c.
  Frejka c.
  gauntlet c.
  Gelocast c.
  hyperextension c.
  Kite metatarsal c.
  Lorenz c.
  Moe modified Cotrel c.
  Neufeld c.
  Orfizip knee c.
  Orthoplast slipper c.
  pantaloon spica c.
  Petrie spica c.
  quadriceps femoris mus-
  cle c.
  Risser turnbuckle c.

cast *(continued)*
    semirigid fiberglass c.
    Sbarbaro spica c.
    spica c.
    c. spreader
    sugar-tong c.
    univalve c.
    Unna boot c.
    Velpeau c.
    windowed c.

Castiglia ankle brace

Castroviejo
    C. needle holder
    C. trephine

catagmatic

Cathcart Orthocentric hip prosthesis

catheter
    SpineCATH intradiscal c.

Catlin amputating knife

cauda
    c. equina
    c. equina syndrome

caudal
    c. lamina resection
    c. retinaculum

caudocephalad

caudocranial

causalgic pain

cauterization
    Bovie c.

cautery
    Aesculap bipolar c.
    BICAP c.
    monopolar c.

Cave
    C.-Rowe ligature carrier
    C.-Rowe shoulder dislocation technique

Cavin osteotome

cavitas
    c. articularis
    c. glenoidalis
    c. medullaris

cavitation

cavity
    absorption c's
    articular c.
    cotyloid c.
    glenoid c.
    joint c.
    marrow c.
    medullary c.
    popliteal c.
    resorption c.
    saclike c.
    sigmoid c. of radius
    sigmoid c. of ulna
    synovial c.

cavoabductovarus deformity

cavocalcaneovalgus deformity

cavoequinovarus

cavovalgus
    pes c.
    talipes c.

cavovarus
    c. deformity
    pes c.
    talipes c.

cavus
    metatarsus c.
    pes c.

CAWO
    closing abductory-wedge osteotomy

CC
    calcaneocuboid
        CC arthrodesis
        CC subluxation

CCD
    central collodiaphyseal angle

CDH
  congenital dislocation of
    the hip
  congenitally dysplastic hip

CDI
  cartilage-derived inhibitor

CE
  capital epiphysis

Celestone Soluspan

celiomyositis

cell
  bone c.
  cartilage c's
  contractile fiber c's
  Gegenbaur c.
  LE c.
  mesenchymal c.
  osseous c.
  osteoclastic giant c.
  osteogenic c.
  osteoprogenitor c's
  sarcogenic c's
  satellite c's
  Schwann c.
  skeletogenous c.
  spindle c.
  synovial c.
  tendon c.

cellulitis
  anaerobic c.

cement
  acrylic bone c.
  arthroplasty c.
  bone c.
  Boneloc c.
  BoneSource hydroxy-
    apatite c.
  CMW bone c.
  DePuy 1 bone c.
  Endurance bone c.
  Howmedica c.
  Implast bone c.
  low-viscosity bone c.
  methyl methacrylate c.

cement *(continued)*
  Norian SRS c.
  Orthocomp c.
  Orthoset c.
  Osteobond copolymer
    bone c.
  Palacos bone c.
  Palacos radiopaque bone c.
  PMMA bone c.
  polymerized bone c.
  polymethyl methacrylate
    bone c.
  prosthetic antibiotic-
    loaded acrylic c.
    (PROSTALAC)
  Protoplast c.
  Refobacin Palacos c.
  Simplex P bone c.
  SRS injectable c.
  Surgical Simplex P bone c.
  Tisseel c.
  Zimmer bone c.
  Zimmer Cibatome C. Eater
  Zimmer low-viscosity
    bone c.

cement dispenser
  Jet vac c. d.

cementless
  c. broach
  c. femoral component
  c. total hip arthroplasty

cementome
  Anspach c.

Centec Propoint knee brace

center
  accessory ossification c. of
    calcaneus
  c. of axial rotation
  c. edge angle of Wiberg
  ossification c.
  splenial c.

central collodiaphyseal angle
  (CCD)

Centralign precoat hip prosthesis

centrum
c. ossificationis
c. ossificationis primarium
c. ossificationis secundarium
c. of vertebra
vertebral c.

cephalad

cephalocaudal

cephaloscapular projection

Ceramion prosthesis

cerclage
Dall-Miles c.
Dall-Miles cable c.
Howmedica c.
c. wire
c. wire fixation

cervical
AOA c. halo traction
c. arthrodesis
c. compaction test
c. corpectomy
c. diskectomy
c. halter traction
c. interbody fusion
c. lordosis
c. radiculitis
c. rotation in extension
c. screw
c. screw insertion
c. spine kyphotic deformity
c. spine laminectomy
c. spine screw-plate fixation
c. spondylolysis
c. spondylotic myopathy
c. sympathectomy
c. synostosis
c. tension myositis
c. trochanteric fracture

Cervical-Stim

cervicocranial

cervicodynia

cervicogenic

cervicooccipital fusion

cervicothoracolumbosacral orthosis (CTLSO)

cervicotrochanteric displaced fracture

Cervi-Fix system

Cervitrak device

CFL
calcaneofibular ligament

C1 fracture

Chaddock sign

chamfer cut

Championnière bone drill

Chance vertebral fracture

Chandler
C. knee retractor
C. patellar advancement
C. unreamed interlocking tibial nail

change
neuromuscular gait pattern c.

Chang-Miltner incision

Chapchal knee arthrodesis

Chaput
C. fracture
C. tubercle

Charcot
C. arthritis
C. arthropathy
C. arthroplasty
C. foot
C. disruption
C. hip arthrodesis
C. joint
C. joint disease
C. spine

Charcot *(continued)*
    C.-Marie-Tooth disease

Charleston scoliosis brace

charley horse

Charnley
    C. acetabular cup prosthesis
    C. ankle arthrodesis
    C. apparatus
    C. brace
    C. brace handle
    C. cemented prosthesis
    C. compression clamp
    C. compression-type knee fusion
    C. curet
    C. deepening reamer
    C. external fixation clamp
    C. femoral condyle drill
    C. femoral condyle radius gauge
    C. femoral inlay aligner
    C. femoral inlay guillotine
    C. implant
    C. low-friction hip arthroplasty
    C. offset-bore cup
    C. pin
    C. pin clamp
    C. pin retractor
    C. prosthesis
    C. reamer
    C. self-retaining retractor
    C. socket gauge
    C. standard-stem component
    C. tibial onlay jig
    C. total hip arthroplasty
    C. total hip replacement
    C. trochanter reamer
    C. wire-holding forceps
    C.-Hastings prosthesis
    C.-Houston shoulder arthrodesis
    C.-Müller hip prosthesis

Charriere
    C. bone saw
    C. saw

Chassaignac
    C. axillary muscle
    C. tubercle

Chatzidakis hinged Vitallium implant prosthesis

Chaves
    C.-Rapp muscle transfer technique
    C.-Rapp paralysis

cheilectomy
    Garceau c.
    Mann-Coughlin-DuVries c.
    Sage c.
    Sage-Clark c.

cheiralgia paresthetica

cheirarthritis

cheiroarthropathy

cheirobrachialgia

cheiromegaly

cheiroplasty

cheiropodalgia

cheirospasm

chelation therapy

chemonucleolysis
    chymopapain c.
    double-needle c.

Cherf
    C. cast stand
    C. leg holder

Cherry
    C. screw extractor
    C.-Austin drill

chest
    alar c.
    barrel c.

chest *(continued)*
    c.-band transmitter
    cobbler c.
    foveated c.
    funnel c.
    keeled c.
    paralytic c.
    pigeon c.
    pterygoid c.
    tetrahedron c.

Chester disease

chevron
    c.-Akin double osteotomy
    c. bunionectomy
    c. hallux valgus correction
    c. osteotomy
    c. osteotomy with rigid
       screw fixation

Cheyne periosteal elevator

Chiari
    C. innominate osteotomy
    C.-Salter-Steel pelvic osteot-
      omy

chiasm
    c. of digits of hand
    tendinous c. of fingers

chiasma
    Camper c.
    c. tendinum digitorum ma-
      nus

Chiba spine system

Chick
    C.-Foster orthopedic bed
    C.-Langren orthopedic table

Childress
    C. ankle fixation technique
    C. duck waddle test

chip
    bone c.
    cancellous c.
    c. fracture

Chiroflow back rest

chiromegaly

chiropodalgia

chisel
    Adson laminectomy c.
    Alexander c.
    ASIF c.
    Ballenger-Hajek c.
    Biomet cement-removal
      hand c.
    box c.
    Brittain c.
    Bruening c.
    Buckley c.
    Caltagirone c.
    Cinelli-McIndoe c.
    Cloward c.
    Cottle c.
    Dautrey c.
    D'Errico lamina c.
    Fomon c.
    Freer c.
    Harmon c.
    Hibbs c.
    Kerrison c.
    Lambert-Lowman c.
    Lexer c.
    Lucas c.
    Metzenbaum c.
    Meyerding c.
    Moore prosthesis-mortis-
      ing c.
    Oratek c.
    Partsch c.
    Passow c.
    Puka c.
    Schwartze c.
    Smillie cartilage c.
    Smillie meniscectomy c.
    Stille bone c.
    Trautmann c.

choline
    c. magnesium trisalicylate
    c. salicylate

cholinergic vagal function

chondral
    c. fragment

chondralgia

chondralloplasia

chondrectomy

chondrification

chondritis
  costal c.
  c. intervertebralis calcanea

chondroblast

chondroblastoma
  benign c.

chondrocalcinosis

chondroclast

chondrocostal

chondrocyte
  autologous cultured c.
  hypertrophic c.
  isogenous c's

chondrodiastasis

chondrodysplasia
  hereditary deforming c.
  metaphyseal c.
  c. punctata

chondrodystrophia
  c. calcificans congenita
  c. congenita punctata
  c. fetalis calcificans

chondrodystrophy
  hyperplastic c.
  hypoplastic c.
  hypoplastic fetal c.

chondroepiphyseal

chondroepiphysitis

chondrofibroma

chondrogenesis

chondrography

chondroid

chondroitan

chondrolipoma

chondrology

chondrolysis

chondroma
  extraskeletal c.
  joint c.
  juxtacortical c.
  periosteal c.
  synovial c.

chondromalacia
  c. patellae

chondromatosis
  synovial c.

chondromatous

chondrometaplasia
  synovial c.
  tenosynovial c.

chondromucin

chondromucoprotein

chondromyoma

chondromyxoma

chondronecrosis

chondroosseous

chondroosteodystrophy

chondropathia
  c. tuberosa

chondropathology

chondropathy

chondrophyte

chondroplasia
  c. punctata

chondroplast

chondroplastic
  c. dwarfism
  c. myotonia

chondroplasty
  arthroscopic abrasion c.

chondroporosis

chondrosarcoma
    central c.
    clear cell c.
    dedifferentiated c.
    differentiated c.
    extraskeletal c.
    juxtacortical c.
    mesenchymal c.
    myxoid c.
    periosteal c.
    peripheral c.

chondrosarcomatosis

chondrosarcomatous

chondrosis

chondroskeleton

chondrosteoma

chondrosternoplasty

chondrotome

chondrotomy

chondrotrophic

chondroxiphoid

Chonstruct chondral repair system

Chopart
    C. ankle dislocation
    C. articulation
    C. brace
    C. hindfoot amputation
    C. midtarsal joint
    C. operation

chorda
    c. magna
    c. obliqua membranae interosseae antebrachii

chordotomy

Chow technique

CHPS
    chronic back pain syndrome

Chrisman
    C.-Snook procedure
    C.-Snook reconstruction of ankle ligament

Christiansen hip prosthesis

Christmas tree adaptor

chromatolysis

chromium-cobalt alloy implant

chronaxie (*spelled also* chronaxy)

CHSD
    congenital hyperphosphatemic skeletal dysplasia

chrysotherapy

Chuinard
    C. autogenous bone graft
    C.-Petersen ankle arthrodesis
    C.-Petersen ankle fusion

Chvostek
    C. sign
    C. test

chymopapain
    c. blocking agent
    c. chemonucleolysis

Cicherelli bone rongeur

Cincinnati ACL brace

cinearthrography

Cinelli
    C. osteotome
    C.-McIndoe chisel

cineplastics

cineplasty

cinesalgia

cingulotomy

cingulum
    c. membri inferioris
    c. membri superioris

cingulum *(continued)*
    c. pectorale
    c. pelvicum

cingulumotomy

cinology

cinometer

Cintor knee prosthesis

CircOlectric bed

circumduction maneuver

circumference
    articular c.
    calf c.
    pelvic c.

circumferentia
    c. articularis
    c. articularis capitis radii
    c. articularis capitis ulnae
    c. articularis capituli ulnae

circumscripta
    calcinosis c.

Citelli
    C. angle
    C. punch forceps

clamp
    Acland c.
    Aesculap c.
    Allen-Kocher c.
    Allis c.
    ASSI Lalonde dynamic compression bone c.
    Auvard c.
    Backhaus towel c.
    Backhaus-Jones towel c.
    Bailey-Cowley c.
    Bailey-Morse c.
    Balfour c.
    Ballantine c.
    bar-to-bar c.
    Berens muscle c.
    Berke c.
    Bernhard c.
    Bethune c.
    Bircher bone-holding c.
    Bishop bone c.

clamp *(continued)*
    Blalock c.
    Böhler c.
    bone extension c.
    bone-holding c.
    Bonney c.
    Borge c.
    Boyes muscle c.
    bulldog c.
    cartilage c.
    C c.
    Charnley bone c.
    Charnley compression c.
    Charnley external fixation c.
    Charnley pin c.
    Cooley graft c.
    Cooley multipurpose angled c.
    Davidson muscle c.
    Diethrich bulldog c.
    exclusion c.
    Ferguson bone c.
    Frahur cartilage c.
    Frazier-Adson osteoplastic flap c.
    Friedrich c.
    Halifax interlaminar c.
    Hoen c.
    Jackson bone c.
    Jacobson bulldog c.
    Jameson muscle c.
    Jarit cartilage c.
    Jarit meniscal c.
    Johns Hopkins bulldog c.
    Kern bone-holding c.
    Lalonde bone c.
    Lambotte bone-holding c.
    Lamis patellar c.
    Locke bone c.
    Masterson cervical c.
    Masterson straight c.
    meniscal c.
    mini-Ulrich bone c.
    patellar cement c.
    patellar reduction c.
    Péan c.
    pedicle c.
    Pemberton spur-crushing c.

clamp *(continued)*
> Rush bone c.
> Seidel bone-holding c.
> Slocum meniscal c.
> Steinhauser bone c.
> Universal wire c.
> Verbrugge bone c.
> Walton meniscal c.
> Wells pedicle c.
> Wester meniscal c.
> Wylie lumbar bulldog c.
> X c.
> Zimmer cartilage c.

Clancy
> C. cruciate ligament reconstruction
> C. lateral compartment

Clarke arch angle

class
> Aitken hip c.

classification
> acromioclavicular injury c.
> Aitken c. of epiphyseal fracture
> Anderson tibial pseudarthrosis c.
> Anderson-D'Alonzo odontoid fracture c.
> AO c.
> AO c. of ankle fracture
> Bado c.
> Bauer-Jackson c.
> Bayne c. of radial agenesis
> Berndt-Hardy c. of transchondral fracture
> Copeland-Kavat c. of metatarsophalangeal dislocation
> Daseler-Anson c. of plantaris muscle anatomy
> Delbert hip fracture c.
> DeLee c.
> Denis c. of compression fractures *(types A, B, C, D)*
> Dickaut-DeLee c. of discoid meniscus
> El-Ahwany c. of humeral supracondylar fracture

classification *(continued)*
> Evans intertrochanteric fracture c.
> Fielding-Magliato c. of subtrochanteric fracture
> Hawkins c. of talar fracture
> Ideberg glenoid fracture c.
> Jahss ankle dislocation c.
> Johner-Wruhs tibial fracture c.
> Jones-Barnes-Lloyd-Roberts c.
> Kelikian nail deformity c.
> LaGrange humeral supracondylar fracture c.
> Melone distal radius fracture c.
> Modic c. of disk abnormality (1, 2, 3, 4, 4A, 4B *and* 4C)
> Neviaser c. of frozen shoulder
> Papavasiliou olecranon fracture c.
> Ranawat c.
> Steinbrocker c. of rheumatoid arthritis
> Universal distal radius fracture c.
> Universal spine c.
> Vostal c. of radial fracture
> Wagner c.
> Watanabe c. of discoid meniscus
> Watson-Jones c. of tibial tubercle avulsion fracture
> Watson-Jones spinal fracture c.
> Weber c.
> Weber-Danis ankle injury c.
> Winquist femoral shaft fracture c.
> Woofry-Chandler c. of Osgood-Schlatter lesion
> Young pelvic fracture c.

claudication
> jaw c.
> neurogenic c.

claudicatory

clavicle

clavicular

clavicectomy

claviculus

clavipectoral triangle

clavulanate

clawfoot

clawhand

Clayton
  C. forefoot arthroplasty
  C. greenstick splint
  C.-Fowler technique

Cleeman sign

cleft
  c. closure
  c. foot
  c. hand
  intergluteal c.
  interinnominoabdominal c.
  retropharyngeal facial c.
  primary synaptic c.
  secondary synaptic c.
  subneural c.
  synaptic c.

clefting of meniscus

cleidagra

cleidal

cleidarthritis

cleidocostal

cleidomastoid

cleisagra

Cleland ligament

Cleveland
  C. bone rongeur
  C. bone-cutting forceps

click
  hip c.
  Mulder c.
  Ortolani c.

Click'X

clinarthrosis

Clinitron air bed

clinodactyly

clip
  Braun-Yasargil right-
    angle c.

cliseometer

clivus

cloaca

cloacal

clonus
  ankle c.
  patellar c.

Cloquet
  C. fascia
  round ligament of C.
  septum of C.

closed dislocation

closure
  cleft c.

cloverleaf
  c. counterbore
  c. pin extractor

Cloward
  C. anterior spinal fusion
  C. blade retractor
  C. cervical arthrodesis
  C. cervical disk approach
  C. chisel
  C. depth gauge
  C. dowel cutter
  C. drill guide
  C. drill guide cap
  C. fusion diskography
  C. osteophyte elevator
  C. rongeur
  C. spinal fusion osteotome
  C.-Cone curet

clubbing

clubfoot
    arthrogrypotic c.

clubhand
    radial c.
    ulnar c.

Clutton joint

Clyburn Colles fracture fixator

CMC
    carpometacarpal
        Eaton CMC arthrosis
        CMC splint

CMW bone cement

cnemial

cnemis

cnemitis

cnemoscoliosis

coalition
    calcaneocuboid c.
    calcaneonavicular c.
    cubonavicular c.
    lunate-triquetral c.
    naviculocuneiform c.
    talocalcaneal c.
    talonavicular c.
    tarsal c.

coapt

coarctation
    reversed c.

coarticulation

coating
    Porocoat porous c.

Coballoy implant material

cobalt-chromium alloy prosthesis

Coban
    C. dressing
    C. elastic dressing

Cobb
    C. lumbar angle

Cobb *(continued)*
    C. scoliosis angle

Coblation
    C.-based spinal surgery
        system
    C. technology

coccyalgia

coccydynia

coccygalgia

coccygeal

coccygectomy

coccygeus

coccygodynia

coccygotomy

coccyodynia

coccyx

Cocke maxillectomy

Codivilla bone graft

Codman
    C. angle
    C. exercise
    C. sign
    C. triangle
    C. tumor

Cofield shoulder prosthesis

cogener

Cohnheim
    C. areas
    C. fields

Colclough laminectomy rongeur

collagenase
    injectable c.

collagenic

collagenoblast

collagenocyte

collagenogenic

collagenous

collapse
  hindfoot-midfoot c.
  scapholunate advanced c.
  (SLAC)

collar
  Aspen cervical c.
  cervical c.
  Colpack c.
  MAC cervical c.
  Mayo-Thomas c.
  Mayo-Thomas cervical c.
  periosteal bone c.
  Philadelphia c.
  Pneu-trac cervical c.
  Schanz c.
  Thomas c.

Colles
  C. fracture
  C. ligament
  reverse C. fracture
  C. splint

Collet screwdriver adaptor

collicular fracture

Collins dynamometer

Collis
  C. retractor
  C.-Taylor retractor

collodiaphyseal

collodion dressing

collum
  c. anatomicum humeri
  c. chirurgicum humeri
  c. costae
  c. distortum
  c. femoris
  c. ossis femoris
  c. radii
  c. scapulae
  c. tali
  c. valgum

colocutaneous fistula

Colonna
  C. operation
  C. trochanteric arthro-
  plasty
  C.-Ralston ankle approach

Colpack collar

column
  central c.
  dorsal c.
  c. of Kölliker
  muscle c.
  radial c.
  spinal c.
  ulnar c.
  vertebral c.

columna
  c. vertebralis

comminuted
  c. fracture
  c. intrarticular fracture

communicans
  gray ramus c.

communis
  extensor digitorum c.
  flexor digitorum c.
  ligamentum caudale integu-
  menti c.

Comolli sign

compages
  c. thoracis

compartment
  Clancy lateral c.
  muscular c.
  c. fasciotomy
  osseofascial c.
  osteofascial c.
  patellofemoral c.
  posterolateral c.
  c. syndrome

Compere
  C. lengthening
  C. osteotome

Compere *(continued)*
    C. threaded pin
    C. wire
    C.-Thompson arthrodesis

Comperm tubular elastic bandage

complex
    ankle joint c. (AJC)
    arcuate c.
    arcuate-popliteal c.
    atlas-axis c.
    Buford c.
    capulolabral c.
    capuloligamentous c.
    Edinger-Westphal c.
    epiphyseal c.
    fabellofibular c.
    fibrocartilage c.
    gastrocnemius-soleus c.
    Ghon-Sachs c.
    hallux valgus–metatarsus
        primus varus c.
    hindfoot joint c.
    jumped process c.
    lateral quadruple c.
    Lisfranc joint c.
    plantar capsuloligamen-
        tous c.
    semimembranous c.
    soleus c.
    spinal cord–meningeal c.
    c. syndactyly
    talocalcaneonavicular c.
    talonavicular-cuneiform c.
    trialkylphosphine gold c.
    vetebral subluxation c.
        (VSC)
    zygomatic-malar c.

component
    acetabular c.
    AML trial hip c.
    Amstutz femoral c.
    anatomically graduated c.
        (AGC)
    Aufranc-Turner femoral c.
    Bechtol acetabular c.
    Biomet MARS acetabular c.

component *(continued)*
    Black Max mid-size knee c.
    Bombelli-Morscher femor-
        al c.
    chamfered cylinder aceta-
        bular c.
    Charnley standard-stem c.
    DePuy trispiked acetabu-
        lar c.
    Duramer polyethylene c.
    Gustilo-Kyle femoral c.
    Harris-Galante hip replace-
        ment femoral c.
    Infinity femoral c.
    humeral c.
    Lubinus acetabular c.
    Metasul hip joint c.
    Neer II humeral c.
    NexGen c.
    Ogee acetabular c.
    Osteolock Omnifit-HA c.
    porous-coated c.
    Press-Fit femoral c.
    Profix porous femoral c.
    Springlite G foot c.
    Taperloc femoral c.
    Tharies femoral c.
    Ti-Bac acetabular c.
    Tricon-M c.
    uncemented femoral c.
    Universal radial c's
    Vitalock cluster acetabu-
        lar c.
    Zimmer NexGen LPS knee
        femoral c.

compression
    anterior-inferior c.
    axial c. of the foot
    distraction/c.
    interfragmental c.
    spinal cord c.

compressor
    Adair screw c.

Comprifix ankle splint

Compton clavicle pin

compound fracture

Conaxial ankle prosthesis

conchiolinosteomyelitis

Concise compression hip screw

concomitant

concretion
    calculous c.
    tophic c.

conduction
    c. block
    volume c.

conductor
    Bailey c.
    Bozzini light c.

condylar
    c. articulation
    c. implant arthroplasty
    c. notch

condylarthrosis

condyle
    bifid c.
    extensor c. of humerus
    external c. of femur
    external c. of humerus
    external c. of tibia
    femoral c.
    fibular c. of femur
    flexor c. of humerus
    c. of humerus
    internal c. of femur
    internal c. of humerus
    internal c. of tibia
    lateral femoral c.
    lateral c. of femur
    lateral c. of humerus
    lateral c. of tibia
    medial c. of femur
    medial c. of humerus
    medial c. of tibia
    occipital c.
    odontoid c.
    radial c. of humerus
    c. of scapula

condyle *(continued)*
    tibial c. of femur
    ulnar c. of humerus

condylectomy
    DuVries phalangeal c.
    phalangeal c.
    plantar c.

condyli *(plural of* condylus)

condylicus

condylocephalic

condylopatellar sulcus

condylotomy

condylus *pl.* condyli
    c. humeri
    c. lateralis femoris
    c. lateralis humeri
    c. lateralis tibiae
    c. medialis femoris
    c. medialis humeri
    c. medialis tibiae
    c. occipitalis
    c. tibialis femoris

coned-down view

Conform dressing

congener

congeneric

congenerous

congruence
    angle of c.
    patellofemoral c.

congruency
    joint c.

conjoined tendon

Conley pin

connection
    intertendinous c's
    Martin-Gruber c.

connector
    Beurrier c.

connector *(continued)*
    domino spinal instrumentation c.
    intrinsic transverse c.
    tandem c.

conoid
    c. ligament
    c. tubercle

conoideum
    ligamentum conoideum

connexus
    c. intertendinei

Conrad-Bugg trapping

Conradi
    C. disease
    C. syndrome
    C.-Hünermann syndrome

consistency
    boggy c.
    doughy c.

ConstaVac
    C. autoreinfusion system
    C. drainage

construct
    anterior c.
    AO dynamic compression plate c.
    compression instrumentation posterior c.
    double-rod c.
    Edwards modular system bridging sleeve c.
    Edwards modular system distraction-lordosis c.
    Edwards modular system kyphoreduction c.
    Edwards modular system scoliosis c.
    hook-to-screw L4–S1 compression c.
    iliosacral and iliac fixation c.
    pedicle screw c.
    pedicle screw–laminar claw c.

construct *(continued)*
    screw-to-screw compression c.
    segmental compression c.
    spondylo c.
    triplane c.
    TSRH double-rod c.
    upper cervical spine anterior c.
    Wiltse system double-rod c.

Contact
    C. ArthroProbe
    C. SPH cup system

contact
    c. point
    c. shield

Continuum knee system

Contour DF-80 total hip replacement

contour
    double hump c.
    Wiberg type II patellar c.

contractility
    galvanic c.
    idiomuscular c.
    muscle c.
    neuromuscular c.

contraction
    active c.
    carpopedal c.
    concentric c.
    direct c.
    eccentric c.
    extrafusal fiber c.
    c. fasciculation
    fibrillary c's
    idiomuscular c.
    isometric c.
    isotonic c.
    lengthening c.
    lumbrical instrinsic c.
    myotatic c.
    palmar c.
    postural c.
    shortening c.

contraction *(continued)*
    tetanic c.
    tonic c.

contractor
    Bailey-Gibbon rib c.

contracture
    abduction c.
    adduction c.
    burn c.
    clawfoot c.
    digital c.
    Dupuytren c.
    equinus c.
    extension c.
    external rotation c.
    flexion c.
    forearm c.
    gastroc-soleus c.
    hip flexor c.
    intrinsic c.
    ischemic c.
    lumbrical ischemic c.
    opposition c.
    organic c.
    pelvic flexion c.
    postpoliomyelitic c.
    pronation c.
    quadriceps c.
    Skoog procedure for re-
        lease of Dupuytren c.
    spastic intrinsic c.
    supination c.
    valgus c.
    varus c.
    Volkmann c.

contraflexion brace

contrast medium
    Omnipaque c. m.

contrecoup
    fracture by c.
    c. injury

controlled ankle motion (Cam)

conus medullaris syndrome

Cooley
    C. graft clamp

Cooley *(continued)*
    C. multipurpose angled
        clamp

Coombs bone biopsy system

Coonrad-Morrey total elbow ar-
    throplasty

Coonse
    C.-Adams knee approach
    C.-Adams quadricepsplasty

Cooper
    oblique ligament of C.

Coopernail sign

coossification

coossify

Copeland
    C.-Howard scapulothoracic
        fusion
    C.-Kavat classification of
        metatarsophalangeal dis-
        location

copolymer orthotic material

coracoacromial

coracobrachialis

coracoclavicular

coracohumeral

coracoid
    c. fracture

Coraderm dressing

Corbett bone rongeur

cord
    cervical spinal c.
    natatory c.
    oblique c. of elbow joint
    pretendinous c.
    tethered spinal c.
    Weitbrecht c.

Cordase

Cordon-Colles fracture splint

CorIS interference screw

cornu *pl.* cornua
  c. coccygeale
  c. coccygeum
  c. cutaneum
  c. inferius marginis falciformis
  sacral c.
  c. sacrale
  c. superius marginis falciformis

cornuate navicular

corpectomy
  anterior c.
  cervical c.

corporectomy

corpus *pl.* corpora
  c. adiposum infrapatellare
  c. calcanei
  c. claviculae
  c. claviculare
  c. costae
  c. fibulae
  c. humeri
  c. metacarpale
  c. metatarsale
  corpora oryzoidea
  c. ossis ilii
  c. ossis ilium
  c. ossis ischii
  c. ossis metacarpalis
  c. ossis metacarpi
  c. ossis metatarsalis
  c. ossis metatarsi
  c. ossis pubis
  c. phalangis manus
  c. phalangis pedis
  c. radii
  c. sterni
  c. tali
  c. tibiae
  c. tibiale
  c. ulnae
  c. vertebrae
  c. vertebrale

corpuscle
  bone c.

corpuscle *(continued)*
  cartilage c.
  Golgi c.
  paciniform c's
  tendon c's

correction
  chevron hallux valgus c.
  phalangeal malunion c.

corset
  Hoke c.

cortex
  femoral c.

corticocancellous

corticotomy
  DeBastiani c.
  Ilizarov c.

Coryllos
  C. rasp
  C.-Doyen periosteal elevator

costa *pl.* costae
  c. cervicalis
  costae fluctuantes
  costae fluitantes
  c. prima
  c. secunda
  costae spuriae
  costae verae

costal

costalgia

costalis

costectomy

costicervical

costiferous

costiform

costispinal

costocervicalis

costochondral

costoclavicular
  c. maneuver

costolumbar angle

costoscapular

costosternal

costosternoplasty

costotome

costotomy

costotransverse

costotransversectomy
　　Seddon dorsal spine c.

costovertebral
　　c. angle (CVA)

costoxiphoid

Cotrel
　　C. scoliosis
　　C. scoliosis cast
　　Moe modified C. cast
　　C. pedicle screw
　　C.-Dubousset derotation
　　　　operation
　　C.-Dubousset instrumenta-
　　　　tion
　　C.-Dubousset pedicle screw
　　　　instrumentation
　　C.-Dubousset rod

Cottle
　　C. chisel
　　C. osteotome
　　C. saw
　　C.-McKenty elevator

Cotton reduction of elbow dis-
　　location

cotyloid

cotyloplasty

counterbore
　　cloverleaf c.

counterextension

counterrotational splint

countersinking osteotomy

countertraction

coup
　　c. de fouet

coupling
　　excitation-contraction c.

Coventry
　　C. proximal tibial osteot-
　　　　omy
　　C. screw

cover
　　Accu-Flo polyethylene bur
　　　　hole c.
　　Accu-Flo silicone rubber
　　　　bur hole c.

Cowden disease

Cowper
　　C. ligament
　　pubic ligament of C.

coxa
　　c. adducta
　　c. brevis
　　c. flexa
　　c. magna
　　c. plana
　　c. saltans
　　c. senilis
　　c. valga
　　c. vara
　　c. vara luxans

coxalgia

coxarthria

coxarthritis

coxarthrocace

coxarthropathy

coxarthrosis

Cox flexion-distraction tech-
　　nique

coxitis
　　c. fugax
　　senile c.

coxodynia

coxofemoral

Cozen-Brockway Z-plasty

CPPD
 calcium pyrophosphate dihydrate
  CPPD crystals
  CPPD disease

Cracchiolo
 C. forefoot arthroplasty
 C.-Sculco implant arthroplasty
 C.-Sculco implant operation

crack fracture

cradle
 electric c.
 heat c.
 Posey bed c.

Craig-Scott orthosis

Cramer
 C. splint
 C. wire splint

cramp
 accessory c.

Crane shoulder exercise

craniocaudal
 c. guide

craniocervical
 c. plate

craniofacial
 c. dysjunction fracture

craniomandibular
 c. dysfunction

craniotabes

craterization

Crawford
 C. low lithotomy crutch
 C.-Marxen-Osterfeld technique

creaking
 PIP (proximal interphalangeal) flexion c.

cream
 EMLA c.

crease
 flexor skin c.
 palmar c.
 skin c.

Crego
 C. elevator
 C. femoral osteotomy
 C. hip reduction
 C. retractor
 C.-McCarroll pin

crepitans
 peritendinitis c.

crepitation
 patellofemoral c.

crepitus

crescentic
 c. base wedge osteotomy
 c. calcaneal osteotomy

crest
 anterior c. of fibula
 anterior c. of tibia
 deltoid c.
 femoral c.
 gluteal c.
 c. of greater tubercle of humerus
 c. of hypotrochanteric fossa
 iliac c.
 iliopectineal c.
 c. of ilium
 interosseous c.
 intertrochanteric c.
 c. of larger tubercle
 lateral c. of fibula
 c. of lesser tubercle
 medial c. of fibula
 c. of neck of rib
 obturator c.
 pectineal c. of femur
 pubic c.
 c. of pubis

crest *(continued)*
  radial c.
  rough c. of femur
  sacral c.
  c. of smaller tubercle
  c. of spinous processes of
    sacrum
  supinator c.
  supracondylar c. of hu-
    merus
  supraepicondylar c. of hu-
    merus
  tibial c.
  ulnar c.

crista
  c. anterior fibulae
  c. anterior tibiae
  c. capitis costae
  c. capituli costae
  c. colli costae
  c. femoris
  c. iliaca
  c. ilii
  c. interossea fibulae
  c. interossea radii
  c. interossea tibiae
  c. interossea ulnae
  c. intertrochanterica
  c. lateralis fibulae
  c. medialis fibulae
  c. musculi supinatoris
  c. obturatoria
  c. pubica
  c. sacralis articularis
  c. sacralis intermedia
  c. sacralis lateralis
  c. sacralis media
  c. sacralis medialis
  c. sacralis mediana
  c. supracondylaris lateralis
    humeri
  c. supracondylaris medialis
    humeri
  c. supraepicondylaris later-
    alis humeri
  c. supraepicondylaris medi-
    alis humeri
  c. tuberculi majoris

crista *(continued)*
  c. tuberculi minoris
  c. ulnae

criterion *pl.* criteria
  Ackerman criteria for oste-
    omyelitis
  Rome criteria for rheuma-
    toid arthritis

cross-bracing
  spinal rod c.-b.

crosslink
  Edwards modular system
    rod c.
  Galveston fixation with
    TSRH c.

Crowe
  C. congenital hip dysplasia
  C. pilot point

Crow-Fukase syndrome

crown
  Unitek steel c.

cruciate
  anterior c.
  c. condylar knee system
  c. ligament reconstruction

cruciform
  c. anterior spinal hyperex-
    tension orthosis
  c. tibial base plate

crural fascia

crus
  c. inferius marginis falcifor-
    mis
  medial c. of external ingui-
    nal ring
  c. superius marginis falci-
    formis

"crushed eggshell" fracture

crutch
  axillary c.
  Canadian c.
  Crawford low lithotomy c.
  EuroCuff forearm c.

crutch *(continued)*
    Hardy aluminum c.
    iWalkFree hands-free c's
    Lofstrand c.
    triceps c.
    weightbearing c.

Crutchfield drill point

Cruveilhier
    anterior pubic ligament
        of C.
    costovertebral interos-
        seous ligament of C.
    C. joint
    C. ligaments
    transversocostal interos-
        seous ligament of C.

cryoanalgesia

Cryo/Cuff Knee Compression
    Dressing System

cryoepiphysiodesis

cryoprecipitate

cryopreserved cartilage

cryotherapy
    liquid nitrogen c.
    verruca c.

crypt
    synovial c.

cryptococcosis

cryptotic medial border

crystal
    calcium pyrophosphate di-
        hydrate (CPPD) c's
    hydroxyapatite c.

crystal-induced
    c.-i. arthritis
    c.-i. arthrosis
    c.-i. synovitis

crystalloid

C-shaped foot

C-Tek
    C-T. anterior cervical plate

C-Tek *(continued)*
    C-T. anterior cervical plate
        system

CTLSO
    cervicothoracolumbosacral
        orthosis

CTS
    carpal tunnel syndrome

Cubbins
    C. arthroplasty
    C. screw

cubitocarpal

cubitoradial

cubitus *pl.* cubiti
    c. valgus
    c. varus

cuboid

cubonavicular

cucullaris

cuff
    joint distraction c.
    musculotendinous c.
    pneumatic tourniquet c.
    Push-Ease Quad c.
    rotator c. (RC)

Cuff Link orthopedic device

cul-de-sac of Bruger

Culley ulnar splint

cuneatus
    fasciculus c.

cuneiform

cuneocuboid

cuneonavicular

cuneoscaphoid

cup
    AccuPressure heel c.
    acetabular c.
    Arthropor acetabular c.
    Arthropor oblong c. for ac-
        etabular defect

cup (continued)
Aufranc modification of
Smith-Petersen c.
Aufranc-Turner hip c.
Biomet acetabular c.
Buchholz acetabular c.
Charnley offset-bore c.
DePuy bipolar c.
Interseal acetabular c.
Laing concentric hip c.
Müller c.
NEB (New England Baptist)
acetabular c.
Tuli gel-heel c.

Currarino-Silverman syndrome

current
d'Arsonval c.
demarcation c.
galvanic c.
nerve-action c.

curet (spelled also curette)
Acufex c.
angled Scoville c.
bone c.
Brun bone c.
Buck bone c.
Charnley c.
Cloward-Cone c.
Daubenspeck bone c.
Dawson-Yuhl-Cone c.
Faulkner c.
Gillquist suction c.
Halle bone c.
hypophysial c.
Innomed c.
Jansen bone c.
Kerpel bone c.
Kevorkian c.
Lempert bone c.
McCain TMJ c.
Malis c.
Meyhoeffer c.
Moe bone c.
Piffard c.
Schede bone c.
Scoville c.
Spratt bone c.
stout-neck c.

curet (continued)
Volkmann bone c.
Williger bone c.

curette (variant of curet)

Curry
C. hip nail
C. walking splint

curvature
double-kyphotic c.
humpbacked spinal c.
Pott c.

curve
accommodation c.
Barnes c.
calibration c.
cervicothoracic c.
compensatory c.
kyphotic c.
load-deflection c.
lordotic c.
scoliotic c.
strain-stress c.
strength-duration c.
tension c.
thoracolumbar c.
torque c.

curvilinear

Curv/Tek TSR bone drill

Cushing
C. retractor
C. rongeur
C.-Gigli saw guide

cut
chamfer c.
freehand c.
horizontal gantry c.
notch c.

cutter
A-P c.
bone c.
bone plug c.
Breck pin c.
Cloward dowel c.

cutter *(continued)*
    Horsley bone c.
    Howmedica microfixation
        system plate c.
    Jarit pin c.
    Kalish Duredge wire c.
    Kirschner wire c.
    Kleinert-Kutz bone c.
    Midas Rex AMI bone c.
    M-Pact cast c.
    pin c.
    Questus leading edge gras-
        per-c.
    Rochester recipient bone c.
    Roos rib c.
    Sklar pin c.
    Spartan jaw wire c.
    Storz Microsystems plate c.
    Synthes Microsystem
        plate c.
    T-C pin c.
    VersaTor tissue c.
    wire c.
    Wister wire/pin c.

CVA
    costovertebral angle

cyclarthrodial

cyclarthrosis

cylinder
    Arthrotek calibrated c.
    Feldenkrais c.
    Leydig c's

cylindrarthrosis

cyllosis

Cyriax syndrome

cyrtosis

cyst
    aneurysmal bone c. (ABC)
    Baker c.
    bursal c.
    extravasation c.
    ganglionic c.
    hemorrhagic c.
    simple bone c.
    solitary bone c.
    subchondral c.
    subsynovial c.
    thecal c.
    traumatic bone c.
    unicameral bone c.

Czerny
    C. disease
    C. suture

D
dorsal vertebrae (D1–D12)

D/3
distal third

DACO brace

Dacron
D. graft
D.-impregnated silicone rod

dactylitis

dactylogryposis

dactylolysis

dactyly

Dall-Miles
D.-M. cable cerclage
D.-M. cerclage
D.-M. cerclage wire

DANA
designed after natural anatomy

Daniel quadriceps neutral angle test

DarcoGel ankle brace

Darier disease

Darrach
D. periosteal elevator
D. procedure
D. resection
D. retractor
D.-Hughston-Milch fracture
D.-McLaughlin approach

d'Arsonval current

Daseler-Anson classification of plantaris muscle anatomy

Das Gupta
D. G. scapular excision
D. G. scapulectomy

Daubenspeck bone curet

d'Aubigné
d'A. femoral prosthesis

d'Aubigné *(continued)*
d'A. femoral reconstruction
d'A. hip status system
d'A. patellar transplant
d'A. resection reconstruction

Dautrey
D. chisel
D. osteotome

David disease

Davidson muscle clamp

Davis metacarpal splint

Dawbarn sign

Dawson
D.-Yuhl gouge
D.-Yuhl osteotome
D.-Yuhl rongeur forceps
D.-Yuhl-Cone curet
D.-Yuhl-Kerrison rongeur forceps
D.-Yuhl-Key elevator

DDH
developmental dysplasia of the hip

De Anquin test

dearticulation

Deaver retractor

DeBakey prosthesis

de Barsy syndrome

DeBastiani
D. corticotomy
D. distractor
D. femoral lengthening

Debeyre-Patte-Elmelik rotator cuff technique

débridement
Ahern trochanteric d.
arthroscopic d.
bursal d.
cortical d.
diagnostic arthroscopy and d.

débridement *(continued)*
  hemidiaphyseal d.
  irrigation and d.
  Magnuson d.

debris
  fibrin d.
  particulate d.
  polymeric d.

dechondrification

decompression
  Brady-Bishop-Tullos d.
  disk d.
  retroperitoneal d.
  sacral spine d.
  subacromial d.
  vertebral axial d. (VAX-D)

decompressive
  d. acromioplasty
  d. osteotomy

decortication

Decubinex pad

deep
  d. tendon reflex (DTR)
  d. venous thrombosis
    (DVT)

deepening reamer

defect
  cortical d.
  fibrous cortical d.
  intercalary d. of pollical ray
  metaphyseal fibrous d.
  osteoarticular d.

deficiency
  Aitken femoral d.

deformity
  acetabular protrusio d.
  articular d.
  bifid thumb d.
  bone d.
  boutonnière d.
  buttonhole d.
  calcaneocavovarus d.
  cavoabductovarus d.

deformity *(continued)*
  cavocalcaneovalgus d.
  cavovarus d.
  cervical spine kyphotic d.
  composite d.
  cortical d.
  cystic d.
  diaphyseal d.
  digitus flexus d.
  equinocavovarus d.
  equinovalgus d.
  equinovarus hindfoot d.
  flatfoot d.
  forefoot abduction d.
  fusiform d.
  gibbous d. of the spine
  gun stock d.
  Haglund d.
  hallux valgus d.
  llfeld-Holder d.
  Madelung d.
  neuropathic midfoot d.
  osseous d.
  osteochondral d.
  pars d.
  planovalgus d.
  plantar flexion-inversion d.
  recurvatum d.
  rocker-bottom d.
  seal-fin d.
  segmentation d.
  silver fork d.
  spinal coronal plane d.
  splayfoot d.
  Sprengel d.
  swan-neck d.
  thumb-in-palm d.
  ulnar drift d.
  Velpeau d.
  Volkmann d.

Defourmental rongeur

Dega pelvic osteotomy

degeneration
  axon d.
  cartilaginous d.
  joint d.
  reaction of d.

degeneration *(continued)*
    Regnauld d. of MTP joint
    Zenker d.

degloving injury

dehiscence
    wound d.

Dehne cast

Dejerine-Landouzy dystrophy

de Kleyn test

de la Caffinièere trapeziometa-
    carpal prosthesis

delamination

de Lange syndrome

DeLaura knee prosthesis

Delbert hip fracture classifica-
    tion

DeLee classification

Dellon moving two-point dis-
    crimination test

De Lorme
    De L. boot
    De L. exercise

Delrin joint

delta
    d. mesoscapulae
    d. phalanx
    d. tibial nail

Delta Recon nail

deltoid
    d. muscle
    d.-splitting incision

deltopectoral
    d. groove
    d. interval

deltotrapezius fascial ligament

demarcation
    line of d.

DeMarneffe meniscectomy knife

demifacet
    inferior d. for head of rib
    superior d. for head of rib

demineralization
    bone d.

de Morgan spot

DeMuth hip screw

demyelination

Denis
    D. Browne sacral fracture
    D. Browne splint
    D. classification of com-
        pression fractures *(types
        A, B, C, D)*

Dennyson
    D. cervical brace
    D.-Fulford subtalar arthrod-
        esis

dens
    d. anterior screw fixation
    d. axis
    d. epistrophei
    d. fracture

densitometry
    photon d.

density
    bone mineral d.
    fiber d.
    lumbosacral junction
        bone d.

dentate
    d. fracture

Denucé ligament

deossification

DePalma
    D. hip prosthesis
    D. modified patellar tech-
        nique

deposit
    gouty tophaceous d.

deposit *(continued)*
    rotator cuff calcified d.
    tophaceous d.

deposition
    calcium pyrophosphate
        dihydrate d.

depression
    congenital chondroster-
        nal d.
    postactivation d.
    radial d.
    supratrochlear d.

DePuy
    D. awl
    D. bipolar cup
    D. bolt
    D. 1 bone cement
    D. calcar grinder
    D. fracture brace
    D. interference screw
    D. pin
    D. plate
    D. reamer
    D. reducing frame
    D. rod bender
    D. splint
    D. trispiked acetabular
        component

Depuytren diathesis

de Quervain
    de Q. disease
    de Q. fracture
    de Q. Q fracture
    de Q. stenosing tenosynovi-
        tis
    de Q. tendinitis

derangement
    Hey internal d.
    internal d. of the knee
        (IDK)
    structural d.

dermatoarthritis

dermatomal
    d. pattern

dermatome
    Stryker d.

dermatosensory evoked poten-
    tial

derotation
    d. boot
    d. brace
    elongation d. flexion
    oblique osteotomy with d.

D'Errico
    D'E. enlarging drill bur
    D'E. lamina chisel
    D'E. retractor

Desault
    D. sign
    D. wrist dislocation

Descot fracture

designed after natural anatomy
    (DANA)

desmalgia

desmectasis

desmitis

desmodynia

desmogenous

desmography

desmoid
    cortical d.
    d. fibroma
    periosteal d.

desmopathy

desmorrhexis

desmosis

desmotomy

desyndactylization
    Weinstock d.

detritus
    bone d.

Deutschländer disease

deviation
    angular d.
    lateral d.
    radial d.
    ulnar d.

Devic disease

device
    acrylic orthotic d.
    Agee 4-pin fixation d.
    Aggressor d.
    articulated tension d.
    A-V Impulse system foot
        pump DVT prophylaxis d.
    Axer compression d.
    Backbar d.
    Bone Collector d.
    Bovie electrocautery d.
    Buck convoluted trac-
        tion d.
    Cervitrak d.
    Diva d.
    Georgiade fixation d.
    JACE W550 CPM wrist d.
    Kaneda distraction d.
    Ommaya reservoir d.
    Omni-Flexor d.
    Ortholav irrigation and suc-
        tion d.
    PDN (prosthetic disk nu-
        cleus) d.
    Reichert-Mundinger stereo-
        tactic d.
    sequential compression d.
        (SCD)
    Smart-Magnetix prosthetic
        d. for amputees
    Volkov-Oganesian-Povarov
        hinged distraction d.
    Wasserstein fixation d.
    XTB knee flexion d.

DeWald spinal apparatus

Dewar
    D. posterior cervical fusion
    D.-Barrington arthroplasty

Dewar *(continued)*
    D.-Harris paralysis

DEXA
    dual-energy x-ray absorp-
        tiometry
    DEXA scan

dextrorotatory scoliosis

Deyerle
    D. femoral fracture tech-
        nique
    D. fixation apparatus
    D. II pin
    D. plate
    D. screw

diaclasis

diadachokinesis

diagnostic
    d. arthroscopy
    d. arthroscopy and dé-
        bridement
    d. imaging

diameter
    horizontal pedicle d.
    sagittal spinal canal d.
    transverse pedicle d.

diametric pelvic fracture

Diamond-Gould reduction syn-
    dactyly

diaphragm
    Bucky d.
    splinted d.

diaphysary

diaphyseal
    d. aclasis

diaphysectomy

diaphysial

diaphysis *pl.* diaphyses

diaphysitis
    tuberculous d.

diapophysis

diarthric

diarthrodial joint

diarthrosis *pl.* diarthroses
  d. rotatoria

diastasis

diastatic fracture

diastrophic
  d. dwarfism
  d. dysplasia

diathermy
  medical d.
  microwave d.
  short-wave d.
  ultrasound d.

diathesis
  d. of connective tissue
  Depuytren d.
  gouty d.

Dickaut-DeLee classification of
  discoid meniscus

Dick AO Fixateur Interne

dicondylar fracture

Dieffenbach amputation

Diethrich bulldog clamp

digit
  accessory d.
  arthrodesed d.
  congenital trigger d.
  flail d.
  supermumerary d.

digital
  d. aponeurosis
  d. block anesthesia
  d. contracture
  d. extensor mechanism
  d. extensor tendon
  d. flexor tendon
  d. flexor tendinitis
  d. nerve block
  d. photoplethysmography
  d. plethysmography

digital *(continued)*
  d. subtraction angiography
  d. theca

digiti quinti proprius tendon

digitizer
  Amfit d.

digitorum brevis avulsion

digitus
  d. abductus
  d. anularis
  d. flexus deformity
  d. hippocraticus
  d. malleus
  d. medius
  d. minimus manus
  d. minimus pedis
  d. primus (I) manus
  d. primus (I) pedis
  d. quartus (IV) manus
  d. quartus (IV) pedis
  d. quintus (V) manus
  d. quintus (V) pedis
  d. secundus (II) manus
  d. secundus (II) pedis
  d. tertius (III) manus
  d. tertius (III) pedis
  d. valgus
  d. varus

dilator
  Eder-Puestow metal olive d.

Dimon
  D. osteotomy
  D.-Hughston intertrochan-
    teric osteotomy

DIP
  distal interphalangeal
    DIP joint

DIPJ
  distal interphalangeal joint

disarticular amputation

disarticulate

disarticulation
  ankle d.

disarticulation *(continued)*
    Batch-Spittler-McFaddin
      knee d.
    Boyd hip d.
    elbow d.
    hip d.
    joint d.
    knee d.
    Lisfranc d.
    Mazet knee d.
    metatarsophalangeal
      joint d.
    sacroiliac d.
    shoulder d.
    wrist d.

discectomy *(variant of* diskectomy)

discharge
    bizarre high-frequency d.
    bizarre repetitive d.
    complex repetitive d.
    coupled d.
    disruptive d.
    double d.
    grouped d.
    iterative d.
    multiple d.
    myokymic d.
    myotonic d.
    neuromyotonic d.
    neural d.
    paired d.
    repetitive d.
    triple d.

discitis *(variant of* diskitis)

DisCoblator XL

discogenic *(spelled also* diskogenic)

discography *(variant of* diskography)

discoid
    d. lateral meniscus
    d. meniscus

discoligamentous injury

discontinuity
    pelvic d.

discopathy

discrimination
    two-point d.

discus
    d. articularis
    d. articularis articulationis
      acromioclavicularis
    d. articularis articulationis
      radioulnaris distalis
    d. articularis articulationis
      sternoclavicularis
    d. interpubicus
    disci intervertebrales

disdiaclast

disease
    Albers-Schönberg d.
    apatite deposition d.
    Apert d.
    Baastrup d.
    Bamberger-Marie d.
    Beck d.
    Bekhterev (Bechterew) d.
    Berger d.
    Bielschowsky-Janský d.
    Blount d.
    Bornholm d.
    Bourneville d.
    brittle bone d.
    Brodie d.
    Bruck d.
    Buchanan d.
    Buerger d.
    Busquet d.
    Caffey d.
    calcium hydroxyapatite deposition d.
    calcium pyrophosphate deposition d.
    Calvé-Perthes d.
    Camurati-Engelmann d.
    Canavan-van Bogaert-Bertrand d.
    cement d.
    central core d.

disease *(continued)*
    cervical disk d.
    Charcot joint d.
    Charcot-Marie-Tooth d.
    Chester d.
    chronic tophaceous d.
    collagen vascular d.
    Conradi d.
    Cowden d.
    CPPD d.
    Czerny d.
    Darier d.
    David d.
    degenerative disk d.
    degenerative joint d.
    denervation d.
    de Quervain d.
    Deutschländer d.
    Devic d.
    disappearing bone d.
    Duchenne d.
    Duplay d.
    Dupuytren d.
    Durante d.
    Ehrenfeld d.
    Engelmann d.
    Engel-Recklinghausen d.
    Erb-Goldflam d.
    facet joint d. (FJD)
    facioscapulohumeral muscle atrophy d.
    Fazio-Londe d.
    fibromuscular d.
    Fleischner d.
    Forestier d.
    Freiberg d.
    Friedreich d.
    Garré d.
    Gaucher d.
    Gibney d.
    glenohumeral d.
    Gorham d.
    Haglund d.
    Hagner d.
    Hand-Schüller-Christian d.
    Hansen d.
    Hass d.
    Heberden d.

disease *(continued)*
    Henderson-Jones d.
    hip-joint d.
    Hoffa d.
    Horton d.
    hydroxyapatite deposition d.
    hypophosphatemic bone d.
    Iselin d.
    Jaffe-Lichtenstein d.
    Jansen d.
    Kashin-Bek (Kaschin-Beck) d.
    Kawasaki d.
    Kienböck d.
    Köhler bone d.
    Köhler second d.
    Köhler-Pellegrini-Stieda d.
    König d.
    Kümmell d.
    Kümmell-Verneuil d.
    Kussmaul d.
    Kussmaul-Maier d.
    Larsen d.
    Larsen-Johansson d.
    Legg d.
    Legg-Calvé d.
    Legg-Calvé-Perthes d.
    Legg-Calvé-Waldenström d.
    Leriche d.
    Lobstein d.
    Luft d.
    MacLean-Maxwell d.
    Madelung d.
    marble bone d.
    Marie-Bamberger d.
    Marie-Strümpell d.
    metabolic bone d.
    Meyer-Betz d.
    Miller d.
    mixed connective tissue d.
    Mozer d.
    Münchmeyer d.
    Ollier d.
    Osgood-Schlatter d.
    Otto d.
    Paas d.
    Paget d.

disease *(continued)*
Paget d. of bone
Panner d.
Pellegrini d.
Pellegrini-Stieda d.
Perrin-Ferraton d.
Perthes d.
plaster-of-Paris d.
pneumatic hammer d.
policeman's d.
Poncet d.
Pott d.
Preiser d.
pulseless d.
Pyle d.
Quervain d.
Recklinghausen d.
Recklinghausen d. of bone
rheumatoid d.
Rust d.
sacroiliac d.
scapuloperoneal muscle
atrophy d.
Schanz d.
Scheuermann d.
Schlatter d.
Schlatter-Osgood d.
Schmorl d.
Schönlein d.
Sever d.
Sinding-Larsen d.
Sinding-Larsen–Johans-
son d.
skeletal hyperplasia d.
Stieda d.
Still d.
Strümpell-Marie d.
Sudeck d.
Swediaur (Schwediauer) d.
Takayasu d.
Thiemann d.
thoracolumbar degenera-
tive d.
Tietze d.
Trevor d.
Verneuil d.
Verse d.
vibration d.

disease *(continued)*
Volkmann d.
von Recklinghausen d.
Vrolik d.
Waldenström d.
Wartenberg d.
Wegner d.
Werdnig-Hoffmann d.

disinsertion

disjoint

disk
A d.
Amici d.
amphiarthrodial d.
anisotropic d.
anisotropous d.
articular d.
Bowman d's
bulging d.
contained d.
d. decompression
Engelmann d.
epiphyseal d.
extruded d.
fibrocartilaginous d.
growth d.
Hensen d.
herniated d.
d. herniation
I d.
interarticular d.
intermediate d.
interpubic d.
intervertebral d.
intraarticular d's
isotropic d.
J d.
M d.
noncontained d.
protruding d.
Q d.
ruptured d.
sequestered d.
sequestrated d.
slipped d.
thin d.

disk *(continued)*
    transverse d.
    Z d.

diskectomy *(spelled also* discectomy)
    anterior cervical d. and fusion (ACDF)
    automated percutaneous d. (APD)
    automated percutaneous lumbar d. (APLD)
    cervical d.
    d. with Cloward fusion
    laminotomy and d.
    microlumbar d.
    percutaneous lumbar d.
    Wiltse d.

diskitis *(spelled also* discitis)

diskogenic *(variant of* discogenic)

diskography *(spelled also* discography)
    cervical d.
    Cloward fusion d.
    lumbar d.

dislocatio
    d. erecta

dislocation
    acromioclavicular joint d.
    ankle d.
    antenatal d.
    atlantoaxial d.
    atlantooccipital joint d.
    Bankart shoulder d.
    Bell-Dally cervical d.
    Bennet d.
    boutonnière hand d.
    bursting d.
    carpometacarpal joint d.
    Chopart ankle d.
    closed d.
    complete d.
    complicated d.
    compound d.
    congenital d. of the hip (CDH)
    consecutive d.

dislocation *(continued)*
    Desault wrist d.
    divergent d.
    dorsal perilunate d.
    elbow d.
    fracture d.
    frank d.
    glenohumeral joint d.
    habitual d.
    Hill-Sachs shoulder d.
    incomplete d.
    interphalangeal joint d.
    intra-articular d.
    Jahss metatarsophalangeal joint d.
    joint d.
    Kienböck d.
    Lisfranc d.
    lumbosacral d.
    lunate d.
    metacarpophalangeal d.
    metacarpophalangeal joint d.
    metatarsophalangeal d.
    metatarsophalangeal joint d.
    Monteggia d.
    Nélaton d.
    old d.
    open d.
    Otto pelvis d.
    Palmer transscaphoid perilunar d.
    panclavicular d.
    partial d.
    patellar intraarticular d.
    pathologic d.
    pelvis d.
    perilunate carpal d.
    perilunate transscaphoid d.
    peroneal d.
    phalangeal d.
    primitive d.
    proximal tibiofibular joint d.
    recent d.
    recurrent patellar d.
    simple d.
    Smith d.

dislocation *(continued)*
 sternoclavicular joint d.
 subastragalar d.
 subcoracoid d.
 subglenoid d.
 subspinous d.
 traumatic d.
 triquetrolunate d.
 unilateral interfacetal d.
 volar semilunar wrist d.
 wrist d.

dismemberment

dispenser
 cement d.
 Jet vac cement d.

displacement
 atlantoaxial rotary d.
 oblique d.

disrelationship

disruption
 anterior column d.
 Charcot d.
 facet capsule d.
 pedicle cortex d.

dissecans
 osteochondritis d.
 osteochondrosis d.

dissection
 extracapsular d.
 subperiosteal d.

dissector
 Angell-James d.
 Effler-Groves d.
 elevator-d.
 Freer elevator-d.

dissociation
 scapholunate d.

distal
 d. interphalangeal joint
  (DIPJ)
 d. radioulnar joint (DRUJ)
 d. tibiofibular joint

distalward

distortion
 multisegmental spinal d.

distortor
 d. oris

distraction
 d. arthroplasty
 d. bone block arthrodesis
 d./compression
 flexion d.
 d. of fracture
 Guhl d.
 d. instrumentation
 physeal d.
 spinal d.

distractor
 Acufex ankle d.
 AO femoral d.
 DeBastiani d.
 Ilizarov d.
 intramedullary skeletal ki-
  netic d. (ISKD)
 Kessler metacarpal d.
 Orthofix M-100 d.
 Pinto d.
 turnbuckle d.

disuse atrophy

Diva device

divarication

divergence
 angle of d.

diverticulum
 ganglion d.
 synovial d.

Dix-Hallpike maneuver

DJD
 degenerative joint disease

dj Orthopedics

DMI orthopedic bed

DOA
 diagnostic and operative
  arthroscopy

Dobie
  D. globule
  D. layer
  D. line

dolor
  d. coxae

dominant
  left-hand d.
  right-hand d.

DonJoy
  D. ALP brace
  D. Gold Point knee brace
  D. wrist splint

dorsale
  ligamentum calcaneonavi-
    culare dorsale
  ligamentum cuboideonavi-
    culare dorsale
  ligamentum cuneoclavicu-
    lare dorsale
  ligamentum radiocarpale
    dorsale

dorsalgia

dorsal-V osteotomy

dorsalward approach

dorsi
  latissimus d.

dorsiflexion

dorsiflexory wedge osteotomy

dorsispinal

dorsodynia

dorsolateral

dorsolumbar area

dorsomedial

dorsoplantar

dorsoradial

dorsorostral approach

dorsoscapular

dorsoulnar approach

dorsum
  d. of foot
  d. of hand
  d. manus
  d. pedis
  d. of scapula
  d. scapulae

double hump contour

doublet

downbiting rongeur

Down epiphyseal knife

Downey hemilaminectomy retractor

Downing cartilage knife

Doyen
  D. bone mallet
  D. costal rasp
  D. cylindrical bur
  D. periosteal elevator
  D. rib elevator

drain
  Wound-Evac d.

drainage
  ConstaVac d.

Drennan metaphyseal-epiphyseal angle

dressing
  Adaptic d.
  Aeroplast d.
  Alginate d.
  Allevyn wound d.
  Aquaphor gauze d.
  Bioclusive select transpar-
    ent film d.
  Bioclusive transparent
    film d.
  calcium alginate d.
  Coban d.
  Coban elastic d.
  collodion d.
  Conform d.

dressing *(continued)*
    Coraderm d.
    dry sterile d. (DSD)
    DuoDerm d.
    Elastikon d.
    Flexderm wound d.
    hydrocolloid occlusive d.
    Intrasite d.
    Kelikian foot d.
    Kerlix d.
    Kling adhesive d.
    Oasis wound d.
    OpSite wound d.
    PolyWic d.
    Silastic gel d.
    Tegaderm d.
    Tubigrip d.
    Velpeau d.
    Webril d.
    Xeroform gauze d.

Driessen hinged plate

drift
    radial d.
    ulnar d.

drill
    Acra-Cut wire pass d.
    Aesculap d.
    Anspach power d.
    anticavitation d.
    Archimedean d.
    autotome d.
    d. bit
    Brunswick-Mack rotating d.
    Carroll-Bunnell d.
    Championnière bone d.
    Charnley femoral con-
      dyle d.
    Cherry-Austin d.
    Curv/Tek TSR bone d.
    Elan d.
    Fisch d.
    Hall air d.
    Hall Versipower d.
    Jordan-Day d.
    Moore bone d.
    Neurairtome d.
    Pease bone d.
    Portmann d.

drill *(continued)*
    Ralks bone d.
    Raney bone d.
    Raney perforator d.
    Rica bone d.
    Richards pistol-grip d.
    Richter bone d.
    Smedberg hand d.
    Suretac d. and guidewire
    Uniflex calibrated step d.
    Universal two-speed
      hand d.
    Warren-Mack rotating d.
    Wolferman d.
    Wullstein d.
    Xomed d.

drill guide
    acetabular cup peg d. g.
    ACL d. g.
    Adapteur multi-functional
      d. g.
    Adson d. g.
    Cloward d. g.
    d. g. forceps
    glenoid d. g.
    Levin d. g.
    Richards d. g.
    Ulrich d. g.
    Uslenghi d. g.
    wire and d. g.

driver
    d.-extractor
    Küntscher nail d.
    nail d.
    Zimmer d.-extractor

drop
    foot d.
    osseous d.
    d. phalangette
    pronator d.

dropsy
    articular d.

DRUJ
    distal radioulnar joint

Drummond
    D. spinal instrumentation
    D. wire

DSD
дry sterile dressing

DTR
deep tendon reflex

Duchenne
D. disease
D. dystrophy
D. muscular dystrophy
D. test
D.-type muscular dystrophy
D.-Landouzy dystrophy

Dugas
D. sign
D. test

Duhot line

dumbbells of Schäfer

Duncan shoulder brace

Dunn
D.-Brittain triple arthrodesis
D.-Hess trochanteric osteotomy

duocondylar knee prosthesis

DuoDerm dressing

Duo-Drive screw

Duopress
D. guide
D. plate

Duplay disease

Dupuytren
D. amputation
D. contracture
D. contracture release
D. disease
D. exostosis
D. fascia
D. fasciitis
D. fracture
D. operation
D. sign
D. splint
D. test

Duracon
D. knee implant
D. total knee system

DuraGen

dural
d. ectasia
d. ligament

Duramer polyethylene component

Durante disease

Durapatite bone replacement material

Dura-Stick adhesive electrode

Durasul Natural-Knee implant

duToit-Roux arthroplasty

Duverney fracture

DuVries
D. approach
D. arthroplasty
D. hammertoe repair
D. modified McBride hallux valgus operation
D. phalangeal condylectomy
D. technique for overlapping toe
D.-Mann modified Z bunionectomy

DVT
deep venous thrombosis

dwarfism
achondroplastic d.
ateliotic d.
camptomelic d.
chondroplastic d.
diastrophic d.
Laron d.
micromelic d.
phocomelic d.
Russell-Silver d.

Dwyer
D. spinal instrumentation

Dwyer *(continued)*
   D.-Hall plate

Dycor prosthetic foot

DynaGraft implant

Dynagrip blade handle

DynaHeat hot pack

Dyna knee splint

dynametric testing

Dynamic condylar screw

dynamogenesis

dynamogenic

dynamogeny

dynamograph

dynamometer
   Biodex isokinetic d.
   Collins d.
   grip d.
   hand-held d.
   Harpenden d.
   Isobex d.
   Lido isokinetic d.
   Smedley d.
   squeeze d.

dynamometry
   isokinetic d.

Dynaplex knee prosthesis

DynaWell

DyoCam
   D. 550 arthroscopic video
     camera

Dyonics
   D. Access 15 arthroscopic
     fluid irrigation system
   D. arthroplasty bur
   D. arthroscope
   D. cannula
   D. shaver

dysarthria
   spinal d.

dysarthric lesion

dysarthrosis
   patellofemoral d.

dysbaric
   d. osteonecrosis

dyschondroplasia

dyscollagenosis

dyscrasic fracture

dysdiadochokinesia

dysesthesia

dysfunction
   craniomandibular d.
   flexor hallucis longus d.
     (FHLD)
   motor d.

dysgenesis
   alar d.
   epiphyseal d.

dysmetria

dysosteogenesis

dysostosis
   d. enchondralis epiphy-
     saria
   Jansen metaphyseal d.
   metaphyseal d.
   Schmid metaphyseal dyos-
     tosis

dysplasia
   acropectorovertebral d.
   bony d.
   cleidocranial d.
   congenital hip d.
   congenital hyperphospha-
     temic skeletal d. (CHSD)
   cortical fibrous d.
   craniometaphyseal d.
   Crowe congenital hip d.
     (types I–IV)
   developmental d. of the hip
   diaphyseal d.
   diastrophic d.
   epiarticular d.
   epiphyseal d.

dysplasia *(continued)*
　d. epiphysealis hemimelica
　d. epiphysealis multiplex
　d. epiphysealis punctata
　femoral head d.
　fibrous d.
　d. of hip
　intracortical fibrous d.
　metaphyseal d.
　Meyer d.
　Mondini d.
　monostotic fibrous d.
　multiple epiphyseal d.
　Namaqualand hip d.
　oculoauriculovertebral d.
　osteofibrous d.
　patellofemoral d.
　polyostotic fibrous d.
　progressive diaphyseal d.
　rhizomesomelic bone d.
　spondyloepiphyseal d.
　Streeter d.

dysraphism
　spinal d.

dystopia
　shoulder d.

dystrophia
　d. brevicollis

dystrophin

dystrophy
　Albright d.
　Becker muscular d.
　Becker variant of Duchen-
　　ne d.
　Dejerine-Landouzy d.
　distal muscular d.

dystrophy *(continued)*
　Duchenne d.
　Duchenne muscular d.
　Duchenne-type muscular d.
　Duchenne-Landouzy d.
　Emery-Dreifuss muscular d.
　Erb d.
　Erb muscular d.
　facioscapulohumeral mus-
　　cular d.
　Frohlich adipogenital d.
　Fukuyama type congenital
　　muscular d.
　Gowers muscular d.
　humeroperoneal d.
　Kiloh-Nevin ocular form of
　　progressive muscular d.
　Landouzy d.
　Landouzy-Dejerine d.
　Landouzy-Dejerine muscu-
　　lar d.
　Leyden-Möbius muscular d.
　limb-girdle muscular d.
　muscular d.
　myotonic d.
　osseous d.
　pelvifemoral muscular d.
　posttraumatic d.
　progressive muscular d.
　pseudohypertrophic mus-
　　cular d.
　reflex sympathetic d.
　scapulohumeral muscu-
　　lar d.
　scapuloperoneal muscu-
　　lar d.
　Simmerlin d.
　sympathetic d.

Eagle straight-ahead arthroscope

EAST
    external rotation-abduction stress test

Easton cock-up splint

Eaton
    E. closed reduction
    E. CMC (carpometacarpal) arthrosis (*stages I–IV*)
    E. implant arthroplasty
    E. trapezium finger joint replacement prosthesis
    E. volar plate arthroplasty
    E.-Malerich fracture-dislocation operation
    E.-Malerich reduction

Eberle contracture release

EBI Xfix DynaFix System

eburnate

eburnated bone

eburnation
    bony e.
    e. of cartilage

eccentric
    e. access of ankle rotation
    e. contraction
    e. dynamic compression plate (EDCP)

ecchondroma

ecchondrosis

ecchondrotome

Echlin
    E. duckbill rongeur
    E. rongeur forceps

Ecker-Lotke-Glazer patellar tendon repair

EcoNail

ECRB
    extensor carpi radialis brevis
        ECRB muscle

ECRL
    extensor carpi radialis longus
        ECRL muscle

ectasia
    dural e.

ectocondyle

ectocuneiform

ectopectoralis

ectosteal

ectostosis

ECTR
    ectopic carpal tunnel release

ED
    elbow disarticulation

EDB
    extensor digitorum brevis

EDC
    extensor digitorum communis

EDCP
    eccentric dynamic compression plate

Eddowes syndrome

edema
    intracompartmental e.
    nonpitting e.
    pitting e.
    pretibial e.
    rheumatismal e.
    stump e.

Eden-Hybbinette arthroplasty

Eder-Puestow metal olive dilator

Edgarton-Grand thumb adduction

Edinger-Westphal complex

EDL
extensor digitorum longus

EDQ
extensor digiti quinti

Edwards
E. modular system bridging sleeve construct
E. modular system rod crosslink
E. modular system distraction-lordosis construct
E. modular system kypho-reduction construct
E. modular system scoliosis construct

effect
anticholinergic e.
neurophysiologic e.
Orbeli e.
Steindler e.
tenodesis e.
tethered e.

efferent nerve impulse

Effler-Groves dissector

effleurage massage

Eftekhar broken femoral stem technique

Egawa sign

Eggers
E. bone plate
E. contact splint
E. screw
E. tendon transfer
E. tendon transfer technique
E. tenodesis

EHL
extensor hallucis longus
EHL tendon

Ehrenfeld disease

Eicher
E. femoral prosthesis
E. hip prosthesis

EIP
extensor indicis proprius

Ekman
E. syndrome
E.-Lobstein syndrome

El-Ahwany classification of humeral supracondylar fracture

Elan drill

ElastaTrac home lumbar traction system

elasticity
modulus of e.
physical e. of muscle
physiologic e. of muscle
total e. of muscle

Elastikon dressing

elastoma

elastomer
high performance silicone e.
medical e. X7-2320
polyolefin e.
thermoplastic e.

Elastoplast bandage

elbow
e. arthroplasty
baseball pitcher's e.
compound shattered e.
e. disarticulation
e. dislocation
epicondylitis of the e.
e. extension splint
e. extensor tendon
e. flexion splint
Frohse arcade of the e.
golfer's e.
e. jerk reflex test
Little League e.
miners' e.

elbow *(continued)*
    nursemaid's e.
    e. orthosis
    pulled e.
    tennis e.
    triangle of e.
    varus/valgus stress of
        the e.
    wrestler's e.
    e.-wrist-hand orthosis

electrode
    active e.
    bifilar needle e.
    bipolar needle e.
    bipolar stimulating e.
    coaxial needle e.
    concentric needle e.
    Dura-Stick adhesive e.
    Excel Plus e.
    exploring e.
    indifferent e.
    iontophoresis e.
    LSI Easy Stims self-adhe-
        sive e.
    monopolar needle e.
    monopolar stimulating e.
    multilead e.
    needle e.
    recording e.
    reference e.
    single fiber needle e.
    stigmatic e.
    stimulating e.
    surface e.
    Teq-Trode e.
    unipolar needle e.

electrogoniometer
    parallellogram e.

electromyogram

electromyograph

electromyography
    central e.
    dynamic e.
    integrated e.
    single fiber e.
    surface e.

electroneuromyography

electrostimulation

electrotherapist

electrotherapy

electrovibratory massage

Elekta stereotactic head frame
    element

element
    Elekta stereotactic head
        frame e.

elevated rim acetabular liner

elevation
    endosteal e.

elevator
    Adson periosteal e.
    Alexander periosteal e.
    Aufranc periosteal e.
    Bethune periosteal e.
    Bristow periosteal e.
    Brophy periosteal e.
    Buck periosteal e.
    Cameron-Haight perioste-
        al e.
    Campbell periosteal e.
    Carroll-Legg periosteal e.
    Cheyne periosteal e.
    Cloward osteophyte e.
    Coryllos-Doyen perioste-
        al e.
    Cottle-McKenty e.
    Crego e.
    Darrach periosteal e.
    Dawson-Yuhl-Key e.
    e.-dissector
    Doyen periosteal e.
    Doyen rib e.
    Farabeuf periosteal e.
    Fomon periosteal e.
    Freer e.-dissector
    Freer periosteal e.
    Henahan e.
    Herczel rib e.
    Hoen periosteal e.

elevator *(continued)*
    Jannetta duckbill e.
    J-periosteal e.
    Kahre-Williger periosteal e.
    Kocher e.
    Lambotte e.
    Lane periosteal e.
    Langenbeck periosteal e.
    Lempert periosteal e.
    Locke e.
    Malis e.
    Matson-Alexander e.
    McGlamry e.
    Molt periosteal e.
    OSI extremity e.
    osteophyte e.
    Penfield periosteal e.
    periosteal e.
    e.-periosteotome
    Phemister e.
    Presbyterian Hospital staphylorrhaphy e.
    Rhoton e.
    Rochester lamina e.
    Rolyan arm e.
    Sauerbruch rib e.
    Sayre e.
    Sebileau periosteal e.
    Sédillot periosteal e.
    Sisson fracture-reducing e.
    Tegtmeir e.
    Tenzel e.
    Tronzo e.
    von Langenbeck periosteal e.
    Wiberg periosteal e.
    Willauer-Gibbon periosteal e.
    Willliger periosteal e.
    Yankauer periosteal e.
    Yasargil e.

elevatus
    hallux e.
    iatrogenic e.
    metatarsus e.
    metatarsus primus e.

ellipsoid joint

Ellison
    E. fixation staple
    E. iliotibial band tenodesis
    E. lateral knee reconstruction
    E. lateral knee technique

Elmslie
    E. peroneal tendon operation
    E. reconstruction
    E. triple arthrodesis
    E.-Cholmely foot operation
    E.-Trillat peroneal tendon operation

elongation
    e. derotation flexion
    peroneus brevis e.

ELP broach

Ely test

embolization

Emery-Dreifuss muscular dystrophy

Emgel

eminence
    antithenar e.
    bicipital e.
    capitate e.
    coccygeal e.
    cochlear e. of sacral bone
    cuneiform e. of head of rib
    deltoid e.
    gluteal e. of femur
    e. of humerus
    hypothenar e.
    iliopectineal e.
    iliopubic e.
    intercondylar e.
    intercondyloid e.
    intermediate e.
    medial e.
    oblique e. of cuboid bone
    radial e. of wrist
    thenar e.

eminence *(continued)*
    tibial e.
    trochlear e.
    ulnar e. of wrist

eminentia
    e. capitata
    e. carpi radialis
    e. carpi ulnaris
    e. hypothenaris
    e. iliopectinea
    e. iliopubica
    e. intercondylaris
    e. intercondyloidea
    e. intermedia
    e. thenaris

EMLA
    eutectic mixture of local
        anesthetics
            EMLA cream

Emmon osteotomy

empyema

enarthritis

enarthrodial

enarthrosis

enchondral

enchondroma
    e. of bone
    multiple e.
    solitary e.

enchondromatosis
    multiple e.
    skeletal e.

enchondrosis

enclavement
    Regnauld e.

en coin
    fracture en c.

encroachment
    bony e.
    cervical nerve root e.
    foraminal osteophyte e.

encroachment *(continued)*
    osseous foraminal e.

Ender
    E. awl
    E. flexible medullary nail
    E. rod

Endius Endoscopic Access System

endochondral
    e. bone
    e. ossification

endomysial

endomysium

Endopearl

endoprosthesis
    acetabular e.
    Atkinson e.
    Bio-Moore e.
    femoral e.
    nonporous-coated e.
    TPP hip e.

endoprosthetic flange

endoscopy
    laser-assisted spinal e.
        (LASE)

endplate
    e. fragmentation
    e. invagination
    e. ossification
    posterior-superior e.
    e. sclerosis

endosteal
    e. elevation
    e. revascularization

endotendineum

endotenon

Endotrac
    E. blade system
    E. endoscopic carpal tunnel release

Endurance bone cement

Enduron acetabular liner

Engel
  E. angle
  E. plaster saw
  E.-Recklinghausen disease

Engelmann
  E. disease
  E. disk

Engen
  E. extension orthosis
  E. palmar finger orthosis
  E. palmar wrist splint

Engh porous metal hip prosthesis

English anvil nail nipper

enlarging bur

Enneking
  E. knee arthrodesis
  E. knee arthrosis
  E. resection-arthrodesis
  E. rod

enostosis

en rave
  fracture en r.

ensisternum

enthesitis

enthesopathy

entochondrostosis

entocnemial

entocuneiform

entostosis

entrapment
  meniscoid e.

enucleator
  Marino transsphenoidal e.

EpicelSM service

epicondylalgia

epicondylar
  e. avulsion fracture

epicondyle
  femoral e.
  humeral e.
  lateral e.
  medial e.

epicondylectomy
  medial e.

epicondylitis
  e. of the elbow
  lateral e.
  medial e.
  radiohumeral e.

epicoracoid

epicostal

epicritic
  e. pain
  e. receptor

epimysium

epineural

epineurectomy
  interfascicular e.

epineurial
  e. repair

epineurium

epineurolysis

epineurotomy
  anterior e.

epiphyseal
  e. dysgenesis
  e. dysplasia
  e. exostosis
  e. growth plate fracture
  e. ischemic necrosis
  e. osteochondritis
  e. slip fracture
  e. stapling

epiphysiodesis
  Abbott-Gill e.

epiphysiodesis *(continued)*
    Blount e.
    bone peg e.
    Heyman-Herndon e.
    proximal phalangeal e.
    White e.

epiphysiolysis
    femoral e.

epiphysiopathy

epiphysis *pl.* epiphyses
    annular e.
    capital e.
    capital femoral e.
    capitular e.
    clavicular e.
    femoral e.
    humeral e.
    iliac e.
    Perthes e.
    slipped e.
    stippled epiphysiss
    tibial e.
    traction e.

epiphysitis
    e. juvenilis
    vertebral e.

epirotulian

episternal

epistropheus
    tooth of e.

epitendineum

epitenon suture

epithesis

Epitrain active elbow support

epitriquetrum

epitrochlea

epitrochlear

EPL
    extensor pollicus longus

ePTFE
    expanded polytetrafluoro-
      ethylene
        ePTFE graft prosthesis

equina
    cauda e.

equine gait

equinocavovarus deformity

equinovalgus
    e. deformity
    talipes e.

equinovarus
    congenital talipes e.
    e. hindfoot deformity
    talipes e.
    Turco repair of talipes e.

equinus
    ankle e.
    gastrocnemius e.
    gastrosoleal e.
    metatarsus e.
    osseous e.
    pes e.
    talipes e.

equipment
    adaptive e.

Erb
    E. atrophy
    E. dystrophy
    E. muscular dystrophy
    E. palsy
    E. point
    E.-Duchenne palsy
    E.-Goldflam disease

ERE
    external rotation in exten-
      sion

ERF
    external rotation in flexion

ergogenic

ergograph
    Mosso e.

ergonomics

ergoreceptor

ergostat

Erichsen
　E. sign
　E. test

Eriksson
　E. cruciate ligament reconstruction
　E. muscle biopsy cannula

erosion
　osteoclastic e.

erosive arthritis

eschar

escharotic

escharotomy

E-series hip system

ESKA

Eskimo method

Esmarch
　E. bandage
　E. plaster knife
　E. tourniquet

Essex
　E.-Lopresti calcaneal fracture technique
　E.-Lopresti lesion
　E.-Lopresti open reduction

ESSF
　external spinal cord fixator

Esterom

Estersohn osteotomy for tailor's bunion

esquillectomy

Ethrone implant material

etodolac

Euler angle

eulerian angle

EuroCuff forearm crutch

Evans
　E. ankle reconstruction technique
　E. calcaneal lengthening
　E. calcaneal osteotomy
　E. intertrochanteric fracture classification
　E. lateral ankle reconstruction
　E. tenodesis
　E.-Burkhalter protocol

eversion
　ankle e.
　inversion-e.
　e. osteotomy
　e. stress test

Evista

Ewald
　E. capitellocondylar total elbow arthroplasty
　E. elbow arthroplasty
　E. total elbow replacement
　E.-Walker kinematic knee arthroplasty
　E.-Walker knee arthroplasty
　E.-Walker knee implant

EWHO
　elbow-wrist-hand orthosis

Ewing
　E. sarcoma
　E. tumor

Excelart

Excel Plus electrode

excision
　Das Gupta scapular e.
　McKeever-Buck fragment e.
　Ferclot-Thompson e.

exclusion clamp

excoriation

excursion
　hindfoot e.
　range of e.

excrescence
  bony e.

exercise
  active e.
  active-assisted range of
    motion e.
  active range of motion e's
  aerobic e.
  breathing e.
  Buerger-Allen e.
  Calleja e's
  closed kinetic chain pro-
    gressive-resistance e.
  Codman e.
  contracture e.
  Crane shoulder e.
  De Lorme e.
  dynamic stump e.
  eccentric e.
  endurance e.
  external rotation e.
  flexion back e.
  flexion-extension e.
  free e.
  Frenkel e.
  gastric-resistive e.
  hamstring-setting e.
  heel cord stretching e.
  hip adductor strengthen-
    ing e.
  internal rotation e.
  inversion-eversion e.
  isokinetic e.
  isometric e.
  isotonic e.
  kinesthetic e.
  McKenzie extension e.
  muscle-setting e.
  orthokinetic e.
  passive e.
  progressive resistance e.
  progressive resistive e.
  quadriceps-setting e.
  range of motion e.
  Regen flexion e.
  resistive e.
  rotation e.
  Seradge hand e's
  static e.

exercise *(continued)*
  straight leg raising e.
  therapeutic e.
  toe gripping e.
  underwater e.
  volitional e.
  Williams flexion e's

Exeter
  E. bone lavage
  E. cemented hip prosthesis
  E. intramedullary bone
    plug

exhaustion
  postactivation e.
  posttetanic e.
  reaction of e.

Exogen 2000 *(ultrasound)*

exomysium

exostosectomy

exostosis *pl.* exostoses
  blocker's e.
  bony e.
  e. bursata
  e. cartilaginea
  cuneiform-first metatarsal e.
  Dupuytren e.
  epiphyseal e.
  hereditary multiple e.
  hypertrophic e.
  impingement e.
  ivory e.
  marginal e.
  metatarsal cuneiform e.
  metatarsocuneiform joint e.
  multiple e.
  multiple cartilaginous e.
  multiple osteocartilagi-
    nous e.
  osteocartilaginous e.
  retrocalcaneal e.
  subungual e.
  talar neck e.
  talotibial e.
  turret e.

exostotic

Exotec brace

expanding reamer

exsanguinate

Extend total hip system

extender
Rousek e.

extension
active knee e. (AKE)
angle of greatest e. (AGE)
Buck e.
cast with dorsal toe plate e.
cervical rotation in e.
distractive e.
dorsal toe plate e.
Hittenberger halo e.
isokinetic knee e.
Legg-Perthes shoe e.
e. malposition
Maquet table e.
NexGen offset stem e.
e. osteotomy
toe plate e.

extensor
e. brevis
e. brevis arthroplasty
e. carpi radialis
e. carpi radialis brevis
(ECRB)
e. carpi ulnaris
e. digiti minimi
e. digiti quinti (EDQ)
e. digitorum brevis
e. digitorum communis
e. digitorum longus (EDL)
e. digitorum transfer
e. hallucis
e. hallucis brevis
e. hallucis longus
e. hallucis longus (EHL)
tendon
e. hood mechanism
e. indicis proprius (EIP)
knee e.
e. mechanism
e. pollicis brevis
e. pollicis longus (EPL)
e. quinti tendon

extensor (continued)
radial wrist e.
e. retinaculum of foot
e. retinaculum of hand
e. tendon repair
e. tenodesis
e. tenotomy
wrist e.

exteriorization

external
e. alignment compression
jig
e. fixator frame

externum
os tibiale e.

extirpation

extra-articular
e. ankylosis
e. arthrodesis
e. hip fusion
e. pigmented villonodular
synovitis
e. pseudarthrosis
e. subtalar fusion

extrabursal approach

extracapsular
e. ankylosis
e. dissection

extractor
Austin Moore e.
ball e.
Bilos e.
Bilos pin e.
Cherry screw e.
cloverleaf pin e.
driver-e.
femoral trial e.
impactor-e.
Intraflex intramedullary
pin e.
Jewett e.
Küntscher e.
Mark II femoral compo-
nent e.
Mark II tibial component e.

extractor *(continued)*
    Massie e.
    Moreland femoral compo-
      nent e.
    Nicoll e.
    Schneider e.
    Snap Lock wire/pin e.
    Southwick screw e.
    Universal modular femoral
      hip component e.
    Zimmer e.
    Zimmer driver-e.
    Zimmer femoral canal e.

extramedullary
    e. alignment

extraosseous factor

extraperitoneal approach

extrapharyngeal
    e. approach

extratendinous

extravasation

extremitas
    e. acromialis claviculae
    e. sternalis claviculae

extremity
    cartilaginous e. of rib
    external e. of clavicle
    e. mobilization technique
    internal e. of clavicle
    proximal e. of phalanx of
      finger
    proximal e. of phalanx of
      toe
    scapular e. of clavicle

extrusion
    bone graft e.
    disk e.
    extravasation e.

Eyler flexorplasty

Ezeform splint

E-Z Roc anchor

fabella

fabellofibular
f. ligament

fabere
flexion, abduction, external
rotation, extension
fabere sign
fabere test

Fabian screw

facet
f. angle
f. apposition
articular f.
articular f. of atlas
articular f. of dens of axis
articular f's for rib cartilages
clavicular f.
costal f.
f. excision technique
f. fracture
f. fusion
f. joint block
lateral f's of sternum
lateral patellar f.
locked f's of spine
malleolar f. of tibia
medial posterior f. of calcaneus
f. plane
f. replacement
squatting f.
f. subluxation stabilization
wiring
thoracic f.
f. tropism
f. for tubercle of rib

facetectomy
O'Donoghue f.

facies
f. antebrachialis anterior
f. antebrachialis posterior
anterior antebrachial f.
anterior brachial f.
anterior cubital f.
f. anterior lateralis humeri

facies *(continued)*
f. anterior medialis humeri
f. anterior patellae
f. anterior radii
f. anterior scapulae
f. anterior ulnae
f. anterolateralis humeri
f. anteromedialis humeri
f. articularis acromialis
claviculae
f. articularis acromialis
scapulae
f. articularis acromii scapulae
f. articularis anterior calcanei
f. articularis anterior dentis
f. articularis anterior epis-
trophei
f. articularis calcanea anterior tali
f. articularis calcanea media tali
f. articularis calcanea posterior tali
f. articularis capitis costae
f. articularis capitis fibulae
f. articularis capituli costae
f. articularis capituli fibulae
f. articularis carpalis radii
f. articularis carpi radii
f. articularis cuboidea calcanei
f. articularis fibularis tibiae
f. articularis inferior atlantis
f. articularis inferior tibiae
f. articularis inferior vertebrae
f. articularis malleoli lateralis
f. articularis malleoli medialis
f. articularis media calcanei
f. articularis navicularis tali
f. articularis patellae
f. articularis posterior dentis

facies *(continued)*
    f. articularis sternalis clavi-
      culae
    f. articularis superior atlan-
      tis
    f. articularis superior tibiae
    f. articularis superior verte-
      brae
    f. articularis talaris anterior
      calcanei
    f. articularis talaris media
      calcanei
    f. articularis talaris poste-
      rior calcanei
    f. articularis tuberculi cos-
      tae
    f. auricularis ossis ilii
    f. auricularis ossis ilium
    f. auricularis ossis sacri
    f. brachialis anterior
    f. brachialis posterior
    f. costalis scapulae
    f. cruralis anterior
    f. cruralis posterior
    f. cubitalis anterior
    f. cubitalis posterior
    f. digitales
    f. digitales dorsales manus
    f. digitales dorsales pedis
    f. digitales fibulares pedis
    f. digitales laterales manus
    f. digitales laterales pedis
    f. digitales mediales manus
    f. digitales mediales pedis
    f. digitales palmares manus
    f. digitales plantares pedis
    f. digitales radiales manus
    f. digitales tibiales pedis
    f. digitales ulnares manus
    f. digitales ventrales manus
    f. digitales ventrales pedis
    f. dorsales digitorum manus
    f. dorsales digitorum pedis
    f. dorsalis ossis sacri
    f. dorsalis radii
    f. dorsalis scapulae
    f. dorsalis ulnae
    f. femoralis anterior
    f. femoralis posterior

facies *(continued)*
    f. glutealis ossis ilii
    f. glutea ossis ilii
    f. intervertebralis
    f. lateralis fibulae
    f. lateralis radii
    f. lateralis tibiae
    f. lunata acetabuli
    f. malleolaris lateralis tali
    f. malleolaris medialis tali
    f. medialis fibulae
    f. medialis tibiae
    f. medialis ulnae
    f. palmares digitorum ma-
      nus
    f. patellaris femoris
    f. pelvica ossis sacri
    f. pelvina ossis sacri
    f. plantares digitorum pedis
    f. poplitea femoris
    posterior antebrachial f.
    posterior brachial f.
    posterior cubital f.
    f. posterior fibulae
    f. posterior humeri
    f. posterior radii
    f. posterior scapulae
    f. posterior tibiae
    f. posterior ulnae
    f. sacropelvica ossis ilii
    f. sacropelvina ossis ilii
    f. superior trochleae tali
    swan-neck f.
    f. symphyseos ossis pubis
    f. symphysialis ossis pubis
    f. ventralis scapulae
    f. volaris radii
    f. volaris ulnae

facilitation
    convergence f.
    neuromuscular f.
    postactivation f.
    posttetanic f.
    proprioceptive neuromus-
      cular f.

facioscapulohumeral
    f. muscle atrophy disease
    f. muscular atrophy

facioscapulohumeral *(continued)*
   f. muscular dystrophy

F-actin

factor
   extraosseous f.

fadir
   flexion in adduction and internal rotation
      fadir sign
      fadir test

Fahey-Compere pin

failed
   f. back surgery syndrome
   f. back syndrome
   f. femoral osteotomy
   f. joint replacement
   f. triple arthrodesis

Fairbanks
   F. apprehension test
   F. sign

Fallat-Buckholz method

fallopian ligament

Fallopius
   ligament of F.

falx
   aponeurotic f.
   f. aponeurotica
   inguinal f.
   f. inguinalis
   f. ligamentosa
   ligamentous f.

Fanconi syndrome

Farabeuf
   F. forceps
   F. periosteal elevator
   F.-Collin rasp
   F.-Lambotte bone-holding
     forceps

Farrior wire-crimping forceps

fascia
   Abernethy f.
   antebrachial f.
   f. antebrachii
   anterior cervical f.
   axillary f.
   bicipital f.
   brachial f.
   f. brachialis
   f. brachii
   Buck f.
   Camper f.
   cervical f.
   f. cervicalis
   clavipectoral f.
   f. clavipectoralis
   Cloquet f.
   f. colli
   coracoclavicular f.
   f. coracoclavicularis
   coracocostal f.
   cribriform f.
   f. cribrosa
   crural f.
   f. cruris
   deltoid f.
   f. deltoidea
   dorsal f.
   f. dorsalis manus
   f. dorsalis pedis
   Dupuytren f.
   femoral f.
   f. of forearm
   Hesselbach f.
   hypothenar f.
   iliac f.
   f. iliaca
   f. iliopectinea
   iliopectineal f.
   f. lata
   f. of leg
   longitudinal f.
   lumbar f.
   lumbodorsal f.
   f. lumbodorsalis
   f. nuchae
   nuchal f.

fascia *(continued)*
   f. nuchalis
   obturator f.
   f. obturatoria
   palmar f.
   parietal f. of pelvis
   f. pectinea
   pectineal f.
   pectoral f.
   f. pectoralis
   plantar f.
   prevertebral f.
   f. prevertebralis
   quadratus femoris f.
   scalene f.
   semilunar f.
   Sibson f.
   f. of thigh
   f. thoracolumbalis
   thoracolumbar f.
   transversalis f.
   triangular f. of abdomen
   triangular f. of Quain
   volar f.

fasciatome *(variant of* fascio-tome)

fascicle
   popliteomeniscal f.

fascicular
   f. neuropathy

fasciculation
   benign f.
   malignant f.
   f. potential

fasciculus *pl.* fasciculi
   f. cuneatus
   f. exilis
   fibrous f. of biceps muscle
   f. gracilis
   lateral plantar nerve f.
   f. lenticularis
   longitudinal fasciculi of cruciform ligament
   fasciculi longitudinales ligamenti cruciformis atlantis

fasciculus *(continued)*
   fasciculi transversi aponeurosis palmaris
   fasciculi transversi aponeurosis plantaris

fasciectomy
   dermal f.

fasciitis
   Dupuytren f.
   iliotibial band f.
   necrotizing f.
   plantar f.
   recalcitrant plantar f.

fasciodesis

fascio-fat graft

fasciorrhaphy

fasciotome *(spelled also* fasciatome)
   intercompartment f.
   Masson f.
   Moseley f.

fasciotomy
   compartment f.
   decompression f.
   double-incision f.
   Fronet f.
   palmar f.
   percutaneous plantar f.
   plantar f.
   prophylactic f.
   Rorabeck f.
   Skoog f.
   Yount f.

fastener
   Brown-Mueller T-f. set

fatigue
   f. fracture
   metal f.

Faulkner curet

Fay method

Fazio-Londe disease

FBS
    failed back syndrome

FCR
    flexor carpii radialis

FCU
    flexor carpi ulnaris

FDB
    flexor digitorum brevis

FDC
    flexor digitorum communis

FDL
    flexor digitorum longus

FDMA
    first dorsal metatarsal artery

FDP
    flexor digitorum profundus

FDQB
    flexor digiti quinti brevis

FDS
    flexor digitorum sublimis
    flexor digitorum superficialis

Feagin shoulder dislocation test

Feiss line

Feldenkrais cylinder

Felty syndrome

femoral
    f. alignment jig
    f. antetorsion
    f. anteversion
    f. condylar shaving
    f. condyle
    f. cortex
    f. cortical ring allograft
    f. cutaneous nerve
    f. derotation osteotomy
    f. diaphyseal allograft
    f. diaphyseal shortening
    f. endoprosthesis

femoral *(continued)*
    f. epicondyle
    f. epiphysiolysis
    f. epiphysis
    f. impactor
    f. intermedullary guide
    f. intertrochanteric fracture
    f. metaphyseal shortening
    f. neck fracture
    f. neck fracture reduction
    f. notch guide
    f. osteolysis
    f. osteomyelitis
    f. osteoporosis
    f. prosthesis fixation
    f. rasp
    f. retrotorsion
    f. retroversion
    f. shaft malunion
    f. supracondylar fracture
    f. trial extractor
    f. tunnel

femorale
    calcar f.

femoriliac

femoris
    biceps f.
    ligamentum capitis f.
    linea aspera f.
    profunda f.
    quadratus f.
    rectus f.

femorocrural graft

femorodistal
    f. bypass procedure

femoroiliac thrombophlebitis

femoroischial transplantation

femorotibial
    f. angle (FTA)
    f. ligament tenodesis

femur
    adductor tubercle of f.
    distal f.
    popliteal triangle of f.

femur *(continued)*
  proximal f.
  Universal proximal f.

fenestrated
  f. reamer
  f. stem

fenestration

Fenlin total shoulder system

Fenton tibial bolt

Ferclot-Thompson excision

Ferguson
  F. bone clamp
  F. hip reduction
  F. sacral base angle

Fergusson forceps

Ferkel
  F. bipolar release
  F. method for measuring
    scoliosis

Ferran awl

Ferris Smith
  F. S. rongeur
  F. S. rongeur forceps
  F. S.–Kerrison forceps
  F. S.–Spurling disk rongeur

ferromagnetic metal plate

FHB
  flexor hallucis brevis

FHL
  flexor hallucis longus

FHLD
  flexor hallucis longus dys-
    function

fiber
  A-delta f.
  afferent f.
  annular f.
  bone f.
  carbon f.
  f. density

fiber *(continued)*
  extrafusal f.
  fast twitch muscle f's
  Gerdy f.
  intermediate muscle f's
  intrafusal f.
  light f's
  muscle f.
  osteocollagenous f's
  osteogenetic f's
  osteogenic f's
  radiating f's of anterior
    chondrosternal ligaments
  ragged red f's
  red muscle f's
  ring f.
  Sharpey f.
  slow twitch muscle f's
  tendinous f.
  type I muscle f's
  type II muscle f's
  Weissmann f's
  white muscle f's

fibra *pl.* fibrae
  fibrae annulares

fibril
  muscle f.
  muscular f.

fibrillation

fibroblast

fibrocartilage
  circumferential f.
  complex f.
  connecting f.
  cotyloid f.
  elastic f.
  interarticular f.
  intervertebral f's
  semilunar f's
  spongy f.
  stratiform f.
  triangular f.
  white f.
  yellow f.

fibrocartilaginous

fibrocartilago
  fibrocartilagines interverte-
    brales
  f. navicularis

fibrochondrocyte

fibrodysplasia
  f. ossificans progressiva

fibroenchondroma

fibrogenesis
  f. imperfecta ossium

fibroma
  aponeurotic f.
  chondromyxoid f.
  desmoid f.
  desmoplastic f.
  f. molluscum
  nonossifying f.
  nonosteogenic f.
  ossifying f.
  osteogenic f.
  periosteal f.
  periungual f.
  subungual f.

fibromatosis
  f. colli
  congenital general f.
  dermal f.
  irradiation f.
  palmar f.
  plantar f.

fibromyalgia syndrome

fibromyositis
  nodular f.

fibroosseous
  f. ring of Lacroix
  f. sheath

fibrosis
  annular f.

fibrositis
  periarticular f.

fibula
  diastasis f.

fibula (continued)
  dysplastic f.
  f. protibial synostosis
  proximal f.

fibular
  f. anlage
  f. collateral ligament
  f. groove
  f. hemimelia
  f. metaphysis
  f. onlay-inlay graft
  f. ostectomy
  f. osteotomy
  f. pseudarthrosis
  f. sesamoidal ligament
  f. sesamoidectomy
  f. strut graft
  f. transfer

fibularis
  incisura f. tibiae

fibulectomy
  partial f.

fibulocalcaneal ligament

fibulotalar arthrodesis

fibulotalocalcaneal ligament

Ficat-Marcus grading system

field
  f. block
  Cohnheim f's
  pulsating electromagnetic f.

Fielding-Magliato classification
  of subtrochanteric fracture

figure-of-four position

filament
  actin f.
  desmin f's
  muscle f.
  myosin f.
  thick f's
  thin f's

Fillauer
  F. bar foot orthosis
  F. dorsiflexion assist ankle
    joint

Fillauer *(continued)*
  F. night splint
  F. PDC ankle joint
  F. Scottish Rite orthosis kit

filleted graft

filmy adhesion

finger
  adduction stress to f.
  baseball f.
  claw f.
  clubbed f.
  congenital trigger f.
  drop f.
  f. flexion splint
  f. goniometer
  giant f.
  hammer f.
  hippocratic f's
  index f.
  f. joint arthropathy
  little f.
  lock f.
  lumbrical syndrome f.
  mallet f.
  middle f.
  ring f.
  second f.
  snapping f.
  spring f.
  syndactylized f.
  third f.
  trigger f.
  f. tuft
  webbed f.

finish bur

Finkelstein
  F. maneuver
  F. test
  F. test for synovitis

Finney-Flexirod prosthesis

Finochietto
  F. rib retractor
  F. stirrup
  F.-Bunnell test

FIN pin

Finsen-Reya lamp

Fisch drill

Fish cuneiform osteotomy

Fisher brace

fishmouth
  f. amputation
  f. anastomosis
  f. end-to-end suture

fistula *pl.* fistulas, fistulae
  arteriovenous f.
  colocutaneous f.
  enterocutaneous f.
  synovial f.
  vesicocutaneous f.

Fixateur Interne
  Dick AO F. I.
  F. I. fixation system
  F. I. rod
  F. I. screw

fixation
  Ace-Fisher f.
  Ace Unifix f.
  adjunctive screw f.
  Allen-Ferguson Galveston
    pelvic f.
  AMBI f.
  angled blade plate f.
  AO external f.
  arthroscopic screw f.
  axial f.
  bicortical screw f.
  blade plate f.
  cerclage wire f.
  cervical spine internal f.
  cervical spine screw-plate f.
  compression plate f.
  coracoclavicular screw f.
  dens anterior screw f.
  femoral prosthesis f.
  Gallie subtalar f.
  Galveston f. with TSRH
    crosslink
  Georgiade visor halo f.
  Harrington rod f.
  Herbert screw f.

fixation *(continued)*
    humeral supracondylar f.
    Ilizarov external f.
    iliac f.
    intermedullary rod f.
    internal f.
    intersegmental f.
    intraosseous f.
    Kirschner pin f.
    lag screw f.
    lumbar spine segmental f.
    Luque loop f.
    Magerl posterior cervical screw f.
    Matta-Saucedo f.
    medial malleolus f.
    medullary nail f.
    odontoid fracture internal f.
    open reduction and internal f. (ORIF)
    pedicle f.
    pedicle screw f.
    phalangeal fracture f.
    Phemister acromioclavicular pin f.
    pin f.
    plate-screw f.
    posterior screw f.
    posterior segmental f.
    Press-Fit f.
    reduction/f.
    Rogozinski spinal f.
    sacral pedicle screw f.
    sacral spine f.
    sacroiliac extension f.
    sacroiliac flexion f.
    sacrum fusion screw f.
    screw f.
    segmental f.
    spinal f.
    Steinmann pin f.
    strut plate f.
    sublaminar f.
    Sulzer f.
    suprasyndesmotic f.
    suture f.
    tension band f.

fixation *(continued)*
    transarticular wire f.
    transsyndesmotic f.
    TSRH f.
    TSRH rod f.
    Versa-Fx femoral f.
    Volkov-Oganesian external f.
    Ward-Tomasin-Vander Griend f.
    Warner-Farber ankle f.
    Webb f.
    Zickel subtrochanteric f.
    Zickel supracondylar f.

fixator
    Agee WristJack external f.
    articulated external f.
    Clyburn Colles fracture f.
    external f.
    fracture f.
    half-pin external f.
    HTO (high tibial osteotomy) f.
    Jacquet f.
    Manuflex external f.
    Pennig dynamic wrist f.
    Richards-Colles external f.
    spanning external f.
    spinal f.
    Vermont spinal f. (VSF)

FJD
    facet joint disease

flange
    endoprosthetic f.

flap
    adipofascial f.
    advancement f.
    Atasoy triangular advancement f.
    below-knee amputation using long posterior f.
    brachioradialis f.
    buccinator myomucosal f.
    bursal f.
    cutaneous f.
    deltopectoral f.

flap *(continued)*
 dorsalis pedis f.
 free fasciocutaneous f.
 gastrocnemius f.
 gluteus maximus f.
 f. graft
 hemipulp f.
 iliac osteocutaneous f.
 intercostal f.
 Limberg f.
 medial plantar fasciocutaneous f.
 microvascular free f.
 Moberg advancement f.
 muscle f.
 musculocutaneous free f.
 myocutaneous f.
 omental f.
 f. operation
 osteocutaneous free f.
 osteoperiosteal f.
 palmar advancement f.
 pectoralis major f.
 radial-based f.
 remote pedicle f.
 rhomboid f.
 rotational f.
 Schrudde rotational f.
 serratus anterior f.
 sural island f.
 thenar f.
 transposition f.
 triangular advancement f.
 turn-down tendon f.
 vascularized free f.
 V-Y advancement f.
 V-Y Kutler f.

flat-bottomed Kerrison rongeur

flatfoot
 calcaneovalgus f.
 f. deformity
 flaccid f.
 Kidner f.
 pronated straight f.
 rocker-bottom f.
 spastic f.

Flatt recess

flaval ligament

flavum *pl.* flava
 ligamentum f.

Fleischner disease

flex

Flexderm wound dressing

Flex-foot

flexion
 f.-adduction
 f. angle
 angle of greatest f. (AGF)
 f. body cast
 f.-burst fracture
 compression f.
 f. contracture
 f. distraction
 dorsiflexion-f.
 elongation derotation f.
 external rotation in f.
 hip f.
 f. osteotomy
 palmar f.
 plantar f.
 spine f.
 standing f.

Flexisplint flexed armboard

flexor
 f. carpi quinti brevis
  (FDQB)
 f. carpi radialis (FCR)
 f. carpi ulnaris (FCU)
 f. digitorum brevis (FDB)
 f. digitorum communis
  (FDC)
 f. digitorum longus (FDL)
 f. digitorum profundus
  (FDP)
 f. digitorum slip
 f. digitorum sublimus (FDS)
 f. digitorum superficialis
  (FDS)
 f. groove
 f. hallucis brevis (FHB)

flexor *(continued)*
    f. hallucis longus (FHL)
    f.–hallucis longus tendon release
    f. hinge hand splint
    f. hinge hand orthosis
    f. hinge orthosis
    f. hinge splint
    f. mechanism
    f. plate
    f. pollicis brevis (FPB)
    f. pollicis longus (FPL)
    f. profundus tendon
    f.-pronator origin release
    f. pronator slide
    f. retinaculum
    f. retinaculum of foot
    f. retinaculum of hand
    f. skin crease
    f. tendon anastomosis
    f. tendon laceration
    f. tendon repair
    f. tendon rupture
    f. tendon sheath
    f. tenosynovectomy
    f. tenotomy
    f. wad

flexorplasty
    Bunnell modification of Steindler f.
    Eyler f.
    Steindler f.

flexure
    lumbar f.

Flip-Flop pillow

FLOAM ankle stirrup brace

flocculent foci of calcification

Floegel layer

Flood ligament

floor
    f. of acetabulum
    f. of pelvis
    f.-reaction ankle-foot orthosis

florid
    f. callus
    f. synovitis

Florida
    F. back brace
    F. contraflexion brace
    F. hyperextension brace

fluid
    bursal f.
    f. homeostasis
    interstitial f.
    synovial f.

fluoroscope
    C-arm f.
    XiScan f.

Flynn femoral neck fracture reduction

foam
    Plastizote f.

focus *pl.* foci
    flocculent foci of calcification

fold
    alar f's
    asymmetric skin f.
    Bartlett nail f.
    infrapatellar synovial f.
    interarticular f. of hip
    mediopatellar synovial f.
    nail f.
    patellar synovial f.
    suprapatellar synovial f.
    synovial f.
    synovial f. of hip

fomentation therapy

Fomon
    F. chisel
    F. periosteal elevator
    F. periosteotome

Fonar Stand-Up MRI

foot
    ball of the f.

foot *(continued)*
    broad f.
    calcaneocavus f.
    calcaneovalgus f.
    Charcot f.
    cavus f.
    cleft f.
    club f.
    C-shaped f.
    Dycor prosthetic f.
    flat f.
    Flex-F.
    forced f.
    Friedreich f.
    insensate f.
    f. ischemia
    Morton f.
    multiaxis f.
    neuroarthropathic f.
    plantigrade f.
    pronation of the f.
    reel f.
    rocker-bottom f.
    SACH f.
    sag f.
    Seattle f.
    supination of the f.
    spread f.
    tabetic f.
    taut f.
    tripod f.
    valgus f.
    weak f.
football knee
footdrop
footplate
    metal f.
forage procedure
foramen *pl.* foramina
    anterior sacral foramina
    arcuate f.
    f. costotransversarium
    costotransverse f.
    cotyloid f.
    dorsal sacral foramina
    greater ischiadic f.

foramen *(continued)*
    greater sciatic f.
    Hartigan f.
    infrapiriform f.
    internal sacral foramina
    intersacral foramina
    intervertebral f.
    f. intervertebrale
    foramina intervertebralia ossis sacri
    f. ischiadicum majus
    f. ischiadicum minus
    ischiopubic f.
    large sacrosciatic f.
    lesser ischiadic f.
    lesser sciatic f.
    medullary f.
    neural f.
    f. nutricium
    f. nutriens
    nutrient f.
    obturator f.
    f. obturatorium
    f. obturatum
    oval f. of hip bone
    posterior sacral foramina
    f. processus transversi
    f. of sacral canal
    foramina sacralia anteriora
    foramina sacralia dorsalia
    foramina sacralia pelvica
    foramina sacralia pelvina
    foramina sacralia posteriora
    foramina sacralia ventralia
    f. of saphenous vein
    sciatic f.
    f. sciaticum majus
    f. sciaticum minus
    small sacrosciatic f.
    spinal f.
    f. of spinal cord
    suprapiriform f.
    f. transversarium
    f. of transverse process
    ventral sacral foramina
    f. vertebrale
    vertebroarterial f.

foramen *(continued)*
    f. vertebroarteriale
    Weitbrecht f.

foraminal
    f. compression test

foraminotomy
    neural f.

forceplate

forceps
    Acland clamp-applying f.
    Adson drill guide f.
    adventitial f.
    Aesculap f.
    alligator grasping f.
    Allis tissue f.
    angled-down f.
    angled-up f.
    AO reduction f.
    arthroscopy basket f.
    arthroscopy grasping f.
    Asch f.
    Backhaus towel f.
    Baer bone-cutting f.
    Bardeleben bone-holding f.
    basket f.
    Beasley-Babcock f.
    Berens muscle clamp f.
    Boies f.
    bone-biting f.
    bone-cutting f.
    bone-holding f.
    bone-splitting f.
    Brown-Adson f.
    Brown-Cushing f.
    Bulldog clamp-applying f.
    cartilage f.
    Charnley wire-holding f.
    Citelli punch f.
    clamp-applying f.
    Cleveland bone-cutting f.
    coagulating f.
    cupped grasping f.
    curved basket f.
    cutting f.
    Dawson-Yuhl rongeur f.
    Dawson-Yuhl-Kerrison rongeur f.

forceps *(continued)*
    drill guide f.
    Echlin rongeur f.
    ethmoid f.
    Farabeuf f.
    Farabeuf-Lambotte bone-holding f.
    Farrior wire-crimping f.
    Fergusson f.
    Ferris Smith rongeur f.
    Ferris Smith–Kerrison f.
    Gardner bone f.
    glenoid-reaming f.
    Hartmann mosquito f.
    Hibbs bone-cutting f.
    Hirsch hypophysis punch f.
    Hoen f.
    Horsley bone-cutting f.
    Howmedica microfixation system f.
    Hurd bone cutting f.
    Jackson broad-angle staple f.
    Jackson broad-blade staple f.
    Jackson tendon-seizing f.
    Jacobson mosquito f.
    Jansen monopolar f.
    Jarell f.
    Jarit tendon-pulling f.
    jeweler's bipolar f.
    Juers-Lempert rongeur f.
    Kleinert-Kutz tendon f.
    knotting f.
    Kocher f.
    Lalonde bone f.
    Lalonde hook f.
    Lambotte bone-cutting f.
    Lane bone-holding f.
    Lane screw-holding f.
    Lane self-retaining bone holding f.
    Lempert rongeur f.
    Love-Kerrison rongeur f.
    Malis jeweler bipolar f.
    McIndoe rongeur f.
    meniscus f.
    mosquito-tip grasping f.

forceps *(continued)*
  Nicola f.
  Niro bone cutting f.
  Niro wire-twisting f.
  Overholt clip-applying f.
  Perman cartilage f.
  plate-holding f.
  Raimondi hemostatic f.
  rib f.
  rongeur f.
  Ruskin-Liston bone cut-
    ting f.
  Samuels f.
  Sauerbruch rib f.
  Schwartz clip-applying f.
  screw-holding f.
  Selverstone rongeur f.
  sequestrum f.
  side-cutting basket f.
  Spence rongeur f.
  sponge-holding f.
  Spurling-Kerrison rongeur f.
  staple f.
  Steinmann tendon f.
  Stille-Horsley rib f.
  Stille-Luer rongeur f.
  Storz Microsystems plate-
    holding f.
  Synthes Microsystem plate-
    holding f.
  Takahashi f.
  tenaculum-reducing f.
  tendon f.
  tendon-pulling f.
  tendon-tunneling f.
  tissue f.
  Ulrich bone-holding f.
  upbiting basket f.
  Utrata f.
  Verbrugge bone-holding f.
  Walton-Liston f.
  Walton-Ruskin f.
  Weller cartilage f.
  Wiet cup f.
  Wilde rongeur f.
  wire-cutting f.
  wire-holding f.
  wire-pulling f.

forceps *(continued)*
  Zimmer-Hoen f.

forearm
  f. compartment syndrome
  f. contracture
  distal f.
  f. supination test

forefoot
  f. abduction deformity
  f. abductus
  f. adductovarus
  f. angulation
  f. equinus
  f. valgus
  f. varus

forequarter amputation

Forestier
  F. bowstring sign
  F. disease

formation
  beaklike osteophyte f.
  osteophyte f.
  procallus f.
  rouleaux f.

Formatray mandibular splint

Forrester splint

Fosnaugh nail biopsy

fossa
  acetabular f.
  f. acetabularis
  f. acetabuli
  anconal f.
  anconeal f.
  antecubital f.
  articular f. of atlas, inferior
  articular f. of atlas, supe-
    rior
  articular f. for odontoid
    process of axis
  f. capitis femoris
  condyloid f. of atlas
  f. coronoidea humeri
  f. of coronoid process
  costal f., inferior

fossa *(continued)*
  costal f., superior
  costal f. of transverse process
  cubital f.
  f. cubitalis
  digital f. of femur
  glenoid f. of scapula
  Gruber f.
  f. of head of femur
  f. iliaca
  f. infraspinata
  f. infraspinosa
  infraspinous f.
  intercondylar f. of femur
  intercondylar f. of femur, anterior
  intercondylar f. of tibia, anterior
  intercondylar f. of tibia, posterior
  f. intercondylaris femoris
  f. intercondylica
  intercondyloid f.
  f. intercondyloidea anterior tibiae
  f. intercondyloidea femoris
  f. intercondyloidea posterior tibiae
  ischiorectal f.
  Jobert f.
  f. of lateral malleolus
  f. of little head of radius
  f. malleoli lateralis
  f. olecrani
  olecranon f.
  oval f. of thigh
  f. ovalis femoris
  patellar f. of femur
  patellar f. of tibia
  f. poplitea
  popliteal f.
  popliteal f. of femur
  popliteal f. of tibia
  posterior f. of humerus
  prescapular f.
  prespinous f.
  f. radialis humeri
  semilunar f. of ulna

fossa *(continued)*
  sigmoid f. of ulna
  sigmoid f. of ulna, lesser
  sphenoidal f.
  f. subscapularis
  supracondyloid f.
  f. supraspinata
  f. supraspinosa
  supraspinous f.
  supratrochlear f., posterior
  tibiofemoral f.
  f. trochanterica
  ulnar f.

fossula
  inferior costal f.
  superior costal f.

Foundation
  F. total hip system
  F. total knee system

four
  f.-bar external fixation apparatus
  f.-bar Polycentric knee prosthesis
  f.-hole side plate
  f.-point gait

Fournier test

fovea
  anterior f. of humerus, greater
  anterior f. of humerus, lesser
  articular f. of atlas, inferior
  articular f. of atlas, superior
  articular foveae for rib cartilages
  f. articularis capitis radii
  f. articularis inferior atlantis
  f. articularis superior atlantis
  calcaneal f.
  f. capitis femoris
  f. capituli radii
  f. of coronoid process
  costal f., inferior

fovea *(continued)*
    costal f., superior
    costal f., transverse
    costal foveae of sternum
    f. costalis inferior
    f. costalis processus transversi
    f. costalis superior
    dental f. of atlas
    f. dentis atlantis
    f. of head of femur
    f. for head of radius
    f. of lateral malleolus
    f. of little head of radius
    malleolar f. of fibula, lateral
    supratrochlear f., anterior
    supratrochlear f. of humerus
    f. of talus
    f. of tooth of atlas

foveal fat pad

Fowler
    F. central slip tenotomy
    F. tenodesis
    F.-Philip angle
    F.-Philip approach

Fowles dislocation technique

Fox clavicular splint

FPB
    flexor pollicis brevis

FPL
    flexor pollicus longus

Frac-Sur splint

fractionation

fracture
    abduction-external rotation f.
    acetabular posterior wall f.
    acetabular rim f.
    acute avulsion f.
    adduction f.
    agenetic f.
    Aitken classification of epiphyseal f.
    alveolar bone f.

fracture *(continued)*
    Anderson-Hutchins unstable tibial shaft f.
    angulated f.
    ankle f.
    ankle mortise f.
    anterior calcaneal process f.
    anterolateral compression f.
    AO classification of ankle f.
    apophyseal f.
    articular f.
    Ashhurst-Bromer ankle f.
    Atkin epiphyseal f.
    atlas f.
    atrophic f.
    avulsion f.
    avulsion chip f.
    axial compression f.
    backfire f.
    Bankart f.
    Barton f.
    basal neck f.
    basilar femoral neck f.
    basocervical f.
    bending f.
    Bennett comminuted f.
    bicondylar T-shaped f.
    bimalleolar f.
    bipartite f.
    f. blister
    blow-in f.
    blow-out f.
    bone cyst f.
    boxer's f.
    Broberg-Morrey f.
    bucket-handle f.
    bumper f.
    Burkhalter-Reyes method for phalangeal f.
    burst f.
    bursting f.
    butterfly f.
    buttonhole f.
    C1 f.
    calcaneal avulsion f.
    f. callus
    Canale-Kelly talar neck f.

fracture *(continued)*
    capitellar f.
    capitulum radiale humeri f.
    carpal bone stress f.
    carpal scaphoid bone f.
    carpometacarpal joint f.
    cartwheel f.
    cervical trochanteric f.
    cervicotrochanteric displaced f.
    Chance vertebral f.
    Chaput f.
    chip f.
    chisel f.
    cleavage f.
    closed f.
    coccyx f.
    Colles f.
    collicular f.
    comminuted f.
    comminuted intrarticular f.
    complete f.
    complex simple f.
    complicated f.
    compound f.
    compression f.
    condylar f.
    f. by contrecoup
    coracoid f.
    cortical f.
    crack f.
    craniofacial dysjunction f.
    "crushed eggshell" f.
    cuneiform f.
    Darrach-Hughston-Milch f.
    Denis Browne sacral f.
    dens f.
    dentate f.
    de Quervain f.
    de Quervain Q f.
    Descot f.
    diacondylar f.
    diametric pelvic f.
    diaphyseal f.
    diastatic f.
    dicondylar f.
    direct f.
    dislocation f.
    distal humeral f.

fracture *(continued)*
    distal radius f.
    distraction of f.
    double f.
    Dupuytren f.
    Duverney f.
    dyscrasic f.
    f. en coin
    f. en rave
    epicondylar avulsion f.
    epiphyseal f.
    epiphyseal growth plate f.
    epiphyseal slip f.
    explosion f.
    extracapsular f.
    facet f.
    fatigue f.
    femoral intertrochanteric f.
    femoral neck f.
    femoral supracondylar f.
    fibular diaphyseal f.
    fissure f.
    fissured f.
    f. fixation
    flexion-burst f.
    fourth carpometacarpal f.
    f. frame
    Gaenslen f.
    Galeazzi f.
    glenoid rim f.
    Gosselin f.
    greenstick f.
    grenade-thrower's f.
    Gustilo-Anderson open clavicular f.
    Hahn-Steinthal f. of capitellum
    hairline f.
    hamate tail f.
    hangman's f.
    head-splitting humeral f.
    hemicondylar f.
    Herbert scaphoid bone f.
    Hermodsson f.
    hickory stick f.
    Hill-Sachs f.
    hip f.
    hockey stick f.
    Hoffa f.

fracture *(continued)*
    Holstein f. of humerus
    hoop stress f.
    horizontal f.
    humeral head–splitting f.
    humeral physeal f.
    humeral supracondylar f.
    Hutchinson f.
    hyperflexion f.
    idiopathic f.
    impacted f.
    impacted articular f.
    implant f.
    incomplete f.
    indirect f.
    inflammatory f.
    insufficiency f.
    intercondylar femoral f.
    internally fixed f.
    interperiosteal f.
    intertrochanteric femoral f.
    intra-articular calcaneal f.
    intra-articular proximal ti-
      bial f.
    intracapsular f.
    intraperiosteal f.
    intrascapular f.
    ipsilateral femoral neck f.
    irreducible f.
    Jefferson f.
    joint f.
    Jones f.
    juxtaarticular f.
    Kapandji f. of radius
    Kocher f.
    Kocher-Lorenz f. of capitel-
      lum
    laminar f.
    lateral column calcaneal f.
    lateral malleolus f.
    laterally displaced f.
    lead pipe f.
    Le Fort fibular f.
    Le Fort f. of the maxilla
      (I–III)
    lesser trochanter f.
    linear f.
    Lisfranc f.
    Liston-Key-Horsley rib f.

fracture *(continued)*
    long bone f.
    longitudinal f.
    loose f.
    Maisonneuve fibular f.
    Malgaigne pelvic f.
    malleolar f.
    mallet f.
    malunited radial f.
    mandibular f.
    march f.
    maxillary f.
    metacarpal neck f.
    metaphyseal tibial f.
    metatarsal f.
    middle tibial shaft f.
    midfacial f.
    midfoot f.
    Moberg-Gedda f.
    Monteggia f.
    Montercaux f.
    Moore f.
    Moore tibial plateau f.
    multilevel f.
    multiple f.
    multipartite f.
    multiray f.
    naviculocapitate f.
    neoplastic f.
    neurogenic f.
    neuropathic f.
    neurotrophic f.
    nightstick f.
    noncontiguous f.
    nondisplaced f.
    nonphyseal f.
    nonrotational f.
    nonrotational burst f.
    f. nonunion
    oblique f.
    obturator avulsion f.
    occipital condyle f.
    occult f.
    odontoid condyle f.
    olecranon f.
    open-book f.
    open-break f.
    os calcis f.

fracture *(continued)*
    Pais f.
    paratrooper f.
    parry f.
    pars interarticularis f.
    patellar sleeve f.
    pathologic f.
    pedicle f.
    pelvic avulsion f.
    pelvic ring f.
    pelvic straddle f.
    penetrating f.
    perforating f.
    periarticular f.
    periprosthetic f.
    peritrochanteric f.
    phalangeal f.
    phalangeal diaphyseal f.
    Piedmont f.
    pilon f.
    plafond f.
    Posadas f.
    Pott f.
    pressure f.
    pronation-abduction f.
    pronation-eversion f.
    pronation–external rotation f.
    proximal femoral f.
    proximal humeral f.
    proximal tibial f.
    Quervain f.
    radial head f.
    radial neck f.
    radial styloid f.
    f. reduction
    resecting f.
    reverse Colles f.
    reverse Monteggia f.
    Rolando f.
    rotation f.
    Ruedi f.
    sacral f.
    sagittal slice f.
    Salter f.
    Salter epiphyseal f.
    Salter-Harris f.
    scaphoid f.
    Schatzker tibial plateau f.

fracture *(continued)*
    f. with scoliosis
    seat belt f.
    secondary f.
    segmental f.
    Segond f.
    shaft f.
    shear f.
    Shepherd f.
    short-oblique f.
    silver fork f.
    simple f.
    Skillern f.
    Smith f.
    spinous process f.
    spiral f.
    splintered f.
    spontaneous f.
    sprain f.
    sprinter's f.
    stellate f.
    Stieda f.
    stress f.
    subcapital f.
    subcutaneous f.
    subperiosteal f.
    supination-adduction f.
    supination-eversion f.
    subtrochanteric f.
    supracondylar f.
    talar neck f.
    tarsal bone f.
    temporal bone f.
    thoracic spine f.
    thoracolumbar burst f.
    tibial condyle f.
    tibial tubercle avulsion f.
    tibiofibular f.
    Tillaux f.
    torsion f.
    torus f.
    transcervical f.
    transcondylar f.
    transhamate f.
    transtriquetral f.
    transverse f.
    trapezium f.
    trimalleolar f.
    triplane f.

fracture *(continued)*
    triquetral f.
    trophic f.
    tuft f.
    ulnar f.
    uncinate process f.
    undisplaced f.
    unicondylar f.
    vertebral body f.
    Volkmann f.
    Wagstaffe f.
    Walther f.
    wedge-compression f.
    "Western boot" in open f.
    willow f.
    Y-T f.

fracture-dislocation
    atlantoaxial f.-d.
    Monteggia f.-d. of ulna
    perilunate f.-d.
    thoracolumbar f.-d.
    tibial plateau f.-d.
    transcapitate f.-d.
    transhamate f.-d.
    transtriquetral f.-d.
    volar plate arthroplasty
      technique for f.-d.

fragilitas
    f. ossium

fragility
    hereditary f. of bone

fragment
    avascular f.
    butterfly fracture f.
    capital f.
    chondral f.

fragmental bone

fragmentation
    endplate f.

Frahur cartilage clamp

fraise

frame
    Ace-Colles fracture f.
    Alexian Brothers over-
      head f.

frame *(continued)*
    Balkan f.
    Böhler fracture f.
    Böhler-Braun f.
    Bradford f.
    DePuy reducing f.
    external fixator f.
    fracture f.
    Hibbs f.
    Ilizarov f.
    Janes f.
    Kessler traction f.
    Mayfield fixation f.
    quadriplegic standing f.
    spinal turning f.
    Stryker fracture f.
    Whitman f.
    Zimmer fracture f.

Framer splint

frank dislocation

frayed meniscus

Frazier-Adson osteoplastic flap
    clamp

Freebody
    F. pin
    F.-Steinmann retractor

Freedom splint

Freer
    F. chisel
    F. elevator-dissector
    F. periosteal elevator

Freiberg
    F. disease
    F. infraction
    F. meniscectomy knife

Frejka
    F. cast
    F. pillow
    F. pillow splint

fremitus

French
    F. adaptor
    F. supracondylar fracture
      operation

Frenkel
F. exercise
F. movements
F. treatment

frenum
Macdowel f.

frequency
high f.
recruitment f.

Friatec manual arthroscopy
system

Friedman bone rongeur

Friedreich
F. ataxia
F. disease
F. foot

Friedrich clamp

Fries score for rheumatoid arthritis

frigotherapy

Frohlich adipogenital dystrophy

Frohse
arcade of F.

Froimson
F. splint
F.-Oh repair

Froment paper sign

frond
synovial f.

Fronet fasciotomy

Froriep induration

frozen hand

Fruehevald splint

FTA
femorotibial angle

Fukuda humeral head retractor

Fukuyama
F. syndrome
F. type congenital muscular
dystrophy

Fulkerson
F. osteotomy
F. procedure

full-radius resector

fulminate

function
adrenergic vagal f.

fungoides
mycosis f.

funiculus
ligamentous f.

funis
f. hippocratis

Funsten supination splint

fusion
Adkins spinal f.
ankle f.
anterior cervical f.
anterior cervical body f.
anterior cervical diskec-
tomy and f. (ACDF)
anterior-inferior f. with SSI
anterior interbody f.
atlantoaxial f.
atlantoccipital f.
Austin chevron osteoto-
my f.
Bailey-Badgley cervical spine f.
bony f.
Brooks-Gallie cervical f.
f. cage
calcaneotibial f.
cervical f.
cervical interbody f.
cervical spinal f.
Charnley compression-type
knee f.
Chuinard-Petersen ankle f.
Cloward anterior spinal f.

fusion *(continued)*

    Copeland-Howard scapulo-
thoracic f.

    Dewar posterior cervical f.

    diaphyseal-epiphyseal f.

    diskectomy with Cloward f.

    extra-articular hip f.

    extra-articular subtalar f.

    facet f.

    Gallie cervical f.

    Gallie subtalar ankle f.

    Glissane ankle f.

    Hall facet f.

    Henry-Geist spinal f.

    Hibbs spinal f.

    hip f.

    hyperostotic bony f.

    interbody f.

    intra-articular hip f.

    intra-articular knee f.

    joint f.

    f. of joint

    Kellogg-Speed lumbar spin-
al f.

    knee f.

    lumbar f.

    lumbar spine f.

    lumbosacral f.

    lunotriquetral f.

    Marcus-Balourdas-Heiple
ankle f.

    metatarsocuneiform joint f.

fusion *(continued)*

    metatarsophalangeal
joint f.

    multilevel f.

    naviculocuneiform f.

    occipitoatlantoaxial f.

    pantalar f.

    posterior cervical f.

    f. protein

    radiolunate f.

    radioscaphoid f.

    scaphocapitate f.

    scapulothoracic f.

    scoliosis spinal f.

    Smith-Petersen sacroiliac
joint f.

    Soren ankle f.

    spinal f.

    Steffee plates and screws
for lumbar f.

    talocalcaneal f.

    talocrural f.

    thoracic facet f.

    tibiofibular f.

    triscaphe f.

    two-stage hip f.

    Watkins f.

    Watson scaphotrapeziotra-
pezoidal f.

    Wiltse bilateral lateral f.

Futuro wrist brace

gabapentin

G-actin

gadolinium

Gaenslen
  G. fracture
  G. osteomyelitis
  G. sign
  G. test

Gaffney joint

Gage sign

Gagnon splint

gait
  adductor lurch g.
  g. analysis
  antalgic g.
  appropulsive g.
  apraxic g.
  astasia-abasia g.
  ataxic g.
  cadence of g.
  calcaneal g.
  calcaneus g.
  choreatic g.
  compensated gluteus me-
    dius g.
  dorsiflexor g.
  double step g.
  drag-to g.
  drop-foot g.
  dystrophic g.
  equine g.
  four-point g.
  free-swinging knee g.
  gastrocnemius-soleus g.
  gluteal g.
  gluteus maximus g.
  gluteus medius g.
  heel g.
  heel-toe g.
  hip extensor g.
  hobbling g.
  hyperextended knee g.
  instability g.

gait *(continued)*
  intermittent double-step g.
  intoeing g.
  listing g.
  lurching g.
  maximus g.
  myopathic g.
  narrow-base g.
  Oppenheim g.
  parkinsonian g.
  pigeon-toeing g.
  g. plate
  propulsion g.
  quadriceps g.
  reeling g.
  retropulsion of g.
  shuffling g.
  steppage g.
  g. and station
  stiff-legged g.
  swaying g.
  swing g.
  swing-through g.
  swing-to g.
  tabetic g.
  tandem g.
  three-point g.
  tiptoe g.
  toeing-in g.
  g. training
  Trendelenburg g.
  Tubersitz g.
  two-point g.
  uncompensated gluteus
    medius g.
  uncoordinated g.
  waddling g.
  wide-based g.

Galante hip prosthesis

Galeazzi
  G. fracture
  G. patellar operation
  G. realignment
  G. sign
  G. test

Galen scoliosis

Gallagher rasp

Gallenaugh plate

Gallie
- G. ankle arthrodesis
- G. atlantoaxial arthrodesis
- G. cervical fusion
- G. subtalar ankle fusion
- G. subtalar fixation
- G. wiring technique

galvanic
- g. electrode stimulator
- g. skin response
- g. stimulation

galvanization

galvanocontractility

galvanotherapy

Galveston
- G. fixation with TSRH crosslink
- G. metacarpal brace
- G. splint

gampsodactyly

ganglia (*plural of* ganglion)

gangliectomy

ganglion *pl.* ganglia
- Acrel g.
- compound g.
- g. cyst
- diffuse g.
- dorsal root g.
- intraosseous g.
- periosteal g.
- primary g.
- simple g.
- wrist g.

ganglionectomy

ganglioneuroma

ganglionic

ganglionostomy

gangrene
- dry g.
- gas g.
- ischemic g.
- Meleney synergistic g.
- periosteal g.
- vascular g.
- wet g.

gangrenous necrosis

Ganley
- G. splint
- G. technique

Gant
- G. hip arthrodesis
- G. osteotomy

Garceau
- G. cheilectomy
- G. tendon technique
- G.-Brahms arthrodesis

Gardner
- G. bone forceps
- G.-Wells tongs

garment
- Jobskin pressure g's

Garré
- G. disease
- G. osteitis
- G. osteomyelitis
- G. sclerosing osteomyelitis

Gartland procedure

gastroc
- gastrocnemius
  - gastroc-soleus contracture

gastrocnemius
- g. equinus
- g.-soleus complex
- g.-soleus junction
- g.-soleus tendon
- g. tendon
- g. tendon transfer

gastrosoleal equinus

Gatellier
  G.-Chastang ankle approach
  G.-Chastang approach
  G.-Chastang incision
  G.-Chastang posterolateral approach

Gaucher disease

gauge
  acetabular g.
  aneroid g.
  bone screw depth g.
  Charnley femoral condyle radius g.
  Charnley socket g.
  Cloward depth g.
  isometric strain g.
  screw depth g.
  spanner g.
  strain g.
  tourniquet g.
  Vernier caliper g.

gauntlet
  Jobst g.

GCS
  Glasgow coma score

Gedda-Moberg incision

Gegenbaur cell

Gelocast cast

Gelpi retractor

genicular
  g. artery
  g. neuralgia

geniculum *pl.* genicula

genu
  g. extrorsum
  idiopathic g. valgum
  g. impressum
  g. introrsum
  g. recurvatum
  g. valgum
  g. varum

genus
  ligamenta cruciata g.

Genutrain
  G. knee brace
  G. PE patellar realignment

Georgiade
  G. fixation device
  G. visor cervical traction
  G. visor halo fixation

Gerard prosthesis

Gerbert osteotomy

Gerdy
  G. fiber
  G. ligament

Gerota capsule

Gerzog bone mallet

Ghon
  G. tubercle
  G.-Sachs complex

Ghormley
  G. arthrodesis
  G. shelf procedure

GIA stapler

Giannestras metatarsal oblique osteotomy

gibbous deformity of the spine

Gibney
  G. boot
  G. disease
  G. perispondylitis
  G. strapping

Gibson
  G. splint
  G.-Piggott osteotomy

Gigli
  G. saw
  G. saw blade
  G. saw osteotomy

Gill
  G. posterior bone block

Gill *(continued)*
  G.-Manning-White spondy-
    lolisthesis
  G.-Stein arthrodesis

Gillette joint orthosis

Gillies
  G. bone graft
  G. pollicization
  G. prosthesis

Gillquist
  G. arthroscopy
  G. suction curet

Gimbernat
  reflex ligament of G.

ginglymoarthrodial

ginglymoid joint

ginglymus

girdle
  Cadenza g.
  g. of lower limb
  pectoral g.
  pelvic g.
  shoulder g.
  g. of upper limb

Girdlestone
  G. operation
  G. resection
  G. resection arthroplasty

Glacier Pack

gladiolus

gladiomanubrial

gland
  haversian g's
  mucilaginous g's
  synovial g's

Glasgow
  G. coma score (GCS)
  G. screw

Glass-Bessen transfixion screw

Gleich osteotomy

G-lengthening of semitendinous
  tendon

glenohumeral
  g. adhesive capsulitis
  g. arthrodesis
  g. joint
  g. joint dislocation
  g. ligaments

glenohumeralia
  ligamenta g.

glenoid
  g. cartilage
  g. cavity
  g. drill guide
  g. fixation screw
  g. fossa of scapula
  g. labrum
  g. ligaments of Cruveilhier
  g. ligament of Macalister
  g.-reaming forceps
  g. rim fracture

glenoplasty

glide
  anterior-inferior g.
  patellar g.

Glissane
  G. ankle fusion
  G. arthrodesis
  G. crucial angle
  G. spike

Glisson sling

Global Fx shoulder fracture system

globule
  Dobie g.

glossodynamometer

glossodynia

glue
  cyanoacrylate g.
  gelatin-resorcin-formalin g.

gluteus
  g. maximus flap

gluteus *(continued)*
    g. maximus gait
    g. maximus muscle
    g. medius gait
    g. medius muscle

gold
    g. salt
    g. sodium thiomalate

Goldmar opponensplasty

gonagra

Goldner
    G. reconstruction
    G. spinal arthrodesis

Goldthwait
    G. brace
    G. sign

Golgi
    G. corpuscle
    G. membrane
    G. tendon organ

gonalgia

gonarthritis

gonarthrocace

gonarthromeningitis

gonarthrosis

gonarthrotomy

gonatocele

goneitis

gonial angle

goniometer
    finger g.
    full-circle g.
    orthopedic g.
    Polk finger g.
    Sedan g.
    universal g.
    Zimmer g.

goniometry

gonitis
    fungous g.

gonitis *(continued)*
    g. tuberculosa

gonocampsis

gonycampsis

gonycrotesis

gonyectyposis

gonyocele

gonyoncus

Gooch splint

gooseneck gouge

Gordon
    G. reflex
    G.-Taylor hindquarter amputation

Gore-Tex
    G. anterior cruciate ligament
    G. knee prosthesis
    G. vascular graft
    G. waterproof cast liner

Gorham disease

Gosselin fracture

Gottron
    G. papule
    G. sign

Gouffon hip pin

gouge
    Abbott g.
    Acufex g.
    arthroplasty g.
    Aufranc g.
    bone g.
    Buch-Gramcko g.
    Capner g.
    Dawson-Yuhl g.
    gooseneck g.
    Hoen g.
    Jewett g.
    Kelley g.
    Killian g.

gouge *(continued)*
     Lexer g.
     Metzenbaum g.
     Meyerding g.
     Moe g.
     oscillating g.
     Partsch g.
     Read g.
     Smith-Petersen curved g.
     Smith-Petersen straight g.
     Stille bone g.
     tendon g.
     Watson-Jones bone g.
     Zielke g.
     Zimmer g.

gout
     abarticular g.
     articular g.
     chalky g.
     chronic tophaceous g.
     idiopathic g.
     irregular g.
     latent stage of g.
     masked g.
     oxalic g.
     polyarticular g.
     primary g.
     regular g.
     secondary g.
     tophaceous g.

gouty
     g. arthritis
     g. diathesis
     g. tophaceous deposit
     g. tophus

Gowers
     G. maneuver
     G. muscular dystrophy
     G. phenomenon
     G. sign
     G. syndrome

Goyrand injury

grabber
     arthroscopic g.

Grace plate 4-hole adaptor

Graf stabilization system

graft
     acetabular augmentation g.
     advancement bone g.
     allogenic bone g.
     allogenous bone g.
     antebrachial fascial g.
     anterior sliding tibial g.
     autochthonous g.
     autogenous g.
     autogenous bone g.
     autogenous fibular g.
     autogenous patellar liga-
          ment g.
     autogenous semitendi-
          nosus-gracilis g.
     autologous g.
     Banks bone g.
     bicortical iliac bone g.
     bifid g.
     BioPolyMeric g.
     bone g.
     bone-to-bone g.
     bone chip g.
     bone marrow g.
     bone peg g.
     bone-tendon-bone g.
     bovine collagen g.
     bridge g.
     cadaver bone g.
     Calcitite g.
     cancellous bone g.
     cancellous morselized
          bone g.
     Chuinard autogenous
          bone g.
     Codivilla bone g.
     cortical bone g.
     corticocancellous bone g.
     Dacron g.
     fascio-fat g.
     femorocrural g.
     fibular onlay-inlay g.
     fibular strut g.
     filleted g.
     g. fixation
     flap g.

graft (continued)
full-thickness skin g.
Gillies bone g.
Gore-Tex vascular g.
H-g.
hamstring g.
Hemashield enhanced g.
hemicondylar g.
hemicylindrical bone g.
heterogenous g.
homogenous g.
homologous g.
iliac crest bone g.
iliac strut bone g.
iliotibial band g.
g. impingement
inlay bone g.
interbody g.
isologous g.
Isotec patellar bone g.
Judet g.
Lee bone g.
McFarland bone g.
McMaster bone g.
Matti-Russe bone g.
medullary bone g.
meniscus g.
Meyers quadratus muscle-pedicle bone g.
Moberg dowel g.
morcellized bone g.
Müller patellar tendon g.
Nicoll cancellous bone g.
nonisometric g.
Ollier-Thiersch skin g.
onlay bone g.
onlay cancellous iliac g.
osseous g.
osteoarticular g.
osteocartilaginous g.
osteochondral g.
osteoperiosteal bone g.
Overto dowel g.
Papineau g.
particulate cancellous bone g.
patellar tendon g.
pedicle bone g.
pedicle fat g.

graft (continued)
percutaneous autogenous dowel bone g.
periosteal g.
peroneus brevis g.
Phemister g.
Phemister onlay bone g.
porcine skin g.
PTFE (polytetrafluoroethylene) g.
Russe bone g.
Ryerson bone g.
segmental tendon g.
semitendinosus g.
semitendinosus-gracilis g.
semitendinous g.
sliding wedge local bone g.
Soto-Hall bone g.
split calvarial bone g.
strut g.
Weiland iliac crest bone g.
Whitecloud-LaRocca fibular strut g.
Wolfe-Kawamoto bone g.
Z-plasty local flap g.

Grafton putty

Graham ankle arthrodesis

granule
Kölliker interstitial g's
Pro Osteon g's

granuloma
Mignon eosinophilic g.
pyogenic g.
rheumatic g's
subungual g.
tubercular g.

grasper
Acufex g.

grasper-cutter
Questus leading edge g.-c.

Graves scapula

gravitational
g. proprioception

Green-Reverdin osteotomy

greenstick
  g. fixation
  g. fracture

Greissinger
  G. foot prosthesis
  G. Multi-Axis joint

grenade-thrower's fracture

Grice-Green extra-articular subtalar arthrodesis

grimace test

grinder
  DePuy calcar g.

grip
  dowel g.
  g. dynamometer
  hook g.
  power g.
  precision g.
  ulnar side g.

Grisel syndrome

Gristina-Webb total shoulder
  arthroplasty

Gritti
  G. amputation
  G. operation
  G.-Stokes amputation

groove
  annular g.
  biceps g.
  bicipital g. of humerus
  costal g.
  deltopectoral g.
  femoral g.
  fibular g.
  intercollicular g.
  intercondylar g.
  interosseous g. of calca-
    neus
  intertubercular g. of hu-
    merus
  lateral bicipital g.
  medial bicipital g.
  musculospiral g.

groove *(continued)*
  obturator g.
  paraglenoid g.'s of hip bone
  parasagittal g.
  patellar g.
  patellofemoral g.
  peroneal g.
  preauricular g.'s of ilium
  radial g.
  radial bicipital g.
  g. for radial nerve
  Sibson g.
  spiral g.
  subclavian g.
  g. for subclavian vein
  subcostal g.
  supra-acetabular g.
  g. for tibialis posticus mus-
    cle
  trochlear g.
  ulnar g.
  ulnar bicipital g.
  g. for ulnar nerve
  vertebral g.

Grosse-Kempf locking nail

Grover
  G. meniscotome
  G. meniscus knife

Groves opponensplasty

growth
  appositional g.

Gruber fossa

guard
  pin g.

Guardian femoral screw

Gudas scarf Z-plasty osteotomy

Guhl distraction

guide
  Accu-Line g.
  acetabular cup peg drill g.
  ACL drill g.
  Acufex tibial g.
  Adapteur multi-functional
    drill g.

guide *(continued)*
    Adson drill g.
    alignment g.
    Bailey-Gigli saw g.
    ball-tipped Kuntscher g.
    barrel g.
    Cloward drill g.
    craniocaudal g.
    Cushing-Gigli saw g.
    distal femoral cutting g.
    Duopress g.
    femoral intermedullary g.
    femoral notch g.
    glenoid drill g.
    humeral cutting g.
    Lebsche saw g.
    Levin drill g.
    notch cutting g.
    patellar reamer g.
    pin g.
    g. pin
    PCA cutting g.
    PCA medullary g.
    Richards angle g.
    Richards drill g.
    Synthes wire g.
    tibial reaming g.
    Ulrich drill g.
    Uslenghi drill g.
    wire and drill g.
    XMB tibial reaming g.
    Yasargil ligature g.

guidepin *(written also* guide pin)
    AO g.
    ball-tip g.

guidepin *(continued)*
    calibrated g.
    nonbeaded g.
    Rica wire g.
    threaded g.
    tibial g.

guidewire
    Suretac drill and g.

Guilford cervical brace

Guilland sign

guillotine
    Charnley femoral inlay g.

Guleke
    G. bone rongeur
    G.-Stookey approach

Gunning splint

gun stock deformity

Gunston arthroplasty

Gustilo
    G.-Anderson open clavicular fracture
    G.-Kyle femoral component

gutta-percha

Guttmann subtalar arthrodesis

Guyon
    G. operation
    G. tunnel release

gymnastics
    Swedish g.

H
    H band

HA
    hydroxyapatite
        HA-coated hip implant

Haacker sling

Haas
    H. osteotomy
    H. paralysis

Haber-Kraft osteotomy

Haddad
    H. metatarsal osteotomy
    H. osteotomy
    H.-Riordan arthrodesis

Hagie
    H. hip pin
    H. sliding nail plate

Hagl lesion

Haglund
    H. deformity
    H. disease
    H. spur

Hagner disease

Hahn
    H. nail
    H.-Steinthal fracture of cap-
        itellum

hairline fracture

half-pin external fixator

Halifax interlaminar clamp

halisteresis
    h. cerea

halisteretic

Hall
    H. air drill
    H. bur
    H. facet fusion
    H. modular acetabular
        reamer system

Hall *(continued)*
    H. Versipower drill
    H. Versipower oscillating
        saw
    H. Versipower reamer

Halle bone curet

hallucal sesamoid

hallucis
    h. brevis
    h. brevis tenodesis
    extensor hallucis
    extensor hallucis brevis
    extensor hallucis longus
    flexor h. brevis (FHB)
    flexor h. longus (FHL)
    h. longus
    h. longus laceration

hallux
    h. adductovalgus
    h. dolorosus
    h. dorsiflexion angle
    dynamic h. varus
    h. extensus
    h. flexus
    idiopathic h. varus
    h. interphalangeal joint ar-
        throdesis
    h. malleus
    h. migration
    h. rigidus
    h. valgus
    h. valgus angle
    h. valgus interphalangeus
        angle
    h. varus

halo
    h. brace
    Perry-Nickel cranial h.

halosteresis

Halsted maneuver

hamartoma
    cartilaginous h.
    fibrous h.
    lipofibromatous h.

hamartomatous lesion

hamate
- h. bone
- h. ligament

Hamilton test

hammer
- Berliner percussion h.
- Küntscher h.

Hammond splint

hamstring
- h. graft
- inner h.
- h. lengthening
- outer h.
- h. release
- h. tendon

hamulus
- h. of hamate bone
- h. ossis hamati

Hancock
- H. amputation
- H. operation

hand
- h. amputation
- ape h.
- h. block
- claw h.
- cleft h.
- club h.
- h. cock-up splint
- dorsum of h.
- flexor retinaculum of h.
- flat h.
- frozen h.
- h. grasp strength
- h.-held dynamometer
- h.-held retractor
- hemiplegic h.
- lobster claw h.
- opera-glass h.
- h. orthosis
- skeleton h.
- trench h.

hand *(continued)*
- Volkmann claw h.

handle
- Bard-Parker h.
- Beaver blade h.
- Charnley brace h.
- Dynagrip blade h.
- Ortho-Grip silicone rubber h.
- traction h.

HandPort

Hand-Schüller-Christian disease

Handy Buck traction

hangman's fracture

Hansen disease

Hanslik patellar prosthesis

Hapset

Hara infiltration block

Hardinge
- H. femoral approach
- H. technique

Hardy aluminum crutch

Harmon
- H. cervical approach
- H. chisel
- H. hip reconstruction

Harms cage

Harpenden
- H. caliper
- H. dynamometer

Harrington
- H. compression rod
- H. distraction instrumentation
- H. rod
- H. rod fixation
- H. spreader
- H. total hip arthroplasty

Harris
- H. anterolateral approach

Harris *(continued)*
  H. broach
  H. condylocephalic nail
  H. Hemi-Arm sling
  H. hip nail
  H. medullary nail
  H. plate
  H.-Beath arthrodesis
  H.-Galante hip replacement
    femoral component

Hartigan foramen

Hartmann
  H. bone rongeur
  H. mosquito forceps

harvesting
  Weiland h.

Hass procedure

Hassmann-Brunn-Neer elbow
  technique

Hauser
  H. ambulation index
  H. bunionectomy
  H. heel cord procedure
  H. patellar realignment
    technique
  H. tendo calcaneus lengthening

Hausted orthopedic bed

haversian
  h. canal
  h. canaliculus
  h. glands
  h. vessel

Hawkeye suture needle

Hawkins
  H. classification of talar
    fracture
  H. impingement sign
  H. sign

Hayes retractor

Haygarth node

H band

head
  anterior h. of rectus femoris muscle
  articular h.
  h. of astragalus
  coronoid h. of pronator
    teres muscle
  deep h. of triceps brachii
    muscle
  deep h. of triceps extensor
    cubiti muscle
  femoral h.
  h. of femur
  h. of fibula
  first metatarsal h.
  first h. of triceps brachii
    muscle
  first h. of triceps extensor
    cubiti muscle
  great h. of adductor hallucis muscle
  great h. of triceps brachii
    muscle
  great h. of triceps extensor
    cubiti muscle
  great h. of triceps femoris
    muscle
  humeral h.
  humeral h. of flexor carpi
    ulnaris muscle
  humeral h. of flexor digitorum sublimis muscle
  humeral h. of pronator
    teres muscle
  humeroulnar h. of flexor
    digitorum superficialis
    muscle
  h. of humerus
  infrared h.
  lateral h. of abductor hallucis
  lateral h. of gastrocnemius
    muscle
  lateral h. of triceps brachii
    muscle
  lateral h. of triceps extensor cubiti muscle

head *(continued)*

little h. of humerus
long h. of adductor hallucis
 muscle
long h. of adductor triceps
 muscle
long h. of biceps brachii
 muscle
long h. of biceps femoris
 muscle
long h. of biceps flexor
 cruris muscle
long h. of biceps flexor
 cubiti muscle
long h. of triceps brachii
 muscle
long h. of triceps extensor
 cubiti muscle
long h. of triceps femoris
 muscle
Matroc femoral h.
medial h. of biceps brachii
 muscle
medial h. of biceps flexor
 cubiti muscle
medial h. of gastrocnemius
 muscle
medial h. of triceps brachii
 muscle
medial h. of triceps extensor cubiti muscle
h. of metacarpal
h. of metatarsal
middle h. of triceps brachii
 muscle
middle h. of triceps extensor cubiti muscle
h. of muscle
oblique h. of adductor hallucis muscle
oblique h. of adductor pollicis muscle
h. of phalanx of hand
h. of phalanx of foot
plantar h. of flexor digitorum pedis longus muscle
posterior h. of rectus femoris muscle
pseudometatarsal h.

head *(continued)*

quadrate h. of flexor digitorum pedis longus muscle
radial h. of flexor digitorum
 sublimis muscle
radial h. of flexor digitorum
 superficialis muscle
radial h. of humerus
h. of radius
reflected h. of rectus femoris muscle
h. of rib
scapular h. of triceps brachii muscle
scapular h. of triceps extensor cubiti muscle
second h. of triceps brachii
 muscle
Series II humeral h.
short h. of biceps brachii
 muscle
short h. of biceps femoris
 muscle
short h. of biceps flexor
 cruris muscle
short h. of biceps flexor
 cubiti muscle
short h. of coracoradialis
 muscle
short h. of triceps brachii
 muscle
short h. of triceps extensor
 cubiti muscle
short h. of triceps femoris
 muscle
straight h. of rectus fe-
 moris muscle
h. of talus
terminal h.
transverse h. of adductor
 hallucis muscle
transverse h. of adductor
 pollicis muscle
h. of ulna
ulnar h. of flexor carpi ulnaris muscle
ulnar h. of pronator teres
 muscle
V40 forged femoral h.

head *(continued)*
    Vitox femoral h.
    Ziramic femoral h.
    Zirconia orthopedic pros-
      thetic h.
    Zyranox femoral h.

Healos

heat
    conductive h.
    convective h.
    conversive h.
    h.-cured acrylic femoral
      head prosthesis
    dry h.
    moist h.
    radiant h.
    h. therapy

heave
    parasternal h.

Heberden
    H. disease
    H. nodes
    H. rheumatism
    H. signs

hebosteotomy

hebotomy

Hebra blade

Heck screw

Hector
    tendon of H.

Hedblom rib retractor

heel
    anterior h.
    h. cord advancement
      (HCA)
    h. cord lengthening
    h. equinus
    h. gait
    gonorrheal h.
    painful h.
    prominent h.
    SACH orthopedic h.
    h. spur
    Thomas h.

heel *(continued)*
    h.-toe gait
    h. valgus
    h. varus

Hegge pin

Hein rongeur

Heiple arthrodesis

Helbing sign

helical compound tomography

helicopod

heliotherapy

hemapophysis

hemarthrosis
    acute traumatic h.
    posttraumatic h.

Hemashield enhanced graft

hemiarthroplasty
    Austin Moore h.
    Bateman h.
    Neer h.
    prosthetic h.
    Smith-Petersen h.

hemicondylar
    h. graft

hemicylindrical bone graft

hemidiaphyseal débridement

hemidystonia

hemiimplant

hemijoint arthroplasty

hemiknee
    Savastano h.

hemilaminectomy knife

hemilaminotomy

hemimelia
    fibular h.

hemiparetic

hemipelvectomy

hemiphalangectomy
Johnson h.

hemiplegia

hemiplegic

hemiprosthesis
single-stemmed silicone h.

hemipulp flap

hemiresection interposition arthroplasty

Hemi-Silastic implant

hemivertebra
balanced h.
congenital h.

hemostat
Surgicel fibrillar h.

Henahan elevator

Hench-Rosenberg syndrome

Hendel guided osteotome

Henderson
cannulated H. reamer
H. clamp approximator
H.-Jones disease

Henle
inferior ligament of neck of
rib of H.
H. ligament
superior tubercle of H.
trapezoid bone of H.

Hennessy knee brace

Henning meniscal retractor

Henry
knot of H.
H.-Geist spinal fusion

Henschke-Mauch saw

Hensen
H. disk
H. line
H. plane

Herbert
H. scaphoid bone fracture
H. scaphoid screw
H. screw fixation

Herczel rib elevator

Herendeen phenomenon

Hermes total knee system

Hermodsson
H. fracture
H. internal rotation
H. tangential view

hernia
Birkett h.
synovial h.

herniated disk

herniation
disk h.
h. of intervertebral disk
h. of nucleus pulposus
painful fat h.
synovial h.

Herzenberg bolt

Hesselbach fascia

Hessing brace

heterogenous graft

heterograft

heterotopic
h. bone
h. ossification

heterotrophic ossification
bridging

Heuter-Volkmann law

Hexcelite splint

hexhead
h. bolt

hex screw

Hey
H. amputation

Hey *(continued)*
- H. internal derangement
- H. operation
- H. saw

Heyman-Herndon epiphysiodesis

H-graft

hiatus
- h. adductorius
- h. finalis sacralis
- h. intermedius lumbosacralis
- h. interosseus
- h. lumbosacralis
- h. sacralis
- h. saphenus
- h. tendineus
- h. totalis sacralis

Hibbs
- H. arthrodesis
- H. bone-cutting forceps
- H. chisel
- H. curved osteotome
- H. frame
- H. metatarsocalcaneal angle
- H. operation
- H. osteotome
- H. retractor
- H. spinal fusion
- H. straight osteotome
- H.-type retractor

hickory stick fracture

high
- h.-speed bur
- h.-torque bur

Hilgenreiner angle

Hill
- reverse H.-Sachs lesion
- H.-Rom orthopedic bed
- H.-Sachs fracture
- H.-Sachs shoulder dislocation
- H.-Sachs shoulder lesion

Hill *(continued)*
- H.-Sachs sign

hilum *pl.,* hila

hilus
- neurovascular h.
- h. of tendon

hindfoot
- h. arthrodesis
- h. excursion
- h. joint complex
- h. orthosis
- spastic varus h.
- h. valgus
- varus h.

hinge
- Adjusta-Wrist h.
- Bahler h.

hinged cylinder splint

hip
- h. abduction
- h. arthroplasty
- h. capsule joint
- h. click
- congenitally dysplastic h. (CDH)
- h. disarticulation
- dysplasia of h.
- h. extensor gait
- h. flexor contracture
- h. joint angle (HJA)
- h.-knee-ankle-foot orthosis
- h. orthosis
- h. reduction
- h. rotation
- snapping h.
- h. spica
- h. subluxation

hippocratic
- h. maneuver
- h. method

HipSaver

Hirayama osteotomy

Hirsch
- H. hypophyseal punch

Hirsch *(continued)*
  H. hypophysis punch forceps

Hirschberg reflex

Hirschhorn compression approach

His-Haas muscle transfer

histogenesis
  distraction h.

Hittenberger halo extension

HJD total knee system

HNA
  hypothalamoneurohypophyseal axis

HNP
  herniated nucleus pulposus

Hock-Bowen cement removal system

hockey stick fracture

Hodgen
  H. apparatus
  H. splint

Hodge plane

Hoen
  H. clamp
  H. forceps
  H. gouge
  H. periosteal elevator
  H. retractor
  H. rongeur
  H. skull plate

Hoffa
  H. disease
  H. fracture
  H. operation
  H.-Lorenz operation

Hoffmann
  H. apex fixation pin
  H. approach
  H. atrophy

Hoffmann *(continued)*
  H. metatarsal arch operation
  H. reflex
  H. syndrome
  H. transfixion pin

Hohmann
  H. osteotomy
  H. retractor

Hoke
  H. Achilles tendon lengthening
  H. Achilles tendon lengthening operation
  H. corset
  H. lumbar brace
  H. osteotome
  H. procedure for tibial palsy
  H. triple arthrodesis

Holden line

holder
  Aesculap head h.
  Ayers needle h.
  Barraquer needle h.
  Böhler-Steinman pin h.
  Cherf leg h.
  leg h.
  OSI arthroscopic leg h.
  Yasargil needle h.

hole
  acetabular seating h.

holorachischisis

Holscher knee retractor

Holstein fracture of humerus

Homans
  H. sign
  H. test

homeopathy

homeostasis
  fluid h.

homogenous graft

homologous graft

hook
    Moe alar h.
    Osher irrigating implant h.
    Tyrell h.

hoop stress fracture

Hoover sign

Hoppenfeld-Deboer approach

hormone
    adrenocorticotropic h.
      (ACTH)

horn
    anterior h.
    bone graft shoe h.
    central h.
    coccygeal h.
    cutaneous h.
    inferior h. of falciform mar-
      gin
    posterior h.
    sacral h.
    superior h. of falciform
      margin

Horner syndrome

Horsley
    H. bone cutter
    H. bone-cutting forceps
    H. bone saw

Horton
    H. disease
    H. syndrome

Horwitz-Adams arthrodesis

hose
    Venosan support h.

Houghton law

housemaid's knee

Howmedica
    H. cement
    H. cerclage
    H. Duracon implant

Howmedica *(continued)*
    H. ICS screw
    H. knee system
    H. microfixation system
    H. microfixation system
      drill bit
    H. microfixation system for-
      ceps
    H. microfixation system
      plate cutter
    H. monotube
    H. monotube external rota-
      tor
    H. total ankle system
    H. Vitallium staple

Howse total hip replacement

Howship lacuna

HPS II total hip prosthesis

HTO
    high tibial osteotomy
      HTO fixator
      HTO wedge

Hubbard
    H. tank
    H.-Nylok bolt

hubbed needle

Huber
    H. opponensplasty
    H. transfer of abductor dig-
      iti quinti

Hudson
    H. chuck adaptor
    H. TLSO brace
    H.-Jones knee cap brace

Hueter
    H. line
    H. sign

Hughston
    H. lateral compartment re-
      construction
    H.-Degenhardt reconstruc-
      tion
    H.-Losee jerk test

humeral
   h. canal
   h. component
   h. cutting guide
   h. epicondyle
   h. epiphysis
   h. head
   h. head of flexor carpi ul-
      naris muscle
   h. head of flexor digitorum
      sublimis muscle
   h. head of pronator teres
      muscle
   h. head–splitting fracture
   h. physeal fracture
   h. reamer
   h. supracondylar fixation
   h. supracondylar fracture
   h.-ulnar angle

humeroradial
   h. articulation
   h. joint

humeroscapular

humerothoracic abduction

humeroulnar
   h. articulation
   h. head of flexor digitorum
      superficialis muscle
   h. joint

humerus pl. humeri
   distal h.
   proximal h.
   semicanal of h.
   h. varus

hump
   dowager's h.

humpback

Humphrey
   inferior tubercle of H.
   superior tubercle of H.

Humphry ligament

Hungerford-Krackow-Kenna
   knee arthroplasty

Hunter
   H. canal
   H. Silastic rod

Hurd bone cutting forceps

Hutchinson fracture

HVA
   hallux valgus angle

Hyalgan

hydrarthrosis
   intermittent h.

HydroBlade

HydroBrush

hydrocele
   h. spinalis

Hydrocollator
   H. pack
   H. pad

hydrocolloid
   h. occlusive dressing

hydromassage table

hydropneumogony

hydrops
   h. articuli

hydrotherapy
   AquaMED dry h.

hydrothermal

hydrothermic

hydroxyapatite
   h. bone replacement mate-
      rial
   calcium h.
   h. crystal

hygroma
   cystic h.
   h. praepatellare

hypalgesia

Hypaque contrast medium

hyperabduction
    h. maneuver

hyperalgesia

hyperchondroplasia

hyperdynamic abductor hallucis

hyperesthesia

hyperesthetic

Hyperex
    H. orthosis
    H. thoracic orthosis

hyperextend

hyperextension
    h. brace
    h. cast
    recurrent h.
    segmental h.

hyperflexion
    h. fracture
    h. trauma

hyperkinesis

hyperkyphoscoliosis
    neuropathic h.

hyperkyphosis

hyperlordosis

hypermobility
    compensatory h.
    joint h.

hyperosteoidosis

hyperostosis
    ankylosing spinal h.
    h. corticalis deformans juvenilis
    h. corticalis generalisata
    flowing h.

hyperostosis *(continued)*
    senile ankylosing h. of spine
    h. syndrome
    h. triangularis ilii

hyperostotic bony fusion

hyperreflexia

hyperspongiosis

hyperthenar

hypertonia

hypertrophic
    h. chrondrocyte
    h. exostosis
    h. granulation tissue
    h. synovitis

hypertrophy
    cartilaginous h.
    ligamentous-muscular h.
    uncinate h.

hypnoanalgesia

hypnoanesthesia

hypocycloidal ankle tomography

hypokyphosis
    thoracic h.

hypophalangism
    pedal h.

hypophysial curet

hypothalamoneurohypophyseal axis (HNA)

hypothenar
    h. eminence
    h. fascia
    h. muscles

hypotonia

hypothesis
    sliding-filament h.

I
  I band
  I disk

iatrogenic

I band

ice massage

ICLH double cup arthroplasty

Ideberg glenoid fracture classification

idiopathic
  i. fracture
  i. genu valgum
  i. hallux varus
  i. scoliosis
  i. skeletal hyperostosis syndrome

I disk

IDK
  internal derangement of the knee

Ikuta clamp approximator

Ilfeld
  I. brace
  I. splint
  I. splint orthosis
  I.-Holder deformity

iliac
  i. apophysis
  i. compression test
  i. crest bone graft
  i. epiphysis
  i. osteocutaneous flap
  i. strut bone graft

iliacus
  i. muscle

iliococcygeus
  i. muscle

iliocostal
  i. muscle

iliofemoral
  i. ligament

iliolumbar
  i. ligament

iliopatellar
  i. ligament

iliopsoas
  i. bursitis
  i. tendon

iliosacral
  i. ligament

iliotibial
  i. band (ITB)
  i. band fasciitis
  i. band graft
  i. band tenodesis
  i. tract

ilium

Ilizarov
  I. ankle arthrodesis
  I. apparatus
  I. corticotomy
  I. distractor
  I. external fixation
  I. frame
  I. leg lengthening
  I. limb lengthening
  I. method
  I. screw
  I. wire

IM
  intermetatarsal
    IM joint

image
  axial multiplanar gradient refocused magnetic resonance i.

Image-I analysis software

imaging
  diagnostic i.

imaging *(continued)*
  magnetic resonance i. (MRI)

imbalance
  isokinetic torque i.

imbricate

imbrication

Immix

immobilization
  cast i.
  joint i.
  sling i.

immobilize

immobilizer
  ankle i.
  knee i.
  shoulder i.
  sternal-occipital-mandibu-lar i. (SOMI)
  Velcro i.
  Velpeau i.
  Velpeau shoulder i.
  Watco knee i.
  Westfield acromioclavicu-lar i.
  Zimmer knee i.

impacted
  i. articular fracture
  i. fracture

impactor
  i.-extractor
  femoral i.
  Smith-Petersen i.

impedence
  bioelectrical i.
  i. plethysmography

impingement
  anterior ankle i.
  anterior cord i.
  i. exostosis
  graft i.
  tibiotalar i.

impingement *(continued)*
  ulnocarpal i.

implant
  AO-ASIF orthopedic i.
  i. arthroplasty
  artificial joint i.
  BAK/Proximity interbody fusion i.
  Bannon-Klein i.
  bicompartmental i.
  Biomet custom i.
  bone i.
  bovine collagen i.
  cartilage i.
  Charnley i.
  chromium-cobalt alloy i.
  condylar i.
  dorsal columella i.
  double-stem i.
  Duracon knee i.
  Durasul Natural-Knee i.
  DynaGraft i.
  Ewald-Walker knee i.
  Hemi-Silastic i.
  Howmedica Duracon i.
  Interpore i.
  McCutchen hip i.
  i. metal
  metal-backed patellar i.
  i. metal prosthesis
  NeuFlex metacarpophalan-geal joint i.
  NexGen knee i.
  Niebauer i.
  patellar surfacing i.
  Pro Osteon 200 i.
  Pro Osteon 200R i.
  Pro Osteon 500 i.
  Pro Osteon 500R i.
  SHIP-Shaw rod hammer-toe i.
  supraspinatus i.
  Surgibone i.
  Surgicel i.
  Swanson carpal scaphoid i.
  titanium i.
  tricompartmental i.
  TSRH i.

implant *(continued)*
  Vitallium i.
  Weber hip i.
  Zeichner i.

implantation
  osteoarticular allograft i.

impressio
  i. ligamenti costoclavicu-
  laris

impression
  basilar i.
  i. of costoclavicular ligament
  deltoid i. of humerus
  rhomboid i. of clavicle

impulse
  efferent nerve i.
  nerve i.

incision
  Burns-Haney i.
  Chang-Miltner i.
  deltoid-splitting i.
  Gatellier-Chastang i.
  Gedda-Moberg i.
  Jergeson i.
  J-shaped skin i.
  L-curved i.
  Loeffler-Ballard i.
  Ober i.
  parathenar i.
  Picot i.
  saber-cut i.
  upright-Y i.
  webspace i.

incisura
  i. acetabularis
  i. acetabuli
  i. clavicularis sterni
  incisurae costales sterni
  i. fibularis tibiae
  i. ischiadica major
  i. ischiadica minor
  i. ischialis major
  i. ischialis minor
  i. jugularis sterni
  i. peronea tibiae

incisura *(continued)*
  i. radialis ulnae
  i. scapulae
  i. scapularis
  i. semilunaris tibiae
  i. semilunaris ulnae
  i. trochlearis ulnae
  i. ulnaris radii
  i. vertebralis inferior
  i. vertebralis superior

incisure
  i. of acetabulum
  i. of calcaneus
  clavicular i. of sternum
  costal i's of sternum
  cotyloid i.
  fibular i. of tibia
  greater i. of ischium
  humeral i. of ulna
  iliac i., lesser
  interclavicular i.
  ischiadic i., greater
  ischiadic i., lesser
  ischial i., greater
  ischial i., lesser
  jugular i. of sternum
  lateral i. of sternum
  lesser i. of ischium
  obturator i. of pubic bone
  patellar i. of femur
  peroneal i. of tibia
  popliteal i.
  radial i. of ulna
  i. of scapula
  scapular i.
  semilunar i.
  semilunar i. of radius
  semilunar i. of scapula
  semilunar i. of sternum
  semilunar i. of sternum, superior
  semilunar i. of tibia
  semilunar i. of ulna
  semilunar i. of ulna, greater
  semilunar i. of ulna, lesser
  sigmoid i. of ulna
  sternal i.
  suprascapular i.

incisure *(continued)*
  i. of talus
  thoracic i.
  trochlear i. of ulna
  ulnar i. of radius
  vertebral i., greater
  vertebral i., inferior
  vertebral i., lesser
  vertebral i., superior

Inclan-Ober procedure

inclination
  i. angle
  pelvic i.
  i. of pelvis

index *pl.* indexes, indices
  acetabular i.
  acromial spur i. (ASI)
  ankle-brachial i. (ABI)
  Arthritis Helplessness I.
    (AHI)
  Barthel i.
  cyst i.
  fatigue i.
  Hauser ambulation i.
  metacarpal i.
  talocalcaneal i.
  Western Ontario and Mc-
    Master University
    Osteoarthritis I.

Indiana Tome system

induration
  Froriep i.

infantile tibia vara (ITV)

infarct
  bone i.

infraction
  Freiberg i.

In-Fast bone screw system

infiltration
  root i.

infection
  anaerobic i.

Infinity femoral component

InFix interbody fusion system

inflammation
  bursal i.

infracalcaneal bursitis

infraclavicular triangle

infraglenoid

infrainguinal

inframalleolar

infrapatellar
  i. bursitis
  i. plica
  i. tendinitis

infraspinous fascia

infundibulum
  crural i.
  i. crurale

Inglis triaxial total elbow arthroplasty

inhibition
  reciprocal i.
  i. test

inhibitor
  cartilage-derived i. (CDI)
  shoulder subluxation i.

injectable collagenase

injury
  acceleration/deceleration i.
  axial loading i.
  contrecoup i.
  degloving i.
  eversion i.
  Goyrand i.
  meniscal i.
  perihamate i.
  peripisiform i.
  sciatic nerve i.
  spinal accessory nerve i.
  supination-inversion i.

inlay bone graft

innervation
    reciprocal i.

innominate
    anterior i.

inochondritis

Innomed curet

inomyositis

inophragma

inostosis

inotropic
    negatively i.
    positively i.

Insall
    I. anterior cruciate liga-
      ment reconstruction
    I.-Salvati ratio

inscriptio
    i. tendinea
    inscriptiones tendineae
      musculi recti abdominis

inscription
    tendinous i.
    tendinous i's of rectus ab-
      dominis muscle

insensate foot

insert
    Osteonics Scorpio i.
    silicone gel socket i.

insertion
    anomalous i.
    cervical screw i.
    oblique screw i.
    pedicle screw i.
    percutaneous pin i.

instability
    anterior cruciate i. with
      pivot shift
    anterolateral-anteromedial
      rotary i.

instability *(continued)*
    anterolateral rotary i.
      (ALRI)
    anteromedial-posterome-
      dial rotary i.
    articular i.
    axial i.
    capitate-lunate i.
    complex i. of carpus
    functional i.
    joint i.
    lunotriquetral i.
    multidirectional i.
    patellar i.
    radiocarpal i.
    scapholunate i.
    subtalar i.
    varus-valgus i.

instrument
    activating adjusting i. (AAI)
    Midas Rex pneumatic i.

instrumentation
    Accu-Line knee i.
    Acufex arthroscopic i.
    anterior distraction i.
    anterior Zielke i.
    Apofix cervical i.
    Arthrotek Ellipticut i.
    Caspar anterior i.
    compression U-rod i.
    Cotrel-Dubousset i.
    Cotrel-Dubousset pedicle
      screw i.
    distraction i.
    Drummond spinal i.
    Dwyer spinal i.
    Harrington distraction i.
    Kaneda anterior spinal i.
    Knodt i.
    Luque semirigid segmental
      spinal i.
    Mayfield i.
    Moss i.
    Putti-Platt i.
    sacral spine modular i.
    segmental spinal i. (SSI)
    Sielke i.
    Smith-Richards i.

instrumentation *(continued)*
  spinal i.
  Steffee spinal i.
  Stryker power i.
  TSRH i.
  Universal i.
  VSP plate i.
  Zielke pedicular i.
  Zielke i. for scoliosis spinal
    fusion

insufficiency
  active i.
  capsular length i.
  ligamentous i.
  muscular i.
  vertebrobasilar i.

In-Tac bone-anchoring system

interarticular
  i. disk

interbody
  i. fusion

intercarpal

intercoccygeal

intercondylar
  i. femoral fracture

intercostal

interdigital

interface
  acetabular prosthetic i.

interfascicular

interferon
  i. gamma-1b

interfragmental compression

interlaminar

intermalleolar

Intermedics
  I. natural hip system
  I. Natural-Knee knee pros-
    thesis

intermetacarpal

intermetatarsal

intermittent paresthesias

interosseous

interpediculate

interpeduncular

interphalangeal (IP)
  i. joint (IPJ)
  i. joint dislocation

Interpore implant

interpositional

interscalene block

Interseal acetabular cup

intersectio *pl.,* intersectiones
  i. tendinea
  intersectiones tendineae
    musculi recti abdominis

intersection
  i. syndrome
  tendinous i.

intersegmental

intersesamoid

intersesamoidal

interspace
  atlantoodontoid i.

interspinal
  i. ligaments

interspinalia

intersternal

interstices
  bone i.

intertrochanteric

interval
  acromiohumeral i. (AHI)
  anterior atlantoodontoid i.
  atlas-dens i.
  deltopectoral i.
  interdischarge i.

interval *(continued)*
    interpeak i.
    interpotential i.
    recruitment i.
    scaphocapitate i.
    trapeziodeltoid i.

intervertebral
    i. disk
    i. foramen

intervolar plate ligament

intorsion

intra-articular
    i. calcaneal fracture
    i. dislocation
    i. knee fusion
    i. proximal tibial fracture

intracapsular

Intracone intramedullary reamer

intracortical

intradiscal

Intraflex
    I. intramedullary pin
    I. intramedullary pin extractor

intraepiphyseal
    i. osteotomy

intrafusal
    i. fiber

intramedullary

intrameniscal

intraosseous

intraosteal

Intrasite dressing

intratendinous

intrathecal

invagination
    basilar i.

invagination *(continued)*
    endplate i.

inventory
    West Haven–Yale Multidimensional Pain I. (WHYMPI)

inversion-eversion

Inyo nail

IP
    interphalangeal

IPJ
    interphalangeal joint

I-plate

ipsilateral

irrigation
    i. and débridement
    Water-Pik i.

irrigator
    Baumrucker clamp i.

irritability
    muscular i.
    myotatic i.
    nerve root i.
    soft tissue i.

ischemia
    brachiocephalic i.
    foot i.
    intracompartmental i.
    myoneural i.
    Volkmann i.

ischial
    i. tuberosity
    i. weight-bearing prosthesis

ischiogluteal
    i. bursa

ischiocapsular
    ischiofemoral ligament

ischiofibular

ischiorectal
    i. fossa

ischiosacral

ischiovertebral

ischium
spine of i.

Iselin disease

ISKD
intramedullary skeletal kinetic distractor

Isobex dynamometer

isokinetic
i. dynamometry
i. exercise
i. knee extension
i. torque imbalance

Isola
I. fixation system
I. spinal implant system
eye rod
I. spinal instrumentation
system
I. vertebral screw
I. wire

isologous graft

IsoMed infusion system

isometric
i. exercise
i. resistance
i. strength testing

Isoprene plastic splint

Isotec patellar bone graft

isotonic
i. contraction
i. exercise

isotropic disk

Isseis-Aussies scoliosis operation

isthmic spondylolisthesis

ITB
iliotibial band

ITV
infantile tibia vara

ithycyphos

ithylordosis

ithyokyphosis

iWalkFree hands-free crutches

Iwashi clamp approximator

J
J disk

J-24 cervical orthosis

J-35 hyperextension brace

J-45 contraflexion brace

J-55 postfusion brace

J-59 Florida brace

Jaboulay
J. amputation
J. operation

Jaccoud
J. arthritis
J. arthroplasty
J. syndrome

JACE W550 CPM wrist device

jacket
Boston soft body j.
cervicothoracic j.
halo traction j.
Kydex body j.
Minerva cervical j.
Orthoplast j.
plaster-of-Paris j.
Risser j.
Virathene j.
von Lackum transection
shift j.

Jackson
J. bone clamp
J. broad-angle staple forceps
J. broad-blade staple forceps
J. compression test
J. intervertebral disk ron-
geur
J. tendon-seizing forceps

Jacobs chuck adaptor

Jacobson
J. bulldog clamp
J. mosquito forceps
J. resonator

Jacoby bunion splint

Jacquet fixator

Jaffe
J.-Capello-Averill hip pros-
thesis
J.-Lichtenstein disease

Jahss
J. ankle dislocation classifi-
cation
J. maneuver
J. metatarsophalangeal
joint dislocation

Jameson muscle clamp

James splint

Jamshidi needle

Janecki
J.-Nelson shoulder girdle
resection
J.-Nelson shoulder opera-
tion

Janes frame

Jannetta duckbill elevator

Jansen
J. bone curet
J. disease
J. metaphyseal dysostosis
J. monopolar forceps

Jansey procedure

Japas osteotomy

Jarell forceps

Jarit
J. cartilage clamp
J. meniscal clamp
J. pin cutter
J. tendon-pulling forceps

jaw claudication

Jeanselme nodules

Jebsen assessment of hand
function

Jefferson fracture

Jelanko splint

Jenet sign

Jergeson
J. incision
J. tapered plate

jerk
Achilles j.
ankle j.
biceps j.
knee j.
patellar j.
quadriceps j.
supinator j.
triceps surae j.

jet
Ortholav j.
J. vac cement dispenser

jeweler's bipolar forceps

Jewett
J. contraflexion brace
J. contraflexion orthosis
J. extractor
J. gouge
J. hyperextension orthosis
J. nail
J. nail overlay plate
J. postfusion brace
J. postfusion orthosis
J. thoracolumbosacral or-
thosis
J.-Benjamin cervical brace
J.-Benjamin cervical ortho-
sis

jig
chamfer cut j.
Charnley tibial onlay j.
cutting j.
drill j.
external alignment com-
pression j.
extramedullary tibial alignment j.
femoral alignment j.
intramedullary alignment j.
Miller-Galante j.

jig (continued)
Osteonics j.
Plexiglas j.
tibial j.

Jobert fossa

Job-Glousman capsular shift
procedure

Jobskin pressure garments

Jobst
J. appliance
J. athrombotic pump
J. brassiere
J. gauntlet
J. prosthesis
J. stockings

Joerns orthopedic bed

Johannson
J. hip nail
J. lag screw
J.-Barrington arthrodesis

Johner-Wruhs tibial fracture
classification

Johns Hopkins bulldog clamp

Johnson
J. hemiphalangectomy
J. medial meniscal suturing
J. pronator advancement

joint
AC j.
acromioclavicular j.
j. activated system
adjusted dynamic j.
amphidiarthrodial j.
ankle j.
anterior sternoclavicular j.
anterior tibiofibular j.
apophyseal j.
j. arthrodesis
arthrodial j.
atavistic tarsometatarsal j.
atlantoaxial j.
atlantooccipital j.
atlantoodontoid j.
ball-and-socket j.

joint *(continued)*
    basal j.
    biaxial j.
    bicondylar j.
    bilocular j.
    bleeder's j.
    calcaneocuboid j.
    calcaneonavicular j.
    Cam Lok knee j.
    capitate-hamate j.
    capitate-lunate j.
    carpal-intercarpal j.
    carpal-metacarpal j.
    carpometacarpal j.
    carpophalangeal j.
    cartilaginous j.
    j. cavitation
    cervical j.
    Charcot j.
    chondrosternal j's
    Chopart midtarsal j.
    Clutton j.
    cochlear j.
    condylar j.
    condyloid j.
    j. congruency
    congruent metatarsophal-
      angeal j.
    coracoclavicular j.
    costochondral j.
    costotransverse j.
    costovertebral j.
    coxofemoral j.
    Cruveilhier j.
    cubital j.
    cubonavicular j.
    cuneiform j.
    cuneocuboid j.
    cuneonavicular j.
    Delrin j.
    diarthrodial j.
    DIP (distal interphalan-
      geal) j.
    j. disarticulation
    j. dislocation
    distal interphalangeal j.
      (DIPJ)
    distal radioulnar j. (DRUJ)
    distal tibiofibular j.

joint *(continued)*
    double-stem silicone lesser
      MP j.
    j. effusion
    ellipsoid j.
    enarthrodial j.
    extraarticular subtalar j.
    facet j.
    false j.
    fibrocartilaginous j.
    fibrous j.
    fifth metatarsophalangeal j.
    Fillauer dorsiflexion assist
      ankle j.
    Fillauer PDC ankle j.
    first metatarsophalangeal j.
    flail j.
    fourth metatarsophalan-
      geal j.
    free knee j.
    Gaffney j.
    ginglymoid j.
    glenohumeral j.
    gliding hinge j.
    Greissinger Multi-Axis j.
    hallux IP (interphalageal) j.
    hamate-lunate j.
    hinge j.
    hip capsule j.
    humeroradial j.
    humeroulnar j.
    hypermobile j.
    IM (intermetatarsal) j.
    intercarpal j.
    intermetacarpal j.
    intermetatarsal j.
    interphalangeal j. (IPJ)
    intertarsal j.
    intervertebral j.
    knee j.
    j. laxity
    Lisfranc j.
    LT (lunotriquetral) j.
    lumbosacral j.
    lunotriquetral j.
    j's of Luschka
    manubriosternal j.
    metacarpocapitate j.
    metacarpocarpal j.
    metacarpohamate j.

joint *(continued)*
  metacarpophalangeal j.
    (MPJ)
  Metasul j.
  metatarsal j.
  metatarsocuboid j.
  metatarsocuneiform j.
  metatarsophalangeal
    (MTP) j.
  metacarpotrapezoid j.
  midcarpal j.
  midfoot j.
  midtarsal j.
  mixed j.
  mortise and tenon j.
  MTP (metatarsophalan-
    geal) j.
  multiaxial j.
  multiple axis knee j.
  naviculocuneiform j.
  neuropathic tarsal-metatar-
    sal j.
  neurotrophic j.
  oblique metatarsocunei-
    form j.
  occipital-axis j.
  occipitoatlantoaxial j.
  occlusal j.
  Otto Bock 3R45 modular
    knee j.
  patellofemoral j.
  pisotriquetral j.
  pivot j.
  proximal interphalangeal
    (PIP) j. (PIPJ)
  proximal tibiofibular j.
  radiocapitellar j.
  radiocarpal j.
  radiohumeral j.
  radiolunate j.
  radioscaphoid j.
  radioscapholunate j.
  radioulnar j.
  Regnauld degeneration of
    MTP (metatarsophalan-
    geal) j.
  sacroiliac j.
  saddle j.
  scaphocapitate j.
  scapholunate j.

joint *(continued)*
  scapulothoracic j.
  sesamoidometatarsal j.
  Silastic j.
  Silastic finger j.
  single-axis ankle j.
  sternoclavicular j.
  subtalar j. (STJ)
  synarthrodial j.
  synovial j.
  talocalcaneal j.
  talocalcaneonavicular j.
  talocrural j.
  talofibular j.
  talonavicular j.
  Tamarack flexure j.
  tarsal j.
  tarsometatarsal j.
  temporomandibular j.
    (TMJ)
  tibiofemoral j.
  tibiofibular j.
  tiobtalar j.
  transverse tarsal j.
  trapeziometacarpal j.
  trapeziotrapezoidal j.
  triscaphe j.
  ulnocarpal j.
  ulnohumeral j.
  Ultraflex dynamic j.
  uncovertebral j.
  von Gies j.
  wrist j.
  xiphisternal j.
  zygapophyseal j.

Jolly reaction

Jonas prosthesis

Jonell
  J. counteraction finger
    splint
  J. thumb splint

Jones
  J. brace
  J. cock-up toe operation
  J. compression pin
  J. first-toe repair
  J. fracture
  J. position

Jones *(continued)*
  J. splint
  J.-Barnes-Lloyd-Roberts
    classification
  J.-Brackett technique
  J.-Ellison ACL (anterior cruciate ligament) reconstruction

Joplin bunionectomy

JOR
  jaw opening reflex

Jordan-Day drill

Joseph splint

J-periosteal elevator

JPS
  joint position sense

J-shaped skin incision

Judet
  J. graft
  J. quadricepsplasty

Juers-Lempert rongeur forceps

jugal suture

junctio
  j. neurocentralis

junction
  atlantooccipital j.
  beaked cervicomedullary j.
  cervicothoracic j.
  craniovertebral j.
  gastrocnemius-soleus j.
  lumbosacral j.
  manubriogladiolar j.
  meniscocapsular j.
  meniscosynovial j.
  metaphyseal-diaphyseal j.
  musculotendinous j.

junction *(continued)*
  myotendinal j.
  neuromuscular j.
  occipitocervical j.
  tarsometatarsal j.
  thoracolumbar j.

junctura *pl.* juncturae
  j. cartilaginea
  juncturae cinguli membri
    inferioris
  juncturae cinguli membri
    superioris
  juncturae cinguli pectoralis
  juncturae cinguli pelvici
  juncturae columnae vertebralis
  j. fibrosa
  j. lumbosacralis
  juncturae membri inferioris
  juncturae membri inferioris
    liberi
  juncturae membri superioris
  juncturae membri superioris liberi
  j. sacrococcygea
  j. synovialis
  juncturae tendinum
  juncturae zygapophyseales

Juvara
  J. foot operation
  J. procedure

juvenilis
  osteochondritis j.

juxta-articular
  j. fracture

juxta-articulation

juxtacortical

juxtacubital reconstruction

Kadian capsule

Kahre-Williger periosteal elevator

Kalish
  K. Duredge wire cutter
  K. osteotomy

Kambin triangular working zone

Kanavel
  K. cock-up splint
  K. sign
  K. triangle

Kaneda
  K. anterior spinal instrumentation
  K. distraction device
  K. rod

Kapandji fracture of radius

Kapel elbow dislocation technique

Kaplan
  K. open reduction
  K.-Meier analysis

Kaposi sarcoma

Kaschin-Beck (*variant of* Kashin-Bek)

Kasdan retractor

Kashin-Bek disease (*spelled also* Kaschin-Beck)

KASS

Kast syndrome

Kaufmann technique

Kawamura
  K. dome osteotomy
  K. pelvic osteotomy

Kawasaki disease

Kazanjian splint

K-Centrum

Kearns-Sayre syndrome

Keck and Kelly osteotomy

Keen sign

Keesay treatment

Kehr sign

Kelikian
  K. foot dressing
  K. modified Z bunionectomy
  K. modified Z osteotomy
  K. nail deformity classification
  K.-McFarland procedure
  K.-Riashi-Gleason patellar tendon repair

Keller
  K. bunionectomy
  K. hallux valgus operation
  modified K. resection arthroplasty
  K. operation
  K. resection arthroplasty
  K.-Blake splint

Kelley gouge

Kellogg
  K.-Speed fusion technique
  K.-Speed lumbar spinal fusion

Kelly-Keck osteotomy

Kelvin body

Kempf-Grosse-Abalo Z-step osteotomy

kenotoxin

keratome
  Automated Disposable K. (ADK)

keratosis
  actinic k.

Kerlix
  K. cast pad

Kerlix *(continued)*
    K. dressing

Kern bone-holding clamp

Kernig sign

Kerpel bone curet

Kerrison
    K. chisel
    K. downbiting rongeur
    flat-bottomed K. rongeur
    K. punch

Kessel plate

Kessler
    K. metacarpal distractor
    K. metacarpal lengthening
    K. posterior tibial tendon
        transfer operation
    K. traction frame

Kevorkian curet

Kickaldy-Willis arthrodesis

Kidner
    K. flatfoot
    K. lesion

Kiel bone

Kienböck
    K. disease
    K. dislocation

Kilian line

Killian gouge

Kiloh-Nevin ocular form of pro-
    gressive muscular dystrophy

kinesalgia

kinesialgia

kinesiatrics

kinesigenic

kinesimeter

kinesiology

kinesiometer

kinesiotherapy

kinesitherapy

kinetic

kinetism

kinetogenic

kinetoscope

King
    K. open reduction
    K.-Moe scoliosis

kinology

kinomometer

Kirk
    K. amputation
    K. distal thigh operation

Kirschner
    K. apparatus
    K. pin fixation
    K. wire (K-wire)
    K. wire cutter
    K. wire pin
    K. wire splint

Kistler force platform

kit
    Fillauer Scottish Rite or-
        thosis k.

Kite
    K. angle
    K. metatarsal cast

Klapp creeping treatment

Kleinert
    K. postoperative traction
        brace
    K. repair
    K. splint
    K.-Kutz bone cutter
    K.-Kutz clamp approxima-
        tor
    K.-Kutz synovectomy ron-
        geur

Kleinert *(continued)*
    K.-Kutz tendon forceps

Klenzak spring brace

Kling adhesive dressing

Klippel-Feil syndrome

kliseometer

Klumpke
    K. palsy
    K. paralysis

kneading massage

knee
    anatomic modular k.
    k.-ankle-foot orthosis
    k. arthrodesis
    k. arthroplasty
    back k.
    beat k.
    k. brace
    Brodie k.
    cadaveric k.
    k. cage brace
    deficient k.
    k. disarticulation
    dislocated k.
    k. extension orthosis
    football k.
    game k.
    housemaid's k.
    k. immobilizer
    k. immobilizer splint
    k. jerk
    k. jerk reflex
    jumper's k.
    knock k.
    locked k.
    neuropathic k.
    k. orthosis
    out k.
    k. prosthesis
    k. rotation
    rugby k.
    septic k.
    k. stability
    trick k.
    valgus k.

knee *(continued)*
    varus k.
    k. valgus-varus

knee brace
    Bauerfeind Comprifix k. b.
    bipivotal hinge k. b.
    Bollinger k. b.
    Centec Propoint k. b.
    DonJoy Gold Point k. b.
    Genutrain k. b.
    Hennessy k. b.
    Korn Cage k. b.
    Lenox Hill derotational k. b.
    Lenox Hill Spectralite k. b.
    Medipedic multicentric
        k. b.
    Neoprene hinged k. b.
    Nextep k. b.
    Omni k. b.
    Os-5/Plus 2 k. b.
    Palumbo k. b.
    ROM k. b.
    k. b. splint
    Tracker k. b.

kneippism

knife
    acetabular k.
    ACL graft k.
    backward-cutting k.
    Ballenger k.
    Bard-Parker k.
    Bircher meniscus k.
    Bovie k.
    Catlin amputating k.
    chondroplasty k.
    DeMarneffe meniscecto-
        my k.
    Down epiphyseal k.
    Downing cartilage k.
    Esmarch plaster k.
    Freiberg meniscectomy k.
    Grover meniscus k.
    hemilaminectomy k.
    Krull acetabular k.
    Langenbeck flap k.
    Langenbeck resection k.
    Liston k.

knife *(continued)*
    Lowe-Breck cartilage k.
    Maltz cartilage k.
    meniscectomy k.
    Midas Rex k.
    Neff meniscus k.
    Salenius meniscus k.
    semilunar cartilage k.
    Smillie cartilage k.
    Smillie meniscal k.
    Smillie-Beaver k.
    Smith cartilage k.
    Stryker cartilage k.
    tenotomy k.
    Weck k.
    Yamada myelotomy k.

Knight brace

knock-knee
    k.-k. brace

Knodt rod

knot
    clove-hitch k.
    k. of Henry
    PDS k.
    Revo k.
    wire k.

knotting forceps

Kocher
    K. elevator
    K. forceps
    K. fracture
    K. maneuver
    K. method
    K. operation
    K. retractor
    K.-Gibson posterolateral
        approach
    K.-Langenbeck approach
    K.-Lorenz fracture of capi-
        tellum
    K.-McFarland hip arthro-
        plasty

Kodel knee sling

Koenig *(see also* König)
    K. metatarsal broach

Koenig *(continued)*
    K. metatarsophalangeal
        joint arthroplasty
    K.-Schaefer medial ap-
        proach

Köhler
    K. bone disease
    K. second disease
    K.-Pellegrini-Stieda disease

koilonychia

Kohnstamm phenomenon

Kölliker
    column of K.
    K. interstitial granules

König *(see also* Koenig)
    K. disease
    K. syndrome

Konstram angle

Korn Cage knee brace

Kotz-Salzer rotationplasty

Krackow point

Krause
    K. line
    K. membrane
    posterior costotransverse
        ligament of K.

Kronner external fixation apparatus

Krukenberg hand reconstruction

Krull acetabular knife

Kuda shaver

Kugelberg
    K. reconstruction
    K.-Welander syndrome

Kühne muscular phenomenon

Kumar spica cast technique

Kümmell
    K. disease
    K. spondylitis

Kümmell *(continued)*
  K.-Verneuil disease
Küntscher
  K. awl
  closed K. nail
  cloverleaf K. nail
  K. extractor
  K. hammer
  K. humeral prosthesis
  K. medullary nailing
  K. nail
  K. nail driver
  K. pin
  K. reamer
  K. traction apparatus
  K. traction device
Kunzel
  nerve of K.
Kussmaul
  K. disease

Kussmaul *(continued)*
  K.-Maier disease

Kutes arthroplasty

K-wire (Kirschner wire)

Kydex body jacket

kyllosis

kyphos

kyphoscoliosis

kyphosis
  adolescent k.
  k. dorsalis juvenilis
  juvenile k.
  sagittal k.
  Scheuermann k.

kyphotic

kyrtorrhachic

labium *pl.* labia
   l. externum cristae iliacae
   l. internum cristae iliacae
   l. laterale lineae asperae femoris
   l. medialis lineae asperae femoris

labrum
   acetabular l.
   anterior glenoid l.
   l. acetabulare
   l. acetabuli
   l. articulare
   l. glenoidale
   l. glenoidale articulationis coxae
   l. glenoidale articulationis humeri

laceration
   burst-type l.
   flexor tendon l.
   hallucis longus l.
   stellate l.

lacertus
   l. fibrosus musculi bicipitis brachii
   l. medius Weitbrechtii
   l. medius Wrisbergii

Lachman
   active L. test
   L. maneuver
   L. sign
   L. test

laciniate ligament

Lacroix
   fibroosseous ring of L.
   fibrous ring of L.
   osseous ring of L.

lacuna
   absorption l.
   bone l.
   cartilage l.
   Howship l.

lacuna *(continued)*
   l. of muscles
   muscular l.
   l. musculorum
   osseous l.
   resorption l.

lag
   interfragmentary l. screw
   l. screw
   l. screw fixation

LaGrange humeral supracondylar fracture classification

Laing
   L. concentric hip cup
   L. plate

Lalonde
   L. bone clamp
   L. bone forceps
   L. hook forceps
   L. tendon approximator

lambdoid suture

Lambert
   L. cosine law
   L.-Lowman chisel

Lambotte
   L. bone-cutting forceps
   L. bone-holding clamp
   L. elevator
   L. osteotome

Lambrinudi
   L. arthrodesis
   L. drop foot operation
   L. osteotomy
   L. splint
   L. technique
   L. triple arthrodesis

lamella *pl.* lamellae
   articular l.
   basic l.
   circumferential l.
   concentric l.
   endosteal l.
   ground l.

lamella *(continued)*
 haversian l.
 intermediate l.
 interstitial l.
 osseous l.
 periosteal l.
 peripheral l.

lamellated bone

lamellation

lamina *pl.* laminae
 l. arcus vertebrae
 cribriform l.
 cribriform l. of transverse
 fascia
 l. elevator
 l. fibrocartilaginea inter-
 pubica
 interpubic l., fibrocartilaginous
 l. prevertebralis fasciae
 cervicalis
 l. superficialis fasciae cervicalis
 l. of vertebra
 l. of vertebral arch

laminaplasty

laminectomy
 cervical spine l.
 multilevel l.
 osteoplastic l.

laminoforaminoplasty

laminoplasty
 Tsudi l.

laminotomy
 l. and diskectomy

Lamisil

Lamis patellar clamp

lamp
 carbon arc l.
 Finsen-Reya l.
 halogen l.
 heat l.

lancinating pain

Landers-Foulks prosthesis

Landouzy
 L. dystrophy
 L.-Dejerine atrophy
 L.-Dejerine dystrophy
 L.-Dejerine muscular dys-
 trophy

Lane
 L. bone-holding forceps
 L. bone screw
 L. periosteal elevator
 L. plates
 L. screwdriver
 L. screw-holding forceps
 L. self-retaining bone hold-
 ing forceps

Lange
 L. Achilles tendon recon-
 struction
 L. bone retractor
 L. hip reduction
 L. tendon lengthening

Langenbeck
 L. amputation
 L. bone saw
 L. flap knife
 L. periosteal elevator
 L. rasp
 L. resection knife
 L. triangle

Langer
 L. axillary arch
 L. muscle

Langoria sign

Lapidus
 L. arthrodesis
 L. bunionectomy
 L. hammertoe technique
 modified L. arthrodesis
 L. operation

LAPOC prosthesis

LaPorte total toe prosthesis

Laron dwarfism

Larrey
  L. amputation
  L. operation

Larsen
  L. disease
  L.-Johansson disease
  L. syndrome

Larson ligament reconstruction

LASE
  laser-assisted spinal endos-
      copy
      LASE probe

Lasègue
  reverse L. test
  L. sign
  L. test

lata
  fascia l.
  tensor fascia l.

Latarjet nerve

latency
  l. of activation
  distal l.
  motor l.
  peak l.
  proximal l.
  residual l.
  terminal l.

lateral
  l. femoral condyle
  l. meniscus

laterolisthesis

lateropulsion

Latranal

Laugier sign

Laurin angle

Lauth ligament

lavage
  Exeter bone l.
  Ortholav jet l.

Lavine reduction

law
  all-or-none l.
  Bowditch l.
  l. of facilitation
  l. of fatigue
  Heuter-Volkmann l.
  Houghton l.
  Lambert cosine l.
  Meyer l.
  Nernst l.
  Ollier l.
  Sherrington l.
  Teevan l.
  Wolff l.

laxity
  ligamentous l.
  radioscapholunate liga-
      ment l.
  l. to varus stress

layer
  capsular l.
  deep l's of cervical fascia
  l's of deep cervical fascia
  Dobie l.
  fibrous l. of articular cap-
      sule
  Floegel l.
  investing l. of cervical fas-
      cia
  investing l. of deep cervical
      fascia
  Ollier l.
  osteogenetic l.
  parietal tendon sheath l.
  superficial l. of cervical fas-
      cia
  superficial l. of deep cervi-
      cal fascia
  superficial investing l. of
      cervical fascia
  synovial l. of articular cap-
      sule

Lazepen-Gamidov anteromedial
  approach

L-curved incision

LE
  lupus erythematosus
    LE cell

Leadbetter
  L. hip manipulation
  L. technique

lead pipe fracture

leakage
  bony slurry l.

LEAP
  Lewis expandable adjust-
    able prosthesis
      LEAP monofilament
        test

Leap chair

Lebsche
  L. rongeur
  L. saw guide
  L. wire saw

LeCocq brace

Le Dentu suture

Lee
  L. bone graft
  L. reconstruction

Le Fort
  Le F. amputation
  Le F. fibular fracture
  Le F. fracture of the maxilla
    (I–III)
  Le F. suture

leg
  badger l.
  baker l.
  bandy l.
  bayonet l.
  bow l.
  l. brace
  l. compartment release
  l. holder
  restless l's

leg *(continued)*
  rider's l.
  scissor l.
  tennis l.

Legg
  L. disease
  L.-Calvé disease
  L.-Calvé-Perthes disease
  L.-Calvé-Perthes syndrome
  L.-Calvé-Waldenström dis-
    ease
  L.-Perthes disease orthosis
  L.-Perthes shoe extension
  L.-Perthes sling

Leibinger titanium plate

Leinbach
  L. olecranon screw
  L. osteotome

Leksell rongeur

Lemmon sternal approximator

Lempert
  L. bone curet
  L. periosteal elevator
  L. rongeur
  L. rongeur forceps

lengthening
  Achilles tendon l.
  aponeurotic l.
  calcaneal l.
  Compere l.
  DeBastiani femoral l.
  distraction l.
  Evans calcaneal l.
  extensor l.
  femoral l.
  gastrocnemius l.
  hamstring l.
  Hauser tendo calcaneus l.
  heel cord l.
  Hoke Achilles tendon l.
  Ilizarov leg l.
  Ilizarov limb l.
  Kessler metacarpal l.
  Lange tendon l.

lengthening *(continued)*
    limb l.
    metacarpal l.
    percutaneous heel cord l.
    sliding-Z l.
    Spencer tendon l.
    subscapularis-capsular l.
    Vulpius-Compere gastroc-
        nemius l.
    Warren White Achilles ten-
        don l.

Lenox Hill
    L. H. derotational knee
        brace
    L. H. knee orthosis
    L. H. Spectralite knee brace

lenticularis
    fasciculus l.

Leone expansion screw

L'Episcopo hip reconstruction

leptodactylous

leptodactyly

Léri
    L. pleonosteosis
    L. sign

Leriche
    L. disease
    L. syndrome

Lerich treatment

Lerman hinge brace

lesion
    anterior labrum perios-
        teum shoulder arthros-
        copic l. (ALPSA)
    articular cartilage l.
    Bankart l.
    Bennett l.
    biceps internal l.
    Brown-Séquard l.
    callosal l.
    cartilaginous l.
    cystic bone l.
    dysarthric l.

lesion *(continued)*
    Essex-Lopresti l.
    fibrous l.
    Hagl l.
    hamartomatous l.
    Hill-Sachs shoulder l.
    impaction l.
    ipsilateral nerve root l.
    juxta-articular l.
    Kidner l.
    labral l.
    lytic l.
    nerve root l.
    occult talar l.
    onionskin l.
    Osgood-Schlatter l.
    osteocartilaginous l.
    osteochondral l.
    Perthes l.
    Perthes-Bankart l.
    retroacetabular l.
    reverse Hill-Sachs l.
    rotator cuff l.
    transient l.
    wire-loop l.
    Wolin meniscoid l.
    Wrisberg l.

Leslie-Ryan anterior axillary ap-
    proach

Letournel
    L. plate
    L.-Joudet approach

Levin drill guide

Levine patellar tendon strap

Levis arm splint

levorotary scoliosis

levoscoliosis

Lewin-Gaenslen test

Lewis expandable adjustable
    prosthesis (LEAP)

Lexer
    L. chisel
    L. gouge

Lexer *(continued)*
  L. osteotome

Leyden
  L.-Möbius muscular dystrophy
  L.-Möbius syndrome

Leydig cylinders

L'hermitte sign

Liddell and Sherrington reflex

Lido isokinetic dynamometer

lift-off
  l.-o. test
  tibial l.-o.
  varus-valgus l.-o.

ligament
  accessory atlantoaxial l.
  accessory collateral l.
  acccessory lateral collateral l.
  accessory l's, palmar
  accessory l's, plantar
  accessory l's, volar
  accessory l. of humerus
  accessory l's of metacarpophalangeal joints
  acromioclavicular l.
  acromiocoracoid l.
  adipose l. of knee (of Cruveilhier)
  alar l's
  alar l's of knee
  annular l.
  annular l., dorsal common
  annular l., inferior
  annular l., internal
  annular l. of ankle, external
  annular l. of ankle, internal
  annular l. of carpus, posterior
  annular l's of digits of foot
  annular l's of digits of hand
  annular l. of femur
  annular l's of fingers
  annular l. of malleolus, external

ligament *(continued)*
  annular l. of malleolus, internal
  anterior pubic l. of Cruveilhier
  annular l. of radius
  annular l. of tarsus, anterior
  annular l's of tendon sheaths of fingers
  annular l's of toes
  annular l. of wrist, dorsal posterior
  anterior cruciate l. (ACL)
  anterior l. of head of fibula
  anterior l. of head of rib
  anterior l. of neck of rib
  anterior l. of radiocarpal joint
  l. of antebrachium (of Weitbrecht)
  l. of apex dentis
  apical l. of dens
  apical dental l.
  arcuate l's
  arcuate l. of knee
  arcuate pubic l.
  arcuate l. of pubis, inferior
  articular l. of vertebrae
  artificial l.
  atlantal transverse l.
  atlantoaxial l.
  atlantooccipital l., anterior
  atlantooccipital l., deep
  atlantooccipital l., lateral
  atlantooccipital l., posterior
  l. augmentation device
  avulsed l.
  avulsion fibular collateral l.
  Barkow l.
  beak l.
  Bellini l.
  Bertin l.
  Bichat l.
  bifurcate l.
  bifurcate l's, deep
  bifurcate l's of Arnold, deep

ligament *(continued)*
    bifurcated l.
    Bigelow l.
    bigeminate l's of Arnold
    l.-bone complex
    Bourgery l.
    brachiocubital l.
    brachioradial l.
    Brodie l.
    l. button
    calcaneoclavicular l.
    calcaneocuboid l.
    calcaneocuboid l., plantar
    calcaneofibular l. (CFL)
    calcaneonavicular l.
    calcaneonavicular l., plantar
    calcaneotibial l.
    Caldani l.
    Campbell l.
    capital l.
    capitular l., volar
    capsular l's
    capsular l., internal
    carpal l., dorsal
    carpal l., radiate
    carpometacarpal l's, anterior
    carpometacarpal l's, dorsal
    carpometacarpal l's, palmar
    carpometacarpal l's, posterior
    carpometacarpal l's, volar
    cervical l., anterior
    cervical l., posterior
    cervical l. of sinus tarsi
    cervicobasilar l.
    CH l.
    check l's of axis
    chondrosternal l., interarticular
    chondroxiphoid l's
    Chrisman-Snook reconstruction of ankle l.
    clavicular l., external capsular
    Cleland l.
    coccygeal l., superior

ligament *(continued)*
    collateral l., anterior
    collateral l., fibular
    collateral l., radial
    collateral l., radial carpal
    collateral l., tibial
    collateral l., ulnar
    collateral l., ulnar carpal
    collateral l. of ankle joint, lateral
    collateral l. of ankle joint, medial
    collateral l. of carpus, radial
    collateral l. of carpus, ulnar
    collateral l's of interphalangeal articulations of foot
    collateral l's of interphalangeal joints of foot
    collateral l's of interphalangeal articulations of hand
    collateral l's of interphalangeal joints of hand
    collateral l's of metacarpophalangeal articulations
    collateral l's of metacarpophalangeal joints
    collateral l's of metatarsophalangeal articulations
    collateral l's of metatarsophalangeal joints
    Colles l.
    common l. of knee (of Weber)
    common l. of wrist joint, deep
    conoid l.
    coracoacromial l.
    coracoclavicular l.
    coracoclavicular l., external
    coracoclavicular l., internal
    coracohumeral l.
    coracoid l. of scapula
    coronary l. of radius
    corporotransverse inferior l.
    corporotransverse superior l.
    costocentral l., anterior

ligament *(continued)*
    costocentral l., interarticular
    costoclavicular l.
    costocoracoid l.
    costosternal l's, radiate
    costotransverse l.
    costotransverse l., anterior
    costotransverse l., lateral
    costotransverse l., posterior
    costotransverse l., superior
    costotransverse l. of Krause, posterior
    costovertebral l.
    costovertebral interosseous l. of Cruveilhier
    costoxiphoid l's
    cotyloid l.
    Cowper l.
    crucial l's of fingers
    crucial l. of foot
    cruciate l. of atlas
    cruciate l's of fingers
    cruciate l's of knee
    cruciate l. of knee, anterior (ACL)
    cruciate l. of knee, posterior
    cruciate l. of leg
    cruciate l's of toes
    cruciform l. of atlas
    crural l.
    Cruveilhier l's
    cubitoradial l.
    cubitoulnar l.
    cuboideometatarsal l's, short
    cuboideonavicular l., dorsal
    cuboideonavicular l., oblique
    cuboideonavicular l., plantar
    cubonavicular l.
    cuboscaphoid l., plantar
    cuneocuboid l., dorsal
    cuneocuboid l., interosseous

ligament *(continued)*
    cuneocuboid l., plantar
    cuneometatarsal l's, interosseous
    cuneonavicular l's, dorsal
    cuneonavicular l's, plantar
    cutaneophalangeal l's
    deltoid l. of ankle
    deltoid l. of ankle joint
    deltoid l. of elbow
    deltotrapezius fascial l.
    Denucé l.
    dorsal l's, carpal
    dorsal l., talonavicular
    dorsal l's of bases of metacarpal bones
    dorsal l's of bases of metatarsal bones
    dorsal l. of radiocarpal joint
    dorsal l's of tarsus
    dorsal l. of wrist
    dural l.
    l. elongation
    external l's of Barkow, plantar
    extra-articular knee l.
    extrinsic l.
    fabellofibular l.
    falciform l.
    fallopian l.
    l. of Fallopius
    fibrous l., anterior
    fibrous l., posterior
    fibular collateral l.
    fibular sesamoidal l.
    fibulocalcaneal l.
    fibulotalocalcaneal l.
    flaval l.
    floating l.
    Flood l.
    FTC l.
    Gerdy l.
    glenohumeral l's
    glenoid l's of Cruveilhier
    glenoid l. of humerus
    glenoid l. of Macalister
    Gore-Tex anterior cruciate l.

ligament *(continued)*

hamate l.
hamatometacarpal l.
l. of head of femoral bone
l. of head of femur
Henle l.
Humphry l.
iliocostal l.
iliofemoral l.
iliolumbar l.
iliopectineal l.
iliopubic l.
iliosacral l., anterior
iliosacral l., interosseous
iliosacral l., long
iliotibial l. of Maissiat
iliotrochanteric l.
inferior l. of neck of rib of Henle
inferior l. of tubercle of rib
inguinal l.
inguinal l., external
inguinal l., internal
inguinal l., reflex
interarticular l.
interarticular l. of articulation of humerus
interarticular l. of head of rib
interarticular l. of hip joint
intercarpal l's, dorsal
intercarpal l's, interosseous
intercarpal l's, palmar
intercarpal l's, volar
interclavicular l.
intercuneiform l's, dorsal
intercuneiform l's, interosseous
intercuneiform l's, plantar
interdigital l.
intermetacarpal l's, anterior proximal
intermetacarpal l., distal
intermetacarpal l's, dorsal
intermetacarpal l's, dorsal transverse
intermetacarpal l's, interosseous

ligament *(continued)*

intermetacarpal l's, palmar
intermetacarpal l's, posterior proximal
intermetacarpal l's, volar transverse
intermetatarsal l., distal plantar
intermetatarsal l's, dorsal proximal
intermetatarsal l's, dorsal transverse
intermetatarsal l's, interosseous
intermetatarsal l's, plantar proximal
intermetatarsal l's, plantar transverse
intermuscular l., fibular
intermuscular l. of arm, external
intermuscular l. of arm, internal
intermuscular l. of arm, lateral
intermuscular l. of arm, medial
intermuscular l. of thigh, external
intermuscular l. of thigh, lateral
intermuscular l. of thigh, medial
internal l. of neck of rib
interosseous l., radioulnar
interosseous l., scapholunate
interosseous l's, transverse metacarpal
interosseous l's of Barkow, internal
interosseous l's of bases of metacarpal bones
interosseous l's of bases of metatarsal bones
interosseous l. of Cruveilhier, costovertebral
interosseous l. of Cruveilhier, transversocostal

ligament *(continued)*

    interosseous l's of knee

    interosseous l. of leg

    interosseous l. of pubis

    interosseous l's of tarsus

    l's of interphalangeal articulations of foot, plantar

    l's of interphalangeal articulations of hand, palmar

    interprocess l.

    interpubic l.

    intersesamoid l.

    interspinal l's

    interspinous l's

    intertarsal l's, dorsal

    intertarsal l's, interosseous

    intertarsal l's, plantar

    intertransverse l's

    intervertebral l.

    intra-articular l. of head of rib

    ischiocapsular l.

    ischiofemoral l.

    ischiosacral l's

    laciniate l.

    laciniate l., external

    lambdoid l.

    lateral l., short

    lateral l. of ankle joint

    lateral l. of carpus, radial

    lateral l. of carpus, ulnar

    lateral l's of joints of fingers

    lateral l's of joints of toes

    lateral l. of knee

    lateral meniscofemoral l.

    lateral l's of metacarpophalangeal joints

    lateral l's of metatarsophalangeal joints

    lateral l. of wrist joint, external

    lateral l. of wrist joint, internal

    Lauth l.

    Lisfranc l.

    longitudinal l., anterior

    longitudinal l., posterior

    lumbocostal l.

ligament *(continued)*

    lumbosacral l.

    lumbotriquetral l.

    l. of Maissiat

    Mauchart l's

    l. of Mayer

    medial l. of ankle

    medial collateral l. (MCL)

    medial l. of elbow joint

    medial l. of wrist

    meniscofemoral l.

    meniscofemoral l., anterior

    meniscofemoral l., posterior

    meniscotibial l.

    metacarpal l., deep transverse

    metacarpal l's, dorsal

    metacarpal l's, interosseous

    metacarpal l's, palmar

    metacarpal l., pisiform

    metacarpal l., superficial transverse

    metacarpoglenoidal l.

    metacarpophalangeal l's, anterior

    metacarpophalangeal l's, palmar

    l's of metacarpophalangeal articulations, palmar

    metacarpotrapezoid l.

    metatarsal l., anterior

    metatarsal l., deep transverse

    metatarsal l's, dorsal

    metatarsal l's, interosseus

    metatarsal l's, interosseous transverse

    metatarsal l's, lateral

    metatarsal l's, lateral proper (of Weber)

    metatarsal l's, lateral (of Weitbrecht)

    metatarsal l's, plantar

    metatarsal l., superficial transverse

    metatarsophalangeal l's, inferior

ligament *(continued)*

l's of metatarsophalangeal articulations, plantar
middle l. of neck of rib
mucous l.
l. of nape
natatory l.
naviculocuneiform l.
navicularicuneiform l's, plantar
nuchal l.
oblique l. of Cooper
oblique l. of forearm
oblique l's of knee
oblique l. of knee, posterior
oblique retinacular l.
oblique l. of scapula
oblique l. of superior radioulnar joint
obturator l., atlantooccipital
obturator l. of atlas
occipitoaxial l.
occipitoodontoid l's
odontoid l., middle
odontoid l's of axis
orbicular l. of radius
palmar l's
palmar l., deep transverse
palmar l. of carpus
palmar l. of radiocarpal joint
patellar l.
patellar l., internal
patellar l., lateral
patellofemoral l.
patellomeniscal l.
patellotibial l.
pelvic l., great posterior
pelvic l., short posterior
petroclinoid l.
pisimetacarpal l.
pisohamate l.
pisometacarpal l.
pisounciform l.
pisouncinate l.
plantar l's
plantar l., long
plantar l., short

ligament *(continued)*

plantar l. of second metatarsal bone
plantar l's of tarsus
popliteal l., arcuate
popliteal l., external
popliteal l., oblique
posterior cruciate l. (PCL)
posterior l. of head of fibula
posterior longitudinal l. (PLL)
posterior oblique l. (POL)
posterior l. of radiocarpal joint
Poupart l.
prismatic l. of Weitbrecht
proper l's of costal cartilages
pubic l., inferior
pubic l., superior
pubic l. of Cowper
pubic l. of Cruveilhier, anterior
pubocapsular l.
pubofemoral l.
quadrate l.
radial l., lateral
radial l. of cubitocarpal articulation
radiate l.
radiate l., lateral
radiate l. of carpus
radiate l. of head of rib
radiate l. of Mayer
radiocapitate l.
radiocarpal l., anterior
radiocarpal l., dorsal
radiocarpal l., palmar
radiocarpal l., volar
radiotriquetral l.
reflex l. of Gimbernat
reinforcing l's
rhomboid l. of clavicle
rhomboid l. of wrist
ring l. of hip joint
Robert l.
round l. of acetabulum
round l. of Cloquet

ligament *(continued)*
    round l. of femur
    round l. of forearm
    sacciform l.
    sacrococcygeal l., anterior
    sacrococcygeal l., deep dorsal
    sacrococcygeal l., deep posterior
    sacrococcygeal l., lateral
    sacrococcygeal l., superficial dorsal
    sacrococcygeal l., superficial posterior
    sacrococcygeal l., ventral
    sacroiliac l., anterior
    sacroiliac l., dorsal
    sacroiliac l., interosseous
    sacroiliac l., long posterior
    sacroiliac l., posterior
    sacroiliac l., short posterior
    sacroiliac l., ventral
    sacrosciatic l., anterior
    sacrosciatic l., great
    sacrosciatic l., internal
    sacrosciatic l., least
    sacrospinal l.
    sacrospinous l.
    sacrotuberal l.
    sacrotuberous l.
    scaphocuneiform l's, plantar
    scapular l.
    l. of Scarpa
    Schlemm l's
    sphenoidal l., external
    sphenoideotarsal l's
    spinal transverse l.
    spinoglenoid l.
    spinosacral l.
    spring l.
    stellate l., anterior
    sternoclavicular l., anterior
    sternoclavicular l., posterior
    sternocostal l's
    sternocostal l., interarticular

ligament *(continued)*
    sternocostal l., intra-articular
    sternocostal l's, radiate
    l. of Struthers
    subflaval l's
    subpubic l.
    superficial l. of carpus
    superior l. of hip
    superior l. of neck of rib, anterior
    superior l. of neck of rib, external
    suprascapular l.
    supraspinal l.
    supraspinous l.
    suspensory l., marsupial
    suspensory l. of axilla
    suspensory l. of axis
    suspensory l. of humerus
    synovial l.
    synovial l. of hip
    talocalcaneal l., interosseous
    talocalcaneal l., lateral
    talocalcaneal l., medial
    l. of talocrural joint, lateral
    talofibular l., anterior
    talofibular l., posterior
    talonavicular l.
    talotibial l., anterior
    talotibial l., posterior
    tarsal l., anterior
    tarsometatarsal l's, dorsal
    tarsometatarsal l's, plantar
    l's of tarsus
    tendinotrochanteric l.
    tibiocalcaneal l.
    tibiocalcanean l.
    tibiofibular l.
    tibiofibular l., anterior
    tibiofibular l., posterior
    tibionavicular l.
    transverse l.
    transverse l. of acetabulum
    transverse l. of atlas
    transverse l. of carpus
    transverse humeral l.
    transverse l. of knee

ligament *(continued)*

    transverse l. of leg

    transverse l. of little head of rib

    transverse l. of scapula, inferior

    transverse l. of scapula, superior

    transverse l. of tibia

    transverse l. of wrist

    transverse l's of wrist, dorsal

    transversocostal l., superior

    transversocostal interosseous l. of Cruveilhier

    trapezoid l.

    triangular l. of abdomen

    triangular l. of pubis, anterior

    triangular l. of scapula

    triangular l. of thigh

    trigeminate l's of Arnold

    triquetral l. of foot

    triquetral l. of scapula

    trochlear l.

    trochlear l's of foot

    trochlear l's of hand

    trochlear l. of little heads of metacarpal bones

    tuberososacral l.

    ulnar l., lateral

    ulnar l. of carpus

    ulnocarpal l.

    ulnocarpal l., palmar

    ulnolunate l.

    ulnotriquetral l.

    vaginal l's of fingers

    l's of vaginal sheaths of fingers

    vaginal l's of toes

    l's of vaginal sheaths of toes

    vertebropleural l.

    l. of Vesalius

    volar l. of carpus, proper

    volar l. of wrist, anterior

    Walther oblique l.

    Weitbrecht l.

ligament *(continued)*

    Winslow l.

    Wrisberg l.

    xiphicostal l's of Macalister

    xiphoid l's

    Y l.

    yellow l's

    zonal l. of thigh

ligamentum

    l. acromioclaviculare

    ligamenta alaria

    ligamenta anularia digitorum manus

    ligamenta anularia digitorum pedis

    l. anulare radii

    l. apicis dentis

    l. apicis dentis epistrophei

    l. atlantooccipitale anterius

    l. atlantooccipitale laterale

    l. bifurcatum

    l. calcaneocuboideum

    l. calcaneocuboideum plantare

    l. calcaneofibulare

    l. calcaneonaviculare

    l. calcaneonaviculare dorsale

    l. calcaneonaviculare plantare

    l. calcaneotibiale

    l. capitis costae intraarticulare

    l. capitis costae radiatum

    l. capitis femoris

    l. capitis fibulae anterius

    l. capitis fibulae posterius

    l. capituli costae radiatum

    ligamenta capituli fibulae

    ligamenta capsularia

    l. carpi dorsale

    l. carpi radiatum

    l. carpi transversum

    l. carpi volare

    ligamenta carpometacarpalia dorsalia

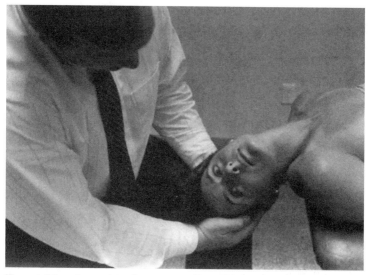
Nonweightbearing vertebral artery test. (From Donatelli, RA, Wooden, MJ: Orthopaedic Physical Therapy, 3rd ed. New York, Churchill Livingstone, 2001.)

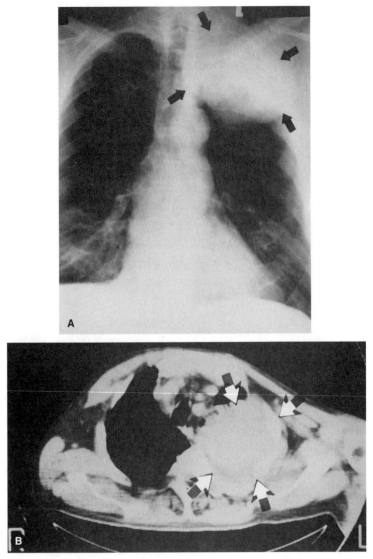

A, Chest radiograph showing Pancoast's tumor *(arrows)*. *B*, Computed tomography scan demonstrating tumor *(arrows)* in the superior pulmonary sulcus. (From Donatelli, RA, Wooden, MJ: Orthopaedic Physical Therapy, 3rd ed. New York, Churchill Livingstone, 2001.)

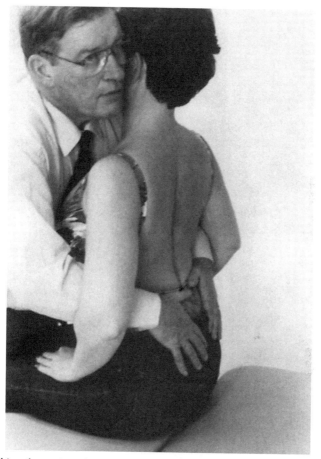

Teaching the patient the proper lumbar lordosis by enhancing an anterior pelvic tilt. An awareness of this tilt is important in learning proper posture. (From Donatelli, RA, Wooden, MJ: Orthopaedic Physical Therapy, 3rd ed. New York, Churchill Livingstone, 2001.)

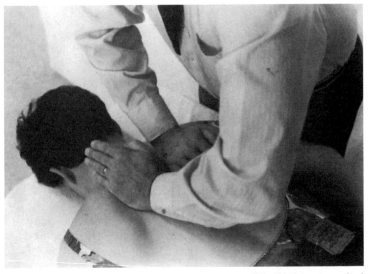

Intervertebral rotatory posteroanterior movements of T1–T4. Force is applied bilaterally through the therapist's hypothenar eminences to the spaces between the spinous processes and the medial borders of the scapulae. A combination of clockwise and counterclockwise movements is applied in a posteroanterior direction. The force may also be directed cephalad, caudad, and laterally. (From Donatelli, RA, Wooden, MJ: Orthopaedic Physical Therapy, 3rd ed. New York, Churchill Livingstone, 2001.)

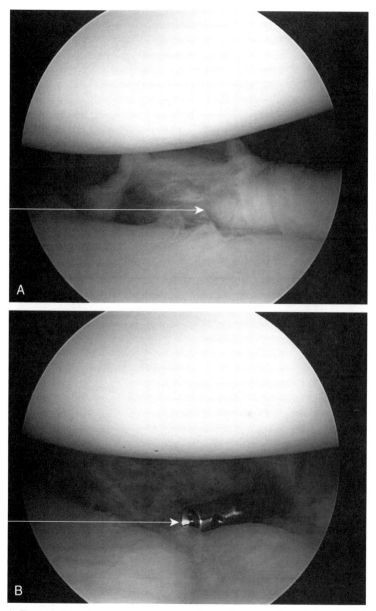

A, Tear of the anterior glenoid labrum. *B*, Surgical resection of the glenoid labrum tear with the holmium laser. (From Donatelli, RA, Wooden, MJ: Orthopaedic Physical Therapy, 3rd ed. New York, Churchill Livingstone, 2001.)

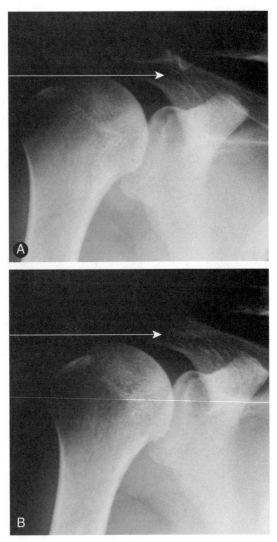

A, Preoperative anteroposterior x-ray of the shoulder with subacromial impingement. *B*, Postoperative anteroposterior x-ray of the shoulder after arthroscopic subacromial decompression and distal clavicle resection. (From Donatelli, RA, Wooden, MJ: Orthopaedic Physical Therapy, 3rd ed. New York, Churchill Livingstone, 2001.)

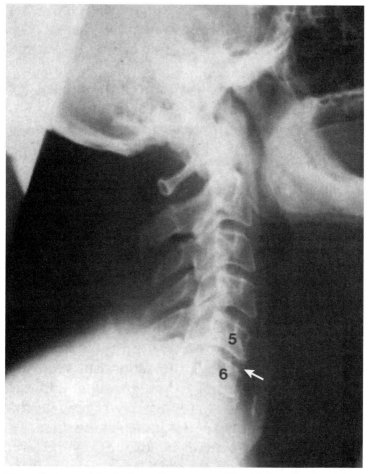

The patient complained of symptoms compatible with lateral epicondylitis. Further interrogation and examination unmasked cervical pathology. The radiograph confirmed C5–C6 degenerative changes *(arrow)*. Although local injection ended the elbow problem, recurrence is likely unless the neck dysfunction is also attended to. (From Donatelli, RA, Wooden, MJ: Orthopaedic Physical Therapy, 3rd ed. New York, Churchill Livingstone, 2001.)

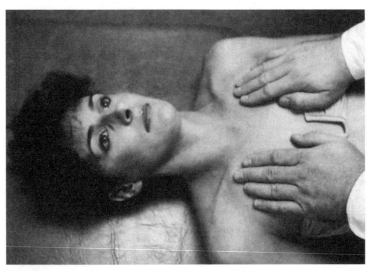

Assessing upper rib cage pump-handle motion. (From Donatelli, RA, Wooden, MJ: Orthopaedic Physical Therapy, 3rd ed. New York, Churchill Livingstone, 2001.)

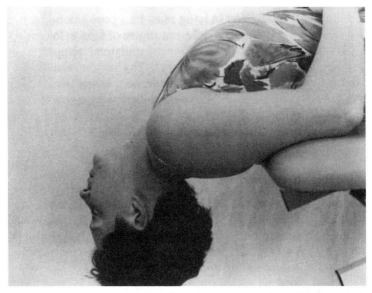

Lower cervical spine extension performed in a lying position. This procedure usually follows retraction in a lying position and usually includes rotations performed at the limit of extension. It is important for the edge of the table to be at the level of T4 to allow for movement in the upper thoracic spine. When returning from extension to neutral position, the patient should lift the head with the hand and not perform the return movement actively. The patient should also rest in the neutral position on the table for about 30 seconds before sitting up. In sitting up, the patient should turn onto one side and sit up sideways to avoid neck flexion instead of sitting straight forward. (From Donatelli, RA, Wooden, MJ: Orthopaedic Physical Therapy, 3rd ed. New York, Churchill Livingstone, 2001.)

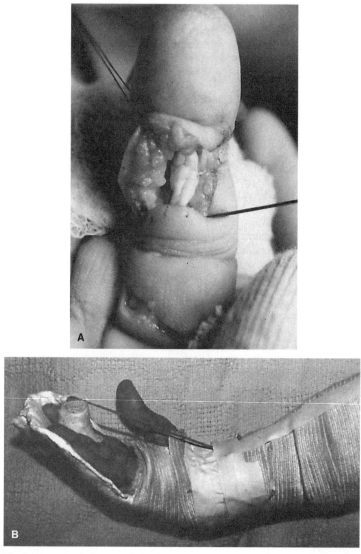

Tendon repair. *A*, Suture of the flexor digitorum profundus after laceration. *B*, Immediate dynamic splinting mobilization for early rehabilitation. (From Donatelli, RA, Wooden, MJ: Orthopaedic Physical Therapy, 3rd ed. New York, Churchill Livingstone, 2001.)

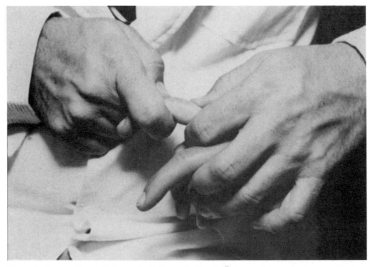

Interphalangeal mediolateral glide and tilt. *Patient position:* supine or sitting. *Contacts:* stabilize the shaft of the proximal humerus; the other hand grasps the medial and lateral aspects of the shaft of the middle phalanx. *Direction of movement:* glide or tilt the middle phalanx in a medial or lateral direction; repeat for all proximal and distal interphalangeal joints. (From Donatelli, RA, Wooden, MJ: Orthopaedic Physical Therapy, 3rd ed. New York, Churchill Livingstone, 2001.)

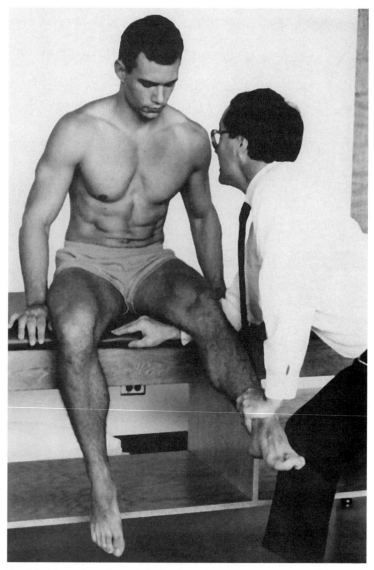

The L3–L4 myotome is evaluated with an isometric contraction of the quadriceps femoris. Care should be taken to make certain that the knee is not locked in full extension. (From Donatelli, RA, Wooden, MJ: Orthopaedic Physical Therapy, 3rd ed. New York, Churchill Livingstone, 2001.)

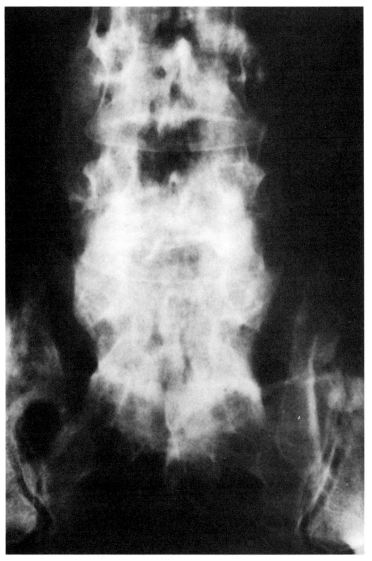

Severe degenerative arthritis of L5 with spinal canal stenosis. The actual canal stenosis is imaged with CT or MRI. (From Donatelli, RA, Wooden, MJ: Orthopaedic Physical Therapy, 3rd ed. New York, Churchill Livingstone, 2001.)

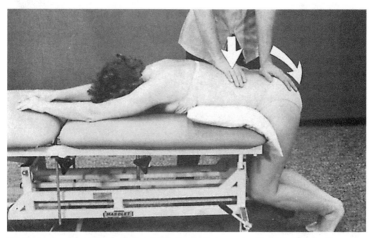

While increasing the flexion of the lumbar spine in the prone position, the therapist stabilizes the T12–L1 segment and presses against the patient's sacrum. Further stretch may be achieved by the therapist pushing downward along the patient's thighs. (From Donatelli, RA, Wooden, MJ: Orthopaedic Physical Therapy, 3rd ed. New York, Churchill Livingstone, 2001.)

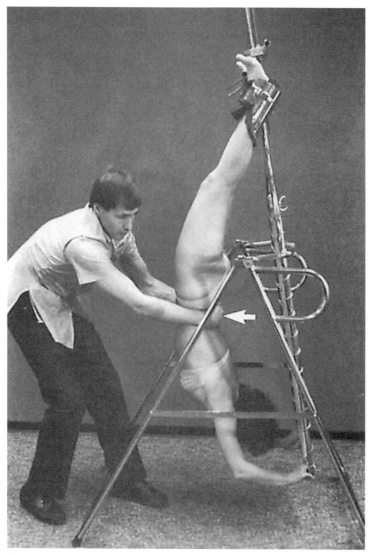

The therapist assists with extension of the lumbar spine with persisting central pain. (From Donatelli, RA, Wooden, MJ: Orthopaedic Physical Therapy, 3rd ed. New York, Churchill Livingstone, 2001.)

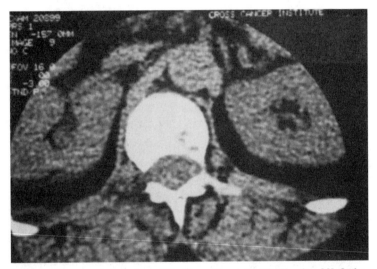

CT scan of a metastatic lesion of L1. (From Donatelli, RA, Wooden, MJ: Orthopaedic Physical Therapy, 3rd ed. New York, Churchill Livingstone, 2001.)

ligamentum *(continued)*
    ligamenta carpometacarpalia palmaria
    ligamenta carpometacarpea dorsalia
    ligamenta carpometacarpea palmaria
    ligamenta collateralia articulationum digitorum manus
    ligamenta collateralia articulationum digitorum pedis
    ligamenta collateralia articulationum interphalangealium manus
    ligamenta collateralia articulationum interphalangealium pedis
    ligamenta collateralia articulationum interphalangearum manus
    ligamenta collateralia articulationum interphalangearum pedis
    ligamenta collateralia articulationum metacarpophalangealium
    ligamenta collateralia articulationum metacarpophalangearum
    ligamenta collateralia articulationum metatarsophalangealium
    ligamenta collateralia articulationum metatarsophalangearum
    l. collaterale carpi radiale
    l. collaterale carpi ulnare
    l. collaterale fibulare
    l. collaterale laterale articulationis talocruralis
    l. collaterale mediale articulationis talocruralis
    l. collaterale radiale
    l. collaterale tibiale
    l. collaterale ulnare
    l. colli costae

ligamentum *(continued)*
    l. conoideum
    l. coracoacromiale
    l. coracoclaviculare
    l. coracohumerale
    l. costoclaviculare
    l. costotransversarium
    l. costotransversarium laterale
    l. costotransversarium superius
    ligamenta costoxiphoidea
    l. cruciatum anterius genus
    l. cruciatum atlantis
    l. cruciatum cruris
    ligamenta cruciata digitorum manus
    ligamenta cruciata digitorum pedis
    ligamenta cruciata genualia
    ligamenta cruciata genus
    l. cruciatum posterius genus
    l. cruciforme atlantis
    l. cuboideonaviculare dorsale
    l. cuboideonaviculare plantare
    l. cuneocuboideum dorsale
    l. cuneocuboideum interosseum
    l. cuneocuboideum plantare
    ligamenta cuneometatarsalia interossea
    ligamenta cuneometatarsea interossea
    ligamenta cuneonavicularia dorsalia
    ligamenta cuneonavicularia plantaria
    l. deltoideum articulationis talocruralis
    l. flavum
    ligamenta extracapsularia
    ligamenta flava
    ligamenta glenohumeralia
    l. iliofemorale
    l. iliolumbale
    l. inguinale
    l. inguinale pouparti
    l. inguinale reflexum

ligamentum *(continued)*
l. inguinale reflexum Collesi
ligamenta intercarpalia dorsalia
ligamenta intercarpalia interossea
ligamenta intercarpalia palmaria
l. interclaviculare
ligamenta intercuneiformia dorsalia
ligamenta intercuneiformia interossea
ligamenta intercuneiformia plantaria
ligamenta interspinalia
ligamenta intertransversaria
ligamenta intracapsularia
l. ischiocapsulare
l. ischiofemorale
l. laciniatum
l. laterale articulationis talocruralis
l. longitudinale anterius
l. longitudinale posterius
l. lumbocostale
l. malleoli lateralis anterius
l. malleoli lateralis posterius
l. mediale articulationis talocruralis
l. meniscofemorale anterius
l. meniscofemorale posterius
ligamenta metacarpalia dorsalia
ligamenta metacarpalia interossea
ligamenta metacarpalia palmaria
l. metacarpale transversum profundum
l. metacarpale transversum superficiale
ligamenta metacarpea dorsalia

ligamentum *(continued)*
ligamenta metacarpea interossea
ligamenta metacarpea palmaria
l. metacarpeum transversum profundum
l. metacarpeum transversum superficiale
ligamenta metatarsalia dorsalia
ligamenta metatarsalia interossea
ligamenta metatarsalia plantaria
l. metatarsale transversum profundum
l. metatarsale transversum superficiale
ligamenta metatarsea dorsalia
ligamenta metatarsea interossea
ligamenta metatarsea plantaria
l. metatarseum transversum profundum
l. metatarseum transversum superficiale
l. mucosum
ligamenta navicularicuneiformia dorsalia
ligamenta navicularicuneiformia plantaria
l. nuchae
ligamenta palmaria articulationum interphalangealium manus
ligamenta palmaria articulationum interphalangearum manus
ligamenta palmaria articulationum metacarpophalangealium
ligamenta palmaria articulationum metacarpophalangearum
l. patellae

ligamentum *(continued)*
l. pisohamatum
l. pisometacarpeum
ligamenta plantaria articulationum interphalangealium pedis
ligamenta plantaria articulationum interphalangearum pedis
ligamenta plantaria articulationum metatarsophalangealium
ligamenta plantaria articulationum metatarsophalangearum
l. plantare longum
l. popliteum arcuatum
l. popliteum obliquum
l. pubicum inferius
l. pubicum superius
l. pubocapsulare
l. pubofemorale
l. quadratum
l. radiocarpale dorsale
l. radiocarpale palmare
l. radiocarpeum dorsale
l. radiocarpeum palmare
l. sacrococcygeum anterius
l. sacrococcygeum dorsale profundum
l. sacrococcygeum dorsale superficiale
l. sacrococcygeum laterale
l. sacrococcygeum posterius profundum
l. sacrococcygeum posterius superficiale
l. sacrococcygeum ventrale
l. sacroiliacum anterius
l. sacroiliacum dorsalis
l. sacroiliacum interosseum
l. sacroiliacum posterius
l. sacroiliacum ventralis
l. sacrospinale
l. sacrospinosum
l. sacrotuberale
l. sacrotuberosum
l. sternoclaviculare

ligamentum *(continued)*
l. sternoclaviculare anterius
l. sternoclaviculare posterius
l. sternocostale interarticulare
l. sternocostale intraarticulare
ligamenta sternocostalia radiata
l. supraspinale
l. talocalcaneare interosseum
l. talocalcaneare laterale
l. talocalcaneare mediale
l. talocalcaneum interosseum
l. talocalcaneum laterale
l. talocalcaneum mediale
l. talofibulare anterius
l. talofibulare posterius
l. talonaviculare
l. talonaviculare [dorsale]
l. talotibiale anterius
l. talotibiale posterius
ligamenta tarsi
ligamenta tarsi dorsalia
ligamenta tarsi interossea
ligamenta tarsi plantaria
ligamenta tarsometatarsalia dorsalia
ligamenta tarsometatarsalia plantaria
ligamenta tarsometatarsea dorsalia
ligamenta tarsometatarsea plantaria
l. teres femoris
l. tibiofibulare anterius
l. tibiofibulare posterius
l. tibionaviculare
l. transversum
l. transversum acetabuli
l. transversum atlantis
l. transversum cruris
l. transversum genuale
l. transversum genus

ligamentum *(continued)*
    l. transversum scapulae inferius
    l. transversum scapulae superius
    l. trapezoideum
    l. tuberculi costae
    l. ulnocarpale palmare
    l. ulnocarpeum palmare
    ligamenta vaginalia digitorum manus
    ligamenta vaginalia digitorum pedis

Ligamentus ankle orthosis

ligature carrier
    Cave-Rowe l. c.

limb
    artificial l.
    ischemic l.
    lower l.
    lower l., free
    plantigrade l.
    upper l.
    upper l., free
    Utah artificial l.

Limberg flap

limbus
    l. acetabuli
    l. annularis

limp
    Trendelenburg l.

LINAC
    linear accelerator
        Boston LINAC

Lindeman procedure

Linder sign

Lindgren oblique osteotomy

Lindholm tendo calcaneus repair

line
    l. of Amici
    anterior axillary l.

line *(continued)*
    anterior gluteal l.
    anterior humeral l.
    anterior intertrochanteric l.
    arcuate l. of ilium
    arcuate l. of pelvis
    Beau l.
    Blumensaat l.
    Brücke l's
    Bryant l.
    cement l.
    coronoid l.
    costoarticular l.
    curved l. of ilium
    l. of demarcation
    Dobie l.
    Duhot l.
    epiphyseal l.
    Feiss l.
    femoral head l.
    fracture l.
    gravitational l.
    Hensen l.
    Holden l.
    Hueter l.
    iliopectineal l.
    inferior curved l. of ilium
    inferior gluteal l.
    intercondylar l.
    intercondyloid l.
    intertrochanteric l.
    Kilian l.
    Krause l.
    lateral supracondylar l.
    medial supracondylar l.
    Meyer l.
    midaxillary l.
    middle curved l. of ilium
    midmalleolar l.
    midspinal l.
    midsternal l.
    muscular l's of scapula
    oblique l. of femur
    oblique l. of fibula
    oblique l. of tibia
    pectineal l.
    popliteal l. of femur
    popliteal l. of tibia

line *(continued)*
>   posterior axillary l. (PAL)
>   posterior gluteal l.
>   posterior intertrochanter-
>   ic l.
>   quadrate l.
>   radiocapitellar l.
>   rough l.
>   sacral arcuate l.
>   sacral horizontal plane l.
>   sesamoid ligament
>   sesamophalangeal ligament
>   soleal l. of tibia
>   spiral l. of femur
>   subscapular l's
>   superior curved l. of ilium
>   terminal l. of pelvis
>   transverse l's of sacral
>   bone
>   transverse l's of sacrum
>   trapezoid l.
>   Trümmerfeld l.
>   Ullmann l.
>   Wagner l.
>   white l. of pelvic fascia
>   Z l.
>   l's of Zahn

linea
>   l. arcuata ossis ilii
>   l. aspera
>   l. aspera femoris
>   l. epiphysialis
>   l. glutea anterior
>   l. glutea inferior
>   l. glutealis anterior
>   l. glutealis inferior
>   l. glutealis posterior
>   l. glutea posterior
>   l. iliopectinea
>   l. innominata
>   l. intercondylaris
>   l. intercondyloidea
>   l. intertrochanterica
>   l. intertrochanterica poste-
>   rior
>   lineae musculares scapulae
>   l. musculi solei

linea *(continued)*
>   l. obliqua fibulae
>   l. obliqua tibiae
>   l. pectinea
>   l. poplitea tibiae
>   l. spiralis
>   l. supracondylaris lateralis
>   l. supracondylaris medialis
>   l. terminalis pelvis
>   lineae transversae ossis
>   sacri
>   l. trapezoidea

linear accelerator *(see* LINAC)

liner
>   acetabular prosthetic l.
>   elevated rim acetabular l.
>   Enduron acetabular l.
>   Gore-Tex waterproof cast l.

lip
>   acetabular l.
>   articular l.
>   external l. of iliac crest
>   external l. of linea aspera
>   of femur
>   fibrocartilaginous l. of ace-
>   tabulum
>   glenoid l.
>   glenoid l. of articulation of
>   hip
>   glenoid l. of articulation of
>   humerus
>   internal l. of iliac crest
>   lateral l. of linea aspera of
>   femur
>   medial l. of linea aspera of
>   femur
>   osteophytic bone l.

lipoarthritis

lipohemarthrosis

lipoma
>   l. arborescens
>   intermuscular l.
>   intramuscular l.
>   intraosseous l.
>   pleomorphic l.

Lippman hip prosthesis

Liprostin

Lipscomb modified McKeever arthrodesis

Lisch nodule

Lisfranc
  L. amputation
  L. arthrodesis
  L. articular set angle
  L. disarticulation
  L. dislocation
  L. fracture
  L. joint complex
  L. joint
  L. ligament
  L. operation
  L. tubercle

Lister tubercle

listhesis
  anterior-inferior l.
  anterior-posterior l.
  lateral l.

Liston
  L. knife
  L. splint
  L.-Key-Horsley rib fracture
  L.-Littauer rongeur

Little League elbow

Littler
  L. opponensplasty
  wing excision of L.

Livingston intramedullary bar

Lloyd
  L. adaptor
  L. adaptor for Smith-Petersen nail
  L.-Roberts-Swann trochanteric advancement

LMB finger splint

L'Nard Multi-Podus orthosis

load
  spinal axial l.

loading
  axial l.
  compression l.
  concentric l.
  sustained l.
  vertical l.

Lobstein
  L. disease
  L. syndrome

lobster claw hand

localization
  pedicle l.

localized nodular synovitis

locator
  Berman-Moorehead metal l.

Locke
  L. bone clamp
  L. elevator

Lodine

Loeffler-Ballard incision

Lofstrand crutch

Logan traction

loge
  l. de Guyon

logrolling maneuver

longus

Looser-Milkman syndrome

lordoscoliosis

lordosis
  cervical l.
  lumbar spine l.
  occipitocervical l.
  thoracic spine l.

lordotic curve

Lorenz
  L. brace
  L. cast
  L. operation
  L. osteotomy

Lorenz *(continued)*
  L. sign

Lorenzo screw

Lottes pin

loupe
  l. magnification

Love-Kerrison rongeur forceps

Lovitt-Uhler modification of
  Jewett postfusion brace

Lowe-Breck cartilage knife

loxarthron

loxarthrosis

loxia

loxotomy

LPPS
  low-pressure plasma spray
    LPPS hydroxyapatite
      fixation

LSI Easy Stims self-adhesive
  electrode

LT
  lunotriquetral
    lunotriquetral joint

Lubinus acetabular component

Lucae bone mallet

Lucas
  L. chisel
  L.-Cottrell osteotomy

Luck-Bishop bone saw

Ludington sign

Ludloff
  L. medial approach
  L. sign

Ludwig plane

Luer bone rongeur

Luft disease

Luhr
  L. miniplate

Luhr *(continued)*
  L. screw

lumbago
  ischemic l.
  l.–mechanical instability
    syndrome

lumbar
  l. fusion
  l. spine
  l. spine fusion

lumbodynia

lumbosacral
  l. fusion

lumbrical
  l. instrinsic contraction
  l. muscle
  l. tendon

lunate
  l. bone
  l. dislocation
  l.-triquetral coalition

lunatomalacia

lunocapitate bone

lunotriquetral (LT)
  l. fusion
  l. joint

lunula *pl.* lunulae
  l. of scapula

Luongo hand retractor

lupus
  drug-induced l.
  l. erythematosus (LE)
  l. erythematosus, cutane-
    ous
  l. erythematosus, discoid
  l. erythematosus, hyper-
    trophic
  l. erythematosus, systemic
  l. erythematosus, systemic,
    ANA-negative
  l. erythematosus, systemic,
    transient neonatal
  l. erythematosus profundus

lupus *(continued)*
    l. erythematosus tumidus
    neonatal l.
    l. profundus

Luque
    L. cerclage wire
    L. loop fixation
    L. pedicle screw
    L. II plate
    L. rod
    L. rod bender
    L. semirigid segmental spi-
      nal instrumentation
    L. wiring

Luschka
    joints of L.

Lutz-Jeanselme nodules

luxatio
    l. coxae congenita
    l. erecta
    l. imperfecta
    l. perinealis

luxation
    atlantoaxial l.
    incomplete l.
    ligamentous l.
    Malgaigne l.
    palmar l.

Lynco foot orthosis

Lyser
    trapezoid bone of L.

lytic bone lesion

M
M band
M disk

Ma
M.-Griffith ruptured Achilles tendon repair
M.-Griffith tendo calcaneus repair

mA
milliampere

McAfee approach

Macalister
glenoid ligament of M.
xiphicostal ligaments of M.

McAtee-Tharias-Blazina arthroplasty

MacAusland lumbar brace

McBride
M. bunionectomy
M. hallux abductovalgus reduction
M. hallux valgus reduction
modified M. bunionectomy
M. operation
M. plate
M.-Moore prosthesis

McCain
M. TMJ cannula
M. TMJ curet

MAC cervical collar

McConnell extensile approach

McCullough retractor

McCune-Albright syndrome

McCutchen hip implant

Macdowel frenum

maceration

Macewen
M. sign
M.-Shands osteotomy

McFarland
M. bone graft
M. technique
M.-Osborne lateral approach

McGee splint

McGehee elbow prosthesis

McGlamry elevator

McIndoe
M. bone rongeur
M. rongeur forceps

McIntire splint

McKee brace

McKee
M. brace
M.-Farrar total hip arthroplasty

McKeever
Lipscomb modified M. arthrodesis
M. metatarsophalangeal arthrodesis
M.-Buck elbow technique
M.-Buck fragment excision
M.-MacIntosh tibial plateau prosthesis

MacKenzie amputation

McKenzie extension exercise

MacKinnon modification
macrobrachia

McKittrick transmetatarsal amputation

McLaughlin
M. acromioplasty
M. carpal scaphoid screw
M. osteosynthesis apparatus

MacLean-Maxwell disease

McLeod padded clavicular splint

McMaster bone graft

McMurray
    M. maneuver for torn knee
      cartilage
    M. sign
    M. test

MacNab
    M. operation
    M. shoulder repair

macrocheiria

macrochiria

macrodactyly

Macrofit hip prosthesis

macronychia

McShane-Leinberry-Fenlin acromioplasty

McWhorter posterior shoulder approach

Madelung
    M. deformity
    M. disease

Maffucci syndrome

MAFO
    molded ankle-foot orthosis

Magerl posterior cervical screw fixation

magnetic resonance imaging (MRI)

magnification
    loupe m.

Magnuson
    M. abduction humeral
      splint
    M. wire
    M.-Stack shoulder arthrotomy

main
    m. en crochet

main *(continued)*
    m. en griffe
    m. en lorgnette
    m. en singe
    m. en squelette

Maisonneuve
    M. amputation
    M. fibular fracture
    M. sign

Maissiat
    M. band
    iliotibial ligament of M.
    ligament of M.
    M. tract

malacia
    metaplastic m.
    myeloplastic m.

malacosteon

malalignment
    radial m.
    rotational m.
    varus m.

Malcolm-Lynn spinal retraction system

malformation
    Arnold-Chiari m.

Malgaigne
    M. amputation
    M. luxation
    M. pelvic fracture

Malibu cervical orthosis

Malis
    M. curet
    M. elevator
    M. jeweler bipolar forceps

malleolar
    m. fracture
    m. osteotomy
    m. screw

malleolus *pl.* malleoli
    external m.
    m. externus
    m. fibulae

malleolus *(continued)*
  fibular m.
  inner m.
  internal m.
  m. internus
  m. lateralis
  m. medialis
  outer m.
  radial m.
  m. radialis
  m. tibiae
  tibial m.
  ulnar m.
  m. ulnaris

Malleotec ankle orthosis

mallet
  Bergman m.
  Doyen bone m.
  m. fracture
  Gerzog bone m.
  Ombrédanne m.
  Steinbach m.
  Wolfe-Böhler m.

Mallory
  M.-Head hip prosthesis
  M.-Head modular calcar
    system

malposed vertebra

malrotation

maltracking patella

Maltz cartilage knife

malum
  m. coxae senilis
  m. vertebrale suboccipitale

malunion
  angulatory m.
  calcaneal m.
  femoral shaft m.
  humeral fracture m.
  talar m.
  varus m.

Mandelbaum-Nartolozzi-Carney
  patellar tendon repair

mandibular
  m. angle
  m. fracture
  m. osteotomy

maneuver
  Adson m.
  Allen m.
  Allis m.
  Barlow m.
  Bárány-Nylen m.
  circumduction m.
  closed manipulative m.
  costoclavicular m.
  Dix-Hallpike m.
  Finkelstein m.
  Gowers m.
  Halsted m.
  hippocratic m.
  hyperabduction m.
  Jahss m.
  Kocher m.
  Lachman m.
  logrolling m.
  McMurray m. for torn knee
    cartilage
  Meyn-Quigley m.
  military m.
  Ortolani m.
  Phalen m.
  rotation-compression m.
  scalene m.
  Slocum m.
  Soto-Hall m.
  Spurling m.
  Valsalva m.

manipulation
  Leadbetter hip m.

Mankin resection

Manktelow pectoralis major
  transfer

Mann
  M. modified McKeever ar-
    throdesis
  M.-Coughlin-DuVries chei-
    lectomy
  M.-DuVries arthroplasty

Mann *(continued)*
  M.-Whitney analysis

Manske-McCarroll oppo-
  nensplasty

manubrium
  m. sterni
  m. of sternum

Manuflex external fixator

manus
  m. cava
  m. extensa
  m. flexa
  m. plana
  m. superextensa
  m. valga
  m. vara

Maquet
  M. advancement
  M. anteromedial osteo-
    plasty
  M. dome osteotomy
  M. procedure
  M. table extension

marche à petits pas

march fracture

Marcus
  M.-Balourdas-Heiple ankle
    fusion
  M.-Balourdas-Heiple trans-
    malleolar arthrodesis

margin
  m. of acetabulum
  anterior m. of fibula
  anterior m. of radius
  anterior m. of scapula
  anterior m. of tibia
  anterior m. of ulna
  axillary m. of scapula
  cartilaginous m. of acetabu-
    lum
  dorsal m. of radius
  dorsal m. of ulna
  external m. of scapula
  falciform m. of white line of
    pelvic fascia

margin *(continued)*
  fibular m. of foot
  interosseous m. of fibula
  interosseous m. of radius
  interosseous m. of tibia
  interosseous m. of ulna
  lateral m. of foot
  lateral m. of humerus
  lateral m. of scapula
  medial m. of foot
  medial m. of humerus
  medial m. of scapula
  medial m. of tibia
  peroneal m. of foot
  posterior m. of fibula
  posterior m. of radius
  posterior m. of ulna
  radial m. of forearm
  superior m. of scapula
  tibial m. of foot
  ulnar m. of forearm
  vertebral m. of scapula
  volar m. of radius
  volar m. of ulna

margo *pl.* margines
  m. acetabularis
  m. acetabuli
  m. anterior fibulae
  m. anterior radii
  m. anterior tibiae
  m. anterior ulnae
  m. axillaris scapulae
  m. dorsalis radii
  m. dorsalis ulnae
  m. fibularis pedis
  m. infraglenoidalis tibiae
  m. interosseus fibulae
  m. interosseus radii
  m. interosseus tibiae
  m. interosseus ulnae
  m. lateralis antebrachii
  margines laterales digito-
    rum pedis
  m. lateralis humeri
  m. lateralis pedis
  m. lateralis scapulae
  m. medialis antebrachii
  margines mediales digito-
    rum pedis

margo *(continued)*
  m. medialis humeri
  m. medialis pedis
  m. medialis scapulae
  m. medialis tibiae
  m. posterior fibulae
  m. posterior radii
  m. posterior ulnae
  m. radialis antebrachii
  m. radialis humeri
  m. superior scapulae
  m. tibialis pedis
  m. ulnaris antebrachii
  m. ulnaris humeri
  m. vertebralis scapulae
  m. volaris radii
  m. volaris ulnae

Marie
  M.-Bamberger disease
  M.-Bamberger syndrome
  M.-Strümpell arthritis
  M.-Strümpell disease
  M.-Strümpell spondylitis

Marino transsphenoidal enucleator

Mark II
  M. II concave total knee retractor
  M. II distal femur retractor
  M. II femoral component extractor
  M. II Kodros radiolucent awl
  M. II lateral collateral ligament retractor
  M. II modular weight retractor
  M. II Sorrells hip arthroplasty
  M. II "S" total knee retractor
  M. II Stulberg leg positioner
  M. II tibial component extractor
  M. II wide PCL knee retractor

Markell brace boot

Markham-Meyerding retractor

Markwalder bone rongeur

marrow
  bone m.
  fat m.
  gelatinous m.
  red m.
  red bone m.
  yellow m.
  yellow bone m.

marsupium *pl.* marsupia
  marsupia patellaris

Martel sign

Martin-Gruber anastomosis

Martorell syndrome

Mary
  angle of M.

Mason splint

mass
  bony m.
  cellular periosteal osteocartilaginous m.
  lateral m. of atlas
  lateral m. of sacrum
  lateral m. of vertebrae
  plantar-hindfoot-midfoot-bony m.

massa
  m. lateralis atlantis
  m. lateralis ossis sacri
  m. lateralis vertebrae

massage
  effleurage m.
  electrovibratory m.
  ice m.
  kneading m.
  Shiatsu m.
  Swedish m.
  vibratory m.

Massie
  M. extractor
  M. plate

Massie
    M. extractor
    M. II nail
    M. sliding nail

Masson fasciotome

massotherapy

Masterson
    M. cervical clamp
    M. straight clamp

Masterstim interferential stimulator

mat
    Airex m.

matchstick fracture

material
    bone replacement m.
    Bonfiglio bone replacement m.
    Coballoy implant m.
    copolymer orthotic m.
    Durapatite bone replacement m.
    Ethrone implant m.
    hydroxyapatite bone replacement m.
    Paladon implant m.
    polyether implant m.
    Porocoat prosthetic m.
    Schepens hollow silicone hemisphere implant m.

Matev sign

matricectomy

matrix pl. matrices
    bone m.
    m.–bone marrow slurry
    demineralized bone m.
    germinal m.
    nail m.
    sarcoplasmic m.

matrixectomy
    phenol m.
    Steindler m.
    Winograd m.

matrixectomy (continued)
    Winograd partial m.
    Zadik total m.

Matroc femoral head

Matson-Alexander elevator

Matta-Saucedo fixation

Matti
    M.-Russe bone graft
    M.-Russe technique

Mattrix spinal cord stimulation system

Mauchart ligaments

Mau osteotomy

maxillectomy
    Cocke m.

maxillofacial bone screw

Maxim knee system

May
    M. anatomical bone plate
    M. plate

May
    M. anatomical bone plate
    M. plate

Mayer
    ligament of M.
    radiate ligament of M.
    M. splint

Mayfield
    M. adaptor
    M. fixation frame
    M. instrumentation

Mayo
    M. hallux valgus modified operation
    M. resection arthroplasty
    M.-Collins retractor
    M.-Thomas cervical collar
    M.-Thomas collar

Mazet knee disarticulation

M band

MCL
  medial collateral ligament

MCP
  metacarpophalangeal

MCS microdebrider

M disk

mean
  m. of consecutive differences
  m. value

Mears-Rubash approach

Meary metarsotalar angle

measurement
  Agliette m.
  arthrometric knee laxity m.

mechanics
  altered intervertebral m.
  body m.

mechanism
  abductor m.
  capsuloligamentous m.
  digital extensor m.
  extensor m.
  extensor hood m.
  flexor m.
  quadriceps m.
  screw-home m.
  tendo Achillis m.
  terminal extensor m.

mecystasis

media (*plural of* medium)

medial
  m. femoral condyle
  m. meniscus

medialization

medial/lateral

median
  m. nerve block
  m. nerve compression
  m. nerve entrapment
  m. parapatellar incision
  m. raphe

median (*continued*)
  m. sagittal plane

Mediloy
  M. implant metal
  M. implant metal prosthesis

mediolateral

mediotarsal

Medipedic multicentric knee brace

mediscalenus

medium *pl.* media
  contrast m.
  Hypaque contrast m.
  Omnipaque contrast m.
  Renografin contrast m.

Medmetric knee ligament arthrometer

Medoff
  M. axial compression screw
  M. sliding plate

Medrol Dosepak

Medtronic spinal stimulation system

medulla
  m. of bone
  m. ossium
  m. ossium flava
  m. ossium rubra

medullary
  m. bone graft
  m. canal reamer
  m. nail fixation
  m. pin
  m. prosthesis

medullitis

medullization

medulloarthritis

medullostomy
  tarsal m.

mefanamic acid

megalocheiria

megalodactylism

megalodactylous

megalodactyly

megalopodia

melagra

melalgia

Meleney synergistic gangrene

melissotherapy

Melnick
    osteodysplasty of M. and
        Needles
    M.-Fraser syndrome

Melone distal radius fracture
    classification

melorheostosis

melosalgia

meloxicam

membrana
    m. atlantooccipitalis ante-
        rior
    m. atlantooccipitalis poste-
        rior
    m. capsularis
    m. fibrosa capsulae articu-
        laris
    m. intercostalis externa
    m. intercostalis interna
    m. interossea antebrachii
    m. interossea antibrachii
    m. interossea cruris
    m. sacciformis
    m. sterni
    m. suprapleuralis
    m. synovialis capsulae arti-
        cularis
    m. tectoria

membrane
    aponeurotic m.

membrane (continued)
    atlantooccipital m., anterior
    atlantooccipital m., poste-
        rior
    basement m.
    capsular m.
    costocoracoid m.
    cribriform m.
    fibrous m. of articular cap-
        sule
    Golgi m.
    ground m.
    intercostal m., external
    intercostal m., internal
    interosseous m., radioulnar
    interosseous m. of leg
    interspinal m's
    Krause m.
    ligamentous m.
    medullary m.
    oblique m. of forearm
    obturator m. of atlas, ante-
        rior
    obturator m. of atlas, pos-
        terior
    occipitoaxial m., long
    periprosthetic m.
    postsynaptic m.
    Preclude Spinal M.
    sternal m.
    suprapleural m.
    synovial m.
    synovial m. of articular
        capsule
    tectorial m.
    tendinous m.

membranous ossification

Memford-Gurd arthroplasty

Mendel
    M.-Bekhterev reflex
    M.-Bekhterev sign

meningoosteophlebitis

meningosis

meniscal
    m. aponeurosis
    m. lateral tear

meniscal *(continued)*
   m. radial tear
   m. repair needle
   m. scissors
   m. spoon
   m. transverse tear

meniscectomy
   arthroscopic m.
   m. knife
   Patel medial m.
   subtotal m.
   total m.

meniscocapsular
   m. junction

meniscofemoral
   m. capsule
   m. ligament

meniscoid
   m. entrapment

meniscoplasty

meniscorrhexis

meniscosynovial junction

meniscotibial
   m. capsule
   m. ligament

meniscotome
   Grover m.

meniscus *pl.* menisci
   m. of acromioclavicular
     joint
   m. articularis
   clefting of m.
   degenerative m.
   discoid m.
   discoid lateral m.
   frayed m.
   m. forceps
   m. graft
   m. of inferior radioulnar
     joint
   joint m.
   lateral m.
   m. lateralis articulationis
     genus

meniscus *(continued)*
   medial m.
   m. medialis articulationis
     genus
   m. of sternoclavicular joint
   resection of the m.
   torn m.
   trapped m.

Mennell sign

meralgia paresthetica

Merchant congruence angle

Merle-d'Aubigné hip score

meromyosin

merorachischisis

merostotic

Mersilene sling

mesocarpal

mesochondrium

mesocuneiform

mesogluteal

mesogluteus

mesophragma

mesorachischisis

mesoscapula

mesosternum

mesotarsal

mesotendon

mesothenar

metacarpal
   m. block
   m. bone
   m. lengthening
   m. ligament
   m. osteotomy

metacarpectomy

metacarpocapitate joint

metacarpocarpal

metacarpoglenoidal ligament

metacarpohamate joint

metacarpophalangeal (MCP)
    m. articulation
    m. joint (MPJ)
    m. ligament

metacarpotrapezoid ligament

metacarpus

metal
    Biotex implant m.
    m. fatigue
    m. footplate
    implant m.
    Mediloy implant m.
    m. pylon
    Vitallium implant m.
    Zimalite implant m.
    Zimaloy implant m.

metaphyseal (*spelled also* meta-
    physial)
    m.-articular nonunion
    m.-diaphyseal angle
    m.-epiphyseal angle
    m. osteotomy
    m. tibial fracture

metaphysial (*variant of* meta-
    physeal)

metaphysis *pl.* metaphyses
    distal m.
    femoral m.
    fibular m.
    tibial m.

metaphysitis

metapodialia

metapophysis

metastasis *pl.* metastases
    calcareous m.
    osteoblastic m.
    spinal m.

metasternum

Metasul
    M. hip joint component
    M. joint
    M. metal-on-metal hip pros-
    thesis

metatarsal
    m. cuneiform exostosis
    m. fracture
    m. head osteotomy
    m. joint
    m. neck
    m. oblique osteotomy
    m. ray
    m. Reverdin osteotomy
    m. V-shaped osteotomy

metatarsalgia
    Morton m.

metatarsectomy

metatarsocalcaneal angle

metatarsocuboid joint

metatarsocuneiform
    m. arthrodesis
    m. articulation
    m. joint orthosis
    m. joint fusion

metatarsophalangeal (MTP)
    m. joint
    m. joint fusion

metatarsus *pl.* metatarsi
    m. adductocavus
    m. adductovarus
    m. adductus
    m. atavicus
    m. brevis
    m. cavus
    m. latus
    m. primus adductus (MPA)
    m. primus atavicus
    m. primus varus (MPV)
    true m. adductovarus
    (TMA)
    true m. adductus (TMA)
    m. varus (MTV)

metazonal region

methacrylate
    antibody-impregnated poly-
      methyl m.
    centrifuged methyl m.
    methyl m.
    polymethyl m.

method
    Abbott m.
    antegrade m.
    Bobath m.
    Borggreve m.
    Brunnstrom m.
    Buck m.
    Burkhalter-Reyes m. for
      phalangeal fracture
    closed-plaster m.
    cup and cone m.
    disk diffusion m.
    dynamic traction m.
    Eskimo m.
    external rotation m.
    Fallat-Buckholz m.
    Fay m.
    Ferkel m. for measuring
      scoliosis
    hippocratic m.
    Ilizarov m.
    immobilization m.
    Kocher m.
    Milch m.
    Mose m.
    Neufeld dynamic m.
    Orr m.
    Palmer m.
    pedicle m.
    proprioceptive neuromus-
      cular facilitation m.
    retrograde m.
    Rood m.
    Stimson m.
    traction-countertraction m.
    Trueta m.

methotrexate

methyl
    m. methacrylate

metmyoglobin

metrostasis

Metzenbaum
    M. chisel
    M. gouge

Meuli arthroplasty

Meyer
    M. law
    M. line
    M.-Betz disease

Meyerding
    M. chisel
    M. curved osteotome
    M. gouge
    M. retractor
    M. straight osteotome

Meyers quadratus muscle-pedi-
    cle bone graft

Meyhoeffer curet

Meyn-Quigley maneuver

MGH osteotome

Miami
    M. fracture brace
    M. TLSO scoliosis brace

Michael Reese articulated pros-
    thesis

Micro-Aire osteotome

microavulsion

microdactyly

microdebrider
    MCS m.

microdiskectomy
    arthroscopic m.
    uniportal arthroscopic m.

microfracture

microgeodic syndrome

microinterlock

microirrigating cannula

microlaminectomy

Microloc knee prosthesis

microlumbar diskectomy

micromelic dwarfism

microscelous

microscrew
Barouk m. with shortening
osteotomy

Microsect shaver

Midas Rex
M. R. acorn
M. R. AMI bone cutter
M. R. bur
M. R. knife
M. R. pneumatic instru-
ment

midaxillary line

midcarpal
m. arthrodesis
m. arthroscopy
m. joint

midfacial fracture

midfoot
m. abductus
m. adductus
m. fracture

midlateral approach

midmalleolar line

midpalmar abscess

midpatellar
m. portal
m. tendon

midsternal line

midtarsal
m. osteoarthritis

Mignon eosinophilic granuloma

migraine
basilar artery m.

migration
hallux m.

Mikhail bone block

Mikulicz
M. angle
M. operation
M. pad

Milch
M. method
M. plate

Milgram test

military maneuver

Milkman syndrome

Millender
M. arthroplasty
M.-Nalebuff arthrodesis

Miller
M. disease
M.-Galante jig

Mills test

Miltex bone saw

Milwaukee
M. brace
M. scoliosis orthosis

Minerva
M. cervical jacket
M. orthosis

mini C-arm
XiScan m. C-a.

miniplate
Luhr m.

ministem shaft

Minkoff-Jaffe-Menendez posterior approach

Minor sign

Mitchell
M. operation
M. step-down osteotomy

Mitek
M. bone saw
M. vapor

Mitek *(continued)*
    M. wire twister

Mittlemeir broach

Miyakawa knee operation

Mize-Bucholz-Grogan approach

Moberg
    M. advancement flap
    M. arthrodesis
    M. dowel graft
    M. osteotome
    M. pickup test
    M. screw
    M. splint
    M.-Gedda fracture
    M.-Gedda open reduction

Mobic

mobility
    symphyseal m.

Modic classification of disk abnormality (1, 2, 3, 4, 4A, 4B, *and* 4C)

modification
    Anderson m. of Berndt-Harty classification
    Aufranc m. of Smith-Petersen cup
    Benyi m. of Lambrinudi triple arthrodesis
    Bonfiglio m.
    Burkhalter m. of Stiles-Bunnell technique
    Lovitt-Uhler m. of Jewett postfusion brace
    MacKinnon m.
    Regnauld m. of Keller arthroplasty
    Seddon m.
    Stauffer m.
    T-plasty m. of Bankart shoulder operation
    Wagner m. of Syme amputation

modified
    m. Boyd amputation of ankle and distal tibial physis

modified *(continued)*
    m. Keller resection arthroplasty
    m. Lapidus arthrodesis

modulator
    selective estrogen receptor m.

modulus of elasticity

Moe
    M. alar hook
    M. bone curet
    M. gouge
    M. intertrochanteric plate
    M. modified Cotrel cast
    M. modified Harrington rod
    M. osteotome
    M. plate
    M. scoliosis operation
    M. scoliosis technique
    M. square-end rod

Mohr finger splint

Moire topographic scoliosis assessment

mold
    Aufranc concentric hip m.

Molesworth
    M. osteotomy
    M.-Campbell elbow approach

mollities
    m. ossium

Molt periosteal elevator

monarthric

monarthritis
    m. deformans

monarticular
    m. synovitis

Mönckeberg sclerosis

monoarticular

monodal

monomelic

monomyositis

monophasic

monopolar
    m. cautery

monostotic

monotube
    Howmedica m.

Monro bursa

Monteggia
    M. dislocation
    M. fracture
    M. fracture-dislocation of
        ulna
    reverse M. fracture

Montenovesi rongeur

Montercaux fracture

Moore
    M. bone drill
    M. femoral neck prosthesis
    M. fixation pin
    M. fracture
    M. hip endoprosthesis sys-
        tem
    M. nail
    M. osteotomy-osteoclasis
    M. posterior approach
    M. prosthesis-mortising
        chisel
    M. sliding nail plate
    M. tibial plateau fracture
    M.-Southern approach

morbus
    m. coxae senilis

morcellate

morcellation

morcellize (*spelled also* morsel-
    lize)

morcellized
    m. bone
    m. bone graft

Moreira plate

Moreland femoral component
    extractor

Morquio sign

Morscher plate

Morrey-Bryan total elbow ar-
    throplasty

morsellize (*variant of* morcel-
    lize)

mortise
    ankle m.
    cuneiform m.

Morton
    M. foot
    M. interdigital neuroma
    M. metatarsalgia
    M. neuroma
    M. neuroma neurolysis
    M. syndrome
    M. test
    M. toe

Mose method

Moseley fasciotome

Moss
    M. instrumentation
    M.-Miami load-sharing spi-
        nal implant system

Mosso ergograph

motion
    accessory m.
    active range of m.
    active-assisted range of m.
    active and passive range
        of m.
    active ankle joint complex
        range of m. (AAROM)
    active integral range of m.
        (AIROM)
    angular m.
    angulation m.
    back range of m. (BROM)
    bucket-handle rib m.
    continuous passive m.
    controlled ankle m. (Cam)

motion *(continued)*
    coupled m.
    distractive m.
    double-flexion knee m.
    intersegmental m.
    limitation of m.
    passive range of m.
    physiologic m.
    plantarflexory m.
    range of m.
    subtalar m.
    triaxial m.
    uninhibited ankle m.
    m. velocity

motofacient

motor
    m. dysfunction
    m. nerve conduction velocity
    m. neuron
    plastic m.

Mould arthroplasty

Moule screw pin

mounding

Mouradian
    M. rod
    M. screw

mouse
    joint m.

mouth
    tapir m.

movement
    active m.
    active range of m.
    adventitious m.
    angular m.
    anterior-inferior m.
    arcuate m.
    atlas-axis m.
    ballistic m's
    compensatory m.
    forced m.
    Frenkel m's
    gliding m.

movement *(continued)*
    hinge m.
    innominate m.
    passive m.
    primary or intentional m.
    range of m. (range of motion)
    sagittal m.
    Swedish m.

mover
    prime m.

Mozer disease

MPA
    metatarsus primus adductus

M-Pact cast cutter

MPJ
    metacarpophalangeal joint

MPV
    metatarsus primus varus

MRI
    magnetic resonance imaging
        Fonar Stand-Up MRI

MTE allograft

MTP
    metatarsophalangeal
        MTP joint
        varus MTP angle

MTV
    metatarsus varus

mucro
    m. sterni

Mudder sign

Mueller (*variant of* Müller)

Mulder
    M. click
    M. sign

Müller (*spelled also* Mueller)
    M. anterolateral femorotibial ligament tenodesis

Müller *(continued)*
    M. arthrodesis
    M. compression apparatus
    M. compression blade
    M. compression blade plate
    M. cup
    M. dual-lock hip prosthesis
    M. hip arthroplasty
    M. intertrochanteric varus
      osteotomy
    M. knee procedure
    M. patellar tendon graft
    M. retractor
    M. total hip replacement
      prosthesis
    M. transposition osteotomy
    M.-Charnley hip prosthesis

multangular

multiarticular

multiaxial

multiaxis foot

multielectrode

multilevel
    m. fracture
    m. fusion
    m. laminectomy

multipartite
    m. fracture
    m. patella

multiplet

multiray fracture

multisegmental spinal stenosis

Münchmeyer disease

Murphy
    M. heel cord advancement
    M. splint

muscle
    abdominal m.
    abductor digiti minimi m.
    abductor digiti quinti m.
    abductor hallucis m.
    abductor m. of great toe
    abductor m. of little finger

muscle *(continued)*
    abductor m. of little toe
    abductor m. of thumb, long
    abductor m. of thumb,
      short
    abductor pollicis brevis m.
    abductor pollicis longus m.
    adductor m., great
    adductor m., long
    adductor m., short
    adductor m., smallest
    adductor m. of great toe
    adductor m. of thumb
    agonist m.
    agonistic m.
    Albinus m.
    anconeus m.
    anconeus m., lateral
    anconeus m., medial
    anconeus m., short
    antagonist m.
    antagonistic m.
    anterior scalene m.
    anterior serratus m.
    anterior tibial m.
    antigravity m's
    appendicular m's
    articular m.
    articular m. of elbow
    articular m. of knee
    BBC m.
    m. belly
    biceps brachialis m.
    biceps brachii m.
    biceps femoris m.
    biceps m. of arm
    biceps m. of thigh
    brachial m.
    brachialis m.
    brachioradial m.
    buccinator m.
    cervical m's
    Chassaignac axillary m.
    coccygeal m.
    coccygeal m's
    m. contracture
    coracobrachial m.
    cricopharyngeal sphinc-
      ter m.

muscle *(continued)*
  cucullaris m.
  deltoid m.
  digastric m.
  dorsal interosseous m.
  m. dysmorphia
  ECRB (extensor carpi radi-
    alis brevis) m.
  ECRL (extensor carpi radi-
    alis brevis) m.
  epitrochleoanconeus m.
  erector m. of spine
  extensor m. of digits, com-
    mon
  extensor m. of fingers
  extensor m. of fifth digit,
    proper
  extensor m. of great toe,
    long
  extensor m. of great toe,
    short
  extensor m. of index finger
  extensor m. of little finger
  extensor m. of thumb, long
  extensor m. of thumb,
    short
  extensor m. of toes, long
  extensor m. of toes, short
  external intercostal m.
  external oblique m.
  femoral m.
  fibular m., long
  fibular m., short
  fibular m., third
  finger flexor m.
  flexor m., accessory
  flexor m. of fingers, deep
  flexor m. of fingers, superfi-
    cial
  flexor m. of great toe, long
  flexor m. of great toe, short
  flexor m. of little finger,
    short
  flexor m. of little toe, short
  flexor m. of thumb, long
  flexor m. of thumb, short
  flexor m. of toes, long
  flexor m. of toes, short
  flexor m. of wrist, radial

muscle *(continued)*
  flexor m. of wrist, ulnar
  gastrocnemius m.
  gastrocnemius m., lateral
  gastrocnemius m., medial
  gastroc-soleus m.
  gemellus m., inferior
  gemellus m., superior
  gluteal m., least
  gluteus maximus m.
  gluteus medius m.
  gracilis m.
  greater rhomboid m.
  hamstring m's
  hypothenar m's
  iliac m.
  iliacus m.
  iliococcygeus m.
  iliocostal m.
  iliopsoas m.
  infraspinous m.
  intercostal m's, external
  intercostal m's, innermost
  intercostal m's, internal
  internal oblique m.
  interosseous m's, palmar
  interosseous m's, plantar
  interosseous m's, volar
  interosseous m's of foot,
    dorsal
  interosseous m's of hand,
    dorsal
  interspinal m's
  interspinal m's of loins
  interspinal m's of neck
  interspinal m's of thorax
  intertransverse m's
  intertransverse m's, ante-
    rior
  intertransverse m's, lateral
    lumbar
  intertransverse m's, medial
    lumbar
  intertransverse m's of
    neck, anterior
  intertransverse m's of
    neck, posterior
  intertransverse m's of tho-
    rax

muscle *(continued)*
intraspinous m.
intrinsic m.
Langer m.
latissimus dorsi m.
levator m's of ribs
levator m's of ribs, long
levator m's of ribs, short
levator m. of scapula
long m. of head
long m. of neck
longissimus m.
longissimus m. of back
longissimus m. of head
longissimus m. of neck
longissimus m. of thorax
longus capitus m.
longus cervicis m.
longus colli m.
m's of lower limb
lumbrical m.
lumbricalis m.
lumbrical m's of foot
lumbrical m's of hand
mesothenar m.
multifidus m's
m's of neck
oblique m. of head, inferior
oblique m. of head, superior
obturator m., external
obturator m., internal
omohyoid m.
oponens digiti quinti m.
oponens pollicis m.
opposing m. of little finger
opposing m. of thumb
palmar interosseous m.
palmar m., long
palmar m., short
palmaris longus m.
paraspinal m.
paravertebral m.
pectineal m.
pectoral m., greater
pectoral m., smaller
pectoralis major m.
m. pedicle bone graft
peroneal m., long

muscle *(continued)*
peroneal m., short
peroneal m., third
peroneus brevis m.
peroneus longus m.
peroneus tertius m.
Phillips m.
piriform m.
plantar m.
plantaris m.
platysma m.
popliteal m.
postaxial m.
posterior deltoid m.
postural m.
preaxial m.
profundus m.
pronator m., quadrate
pronator m., round
psoas m., greater
psoas m., smaller
quadrate m. of sole
quadrate m. of thigh
quadriceps m. of thigh
red m.
rhomboid m., greater
rhomboid m., lesser
rhomboideus major m.
rhomboideus minor m.
rider's m's
rotator m's
rotator m's, long
rotator m's, short
rotator m's of neck
rotator m's of thorax
sacrococcygeal m., anterior
sacrococcygeal m., dorsal
sacrococcygeal m., posterior
sacrococcygeal m., ventral
sacrospinal m.
sartorius m.
scalene m., anterior
scalene m., middle
scalene m., posterior
scalene m., smallest
scalenus anticus m.
scapulohumeral m.
scapulothoracic m.

muscle *(continued)*
   Sebileau m.
   semimembranous m.
   semispinal m.
   semispinal m. of head
   semispinal m. of neck
   semispinal m. of thorax
   semitendinous m.
   serratus m., anterior
   serratus m., inferior posterior
   serratus m., superior posterior
   skeletal m's
   soleus m.
   somatic m's
   spinal m.
   splenius m. of head
   splenius m. of neck
   sternal m.
   sternocleidomastoid m.
   sternohyoid m.
   sternomastoid m.
   sternothyroid m.
   strap m.
   subclavius m.
   subcostal m's
   suboccipital m's
   subscapular m.
   supinator m.
   supraspinous m.
   synergistic m.
   tensor m. of fascia lata
   teres major m.
   teres minor m.
   thenar m's
   tibial m., anterior
   tibial m., posterior
   toe extensor m.
   toe flexor m.
   trachelomastoid m.
   transverse m. of thorax
   transversospinal m's
   trapezius m.
   triad of skeletal m.
   triceps m. of arm
   triceps m. of calf
   triceps surae m.
   m's of upper limb

muscle *(continued)*
   vastus lateralis m.
   vastus medialis m.
   white m.

muscle-tendon

muscular

muscular dystrophy
   Becker m. d.
   Duchenne m. d.
   Duchenne-type m. d.
   Emery-Dreifuss m. d.
   Erb m. d.
   facioscapulohumeral m. d.
   Fukuyama type congenital m. d.
   Gowers m. d.
   Kiloh-Nevin ocular form of progressive m. d.
   Landouzy-Dejerine m. d.
   Leyden-Möbius m. d.
   limb-girdle m. d.
   pelvifemoral m. d.
   progressive m. d.
   pseudohypertrophic m. d.
   scapulohumeral m. d.
   scapuloperoneal m. d.

musculature
   axial m.
   paraspinal m.
   paravertebral m.
   peroneal m.

musculoaponeurotic

musculocutaneous
   m. free flap
   m. nerve block

musculofascial

musculoskeletal

musculotendinous

musculus
   m. abductor digiti minimi manus
   m. abductor digiti minimi pedis
   m. abductor digiti quinti manus

musculus *(continued)*
- m. abductor digiti quinti pedis
- m. abductor hallucis
- m. abductor pollicis brevis
- m. abductor pollicis longus
- m. adductor brevis
- m. adductor hallucis
- m. adductor longus
- m. adductor magnus
- m. adductor minimus
- m. adductor pollicis
- m. anconeus
- m. articularis
- m. articularis cubiti
- m. articularis genus
- m. biceps brachii
- m. biceps femoris
- m. brachioradialis
- musculi cervicis
- musculi coccygei
- m. coccygeus
- musculi colli
- m. coracobrachialis
- m. deltoideus
- musculi dorsi
- m. epitrochleoanconeus
- m. erector spinae
- m. extensor carpi radialis brevis
- m. extensor carpi radialis longus
- m. extensor carpi ulnaris
- m. extensor digiti minimi
- m. extensor digiti quinti proprius
- m. extensor digitorum
- m. extensor digitorum brevis
- m. extensor digitorum communis
- m. extensor digitorum longus
- m. extensor hallucis brevis
- m. extensor hallucis longus
- m. extensor indicis
- m. extensor indicis proprius
- m. extensor pollicis brevis

musculus *(continued)*
- m. extensor pollicis longus
- musculi extremitatis inferioris
- m. fibularis brevis
- m. fibularis longus
- m. fibularis tertius
- m. flexor accessorius
- m. flexor carpi radialis
- m. flexor carpi ulnaris
- m. flexor digiti minimi brevis manus
- m. flexor digiti minimi brevis pedis
- m. flexor digiti quinti brevis manus
- m. flexor digiti quinti brevis pedis
- m. flexor digitorum brevis
- m. flexor digitorum longus
- m. flexor digitorum profundus
- m. flexor digitorum sublimis
- m. flexor digitorum superficialis
- m. flexor hallucis brevis
- m. flexor hallucis longus
- m. flexor pollicis brevis
- m. flexor pollicis longus
- m. gastrocnemius
- m. gemellus inferior
- m. gemellus superior
- m. gluteus maximus
- m. gluteus medius
- m. gluteus minimus
- m. gracilis
- m. iliacus
- m. iliococcygeus
- m. iliocostalis
- m. iliocostalis cervicis
- m. iliocostalis colli
- m. iliocostalis dorsi
- m. iliocostalis lumborum
- m. iliocostalis thoracis
- m. iliopsoas
- m. infraspinatus
- musculi intercostales externi

musculus *(continued)*

musculi intercostales interni

musculi intercostales intimi

musculi interossei dorsales manus

musculi interossei dorsales pedis

musculi interossei palmares

musculi interossei plantares

musculi interossei volares

musculi interspinales

musculi interspinales cervicis

musculi interspinales colli

musculi interspinales lumborum

musculi interspinales thoracis

musculi intertransversarii

musculi intertransversarii anteriores

musculi intertransversarii anteriores cervicis

musculi intertransversarii anteriores colli

musculi intertransversarii laterales

musculi intertransversarii laterales lumborum

musculi intertransversarii mediales

musculi intertransversarii posteriores

musculi intertransversarii posteriores laterales cervicis

musculi intertransversarii posteriores laterales colli

musculi intertransversarii thoracis

m. latissimus dorsi

musculi levatores costarum

musculi levatores costarum breves

musculi levatores costarum longi

musculus *(continued)*

m. levator scapulae

m. longissimus

m. longissimus capitis

m. longissimus cervicis

m. longissimus colli

m. longissimus dorsi

m. longissimus thoracis

m. longus capitis

m. longus cervicis

m. longus colli

musculi lumbricales manus

musculi lumbricales pedis

musculi membri inferioris

musculi membri superioris

musculi multifidi

m. obliquus capitis inferior

m. obliquus capitis superior

m. obturator externus

m. obturator internus

m. obturatorius externus

m. obturatorius internus

m. opponens digiti minimi

m. opponens digiti minimi pedis

m. opponens pollicis

m. opponens digiti quinti manus

m. palmaris brevis

m. palmaris longus

m. pectineus

m. pectoralis major

m. pectoralis minor

m. peroneus brevis

m. peroneus longus

m. peroneus tertius

m. piriformis

m. plantaris

m. popliteus

m. procerus

m. pronator quadratus

m. pronator teres

m. psoas major

m. psoas minor

m. quadratus femoris

m. quadratus lumborum

m. quadratus plantae

m. quadriceps femoris

musculus *(continued)*
  m. rectus abdominis
  m. rectus capitis anterior
  m. rectus capitis lateralis
  m. rectus capitis posterior major
  m. rectus capitis posterior minor
  m. rectus femoris
  m. rhomboideus major
  m. rhomboideus minor
  musculi rotatores
  musculi rotatores breves
  musculi rotatores cervicis
  musculi rotatores longi
  musculi rotatores lumborum
  musculi rotatores thoracis
  m. sacrococcygeus anterior
  m. sacrococcygeus dorsalis
  m. sacrococcygeus posterior
  m. sacrococcygeus ventralis
  m. sacrospinalis
  m. sartorius
  m. scalenus anterior
  m. scalenus medius
  m. scalenus minimus
  m. scalenus posterior
  m. semimembranosus
  m. semispinalis
  m. semispinalis capitis
  m. semispinalis cervicis
  m. semispinalis dorsi
  m. semispinalis thoracis
  m. semitendinosus
  m. serratus anterior
  m. serratus posterior inferior
  m. serratus posterior superior
  musculi skeleti
  m. soleus
  m. spinalis
  m. spinalis capitis
  m. spinalis cervicis
  m. spinalis dorsi
  m. spinalis thoracis

musculus *(continued)*
  m. splenius capitis
  m. splenius cervicis
  m. sternalis
  m. sternocleidomastoideus
  m. subclavius
  musculi subcostales
  musculi suboccipitales
  m. subscapularis
  m. supinator
  m. supraspinatus
  m. tensor fasciae latae
  m. teres major
  m. teres minor
  musculi thoracis
  m. tibialis anterior
  m. tibialis posterior
  musculi transversospinales
  m. transversus abdominis
  m. transversus perinei profundus
  m. transversus perinei superficialis
  m. transversus thoracis
  m. trapezius
  m. triceps brachii
  m. triceps surae
  m. vastus intermedius
  m. vastus lateralis
  m. vastus medialis

mutilans rheumatoid arthritis

myalgia
  m. cervicalis

myatonia

myatony

myatrophy

mycosis fungoides

myectopia

myectopy

myelitic

myelitis

myelocyst

myelodysplasia

myelodysplastic
   m. kyphosis

myelofibrosis
   osteosclerosis m.

myeloid

myeloma
   giant cell m.
   sclerosing m.

myelopathic

myelopathy
   cervical m.
   cervical spondylytic m.
   noncompressive m.
   progressive subacute m.
   spinal stenotic m.
   transverse m.

myeloradiculitis

myeloradiculopathy

myelosclerosis

myelotoxic

myelotoxicity

Myers knee retractor

myoatrophy

myobradia

myocele

myocervical collar

Myochrysine

myocytoma

myodegeneration

myodesis

myodystrophia

myodystrophy

myoedema

myoelectrical

myofasciitis

myofibril

myofibrillar

myofibrositis

myofilament

myofunctional

myogelosis

myogram

myograph

myographic

myography
   acoustic m.

myohypertrophia
   m. kymoparalytica

myoidem

myoidema

myoidism

myokinesis

myokinetic

myolemma

myoma
   m. striocellulare

myomalacia

myomelanosis

myometer

myon

myonecrosis

myonosus

myopachynsis

myopathia
   m. infraspinata

myopathic

myopathy
   acquired m.
   alcoholic m.

myopathy *(continued)*
    central core m.
    centronuclear m.
    cervical spondylotic m.
    distal m.
    late distal hereditary m.
    mitochondrial m.
    myotubular m.
    nemaline m.
    rheumatoid arthritis m.
    rod m.
    thyrotoxic m.
    Welander m.
    Welander distal m.

myophage

myophagism

myoplastic muscle stabilization

myosclerosis

myosin

myositic

myositis
    m. a frigore
    cervical tension m.
    m. fibrosa
    inclusion body m.
    infectious m.
    inflammatory m.
    interstitial m.
    ischemic m.
    multiple m.
    m. ossificans
    m. ossificans circumscripta
    m. ossificans progressiva
    m. ossificans traumatica
    parenchymatous m.
    progressive ossifying m.
    proliferative m.
    m. purulenta
    rheumatoid m.
    m. serosa
    streptococcal m.

myositis *(continued)*
    viral m.

myospasia

myospasm

myosteoma

myosthenic

myosthenometer

myostroma

myosuture

myosynizesis

myotactic

myotasis

myotatic

myotendinous

myotenontoplasty

myotenositis

myotenotomy

myothermic

myotome

myotonia
    m. atrophica
    chondroplastic m.
    chondrodystrophic m.
    m. congenita
    m. dystrophica
    m. hereditaria
    m. tarda

myotronic

myotrophy

myxochondroma

myxoenchondroma

myxoma
    enchondromatous m.

Nafziger test

nail

    Alta tibial n.
    anteroposterior n.
    AO slotted medullary n.
    n. avulsion
    Bailey-Dubow n.
    beak n.
    n. bed graft
    bent n.
    Bickel intramedullary n.
    Brooker intramedullary n.
    Brooker-Wills n.
    cannulated n.
    Chandler unreamed inter-
      locking tibial n.
    closed Küntscher n.
    cloverleaf Küntscher n.
    condylocephalic n.
    Curry hip n.
    delta femoral n.
    Delta Recon n.
    delta tibial n.
    n.-driving guide
    dynamic locking n.
    Ender flexible medullary n.
    n. extender
    flexible intramedullary n.
    flexible medullary n.
    fluted titanium n.
    Grosse-Kempf locking n.
    Hahn n.
    half-and-half n.
    hallux n.
    Harris condylocephalic n.
    Harris hip n.
    Harris medullary n.
    hippocratic n.
    Jewett n.
    Johannson hip n.
    Küntscher n.
    Lloyd adaptor for Smith-Pe-
      tersen n.
    locking n.
    Massie II n.
    Massie sliding n.
    n. matrix

nail *(continued)*

    Moore n.
    Neufeld n.
    noncannulated n.
    nonreamed n.
    OrthoSorb pin n.
    Palmer bone n.
    n. plate apparatus
    n. plate fixation
    Pugh sliding n.
    Recon n.
    ReVision n.
    Rush flexible medullary n.
    Rydell n.
    Sage forearm n.
    Sage tibial n.
    Sampson medullary n.
    Sarmiento n.
    self-broaching n.
    self-locking n.
    Slocum n.
    slotted n.
    Smillie n.
    Smith-Petersen n.
    spring-loaded n.
    Steinmann extension n.
    supracondylar medullary n.
    telescoping n.
    triflanged Lottes n.
    Uniflex humeral n.
    Venable-Stuck n.
    Vitallium Küntscher n.
    V-medullary n.
    Watson-Jones n.
    Webb bolt n.
    Winograd technique for in-
      grown n.
    Y n.
    Z fixation n.
    Zickel subcondylar n.
    Zickel subtrochanteric n.
    Zickel supracondylar med-
      ullary n.
    Zimmer telescoping n.

nailing
    antegrade n.
    blind medullary n.

nailing *(continued)*
  centromedullary n.
  closed medullary n.
  condylocephalic n.
  femoral n.
  interlocking n.
  intermedullary n.
  intramedullary n.
  Küntscher medullary n.
  locked n.
  open medullary n.
  retrograde n.
  static lock n.
  tibiocalcaneal medullary n.
  Vertstreken closed medullary n.
  Zickel n.

Nakamura brace

Nakayama staple

Nalebuff
  N. arthrodesis
  N.-Millender lateral band mobilization technique

Namaqualand hip dysplasia

nape
  region of n.

Naropin

narrow AO dynamic compression plate

natatory
  n. cord
  n. ligament

Natural-Hip
  N.-H. prosthesis
  N.-H. titanium hip stem

Natural-Knee II system

Natural-Lok acetabular cup prosthesis

Naughton-Dunn triple arthrodesis

Nauth traction apparatus

navicular
  accessory n.
  cornuate n.
  n. fracture
  tarsal n.

naviculectomy

naviculocapitate
  n. fracture

naviculocuneiform
  n. fusion
  n. joint
  n. joint arthrodesis
  n. ligament

Navitrack 3-D surgical guidance system

NC-stat nerve conduction monitoring system

nearthrosis

NEB
  New England Baptist
    NEB acetabular cup
    NEB hip arthroplasty
    NEB total hip prosthesis

Nebcin

neck
  anatomical n. of humerus
  n. of ankle bone
  basal n.
  false n. of humerus
  n. of femur
  n. of fibula
  glenoid n.
  n. of humerus
  lateral n. of vertebra
  metacarpal n.
  metatarsal n.
  n. of radius
  n. of rib
  n. of scapula
  phalangeal n.
  radial n.
  supple n.
  surgical n. of humerus

neck *(continued)*
    talar n.
    n. of talus
    true n. of humerus
    n. of vertebra
    n. of vertebral arch
    n. wrap
    wry n.

Neck-Hugger cervical support
  pillow

necrosis
    aseptic n.
    atraumatic n.
    avascular n. (AVN)
    avascular n. of bone
    avascular n. of the femoral
      head (AVNFH)
    bone n.
    corticosteroid-induced
      avascular n.
    epiphyseal ischemic n.
    gangrenous n.
    hyaline n.
    idiopathic avascular n.
    ischemic n. of bone
    Paget quiet n.
    radiographc avascular n.
    septic n.
    skin n.
    superficial n.
    total n.
    Zenker n.

necrotic tissue

necrotizing fasciitis

needle
    Beath n.
    Bergstrom n.
    Bouge n.
    Hawkeye suture n.
    n. holder
    hubbed n.
    meniscal repair n.
    n.-nose vise-grip pliers
    Tuohy n.
    Wangensteen n.

Needles
    osteodysplasty of Melnick
      and N.

Neer
    N. acromioplasty
    N. capsular shift procedure
    N. hemiarthroplasty
    N. II humeral component
    N. open reduction
    N. posterior shoulder re-
      construction

Neff meniscus knife

Nélaton dislocation

Nelson sign

neoarthrosis

Neoprene hinged knee brace

Ne-Osteo bone morphogenetic
  protein

Neotendon

Nernst law

nerve
    abductor digit minimi n.
    accessory n.
    spinal accessory n.
    vagal accessory n.
    anococcygeal n.
    antebrachial cutaneous n.
    anterior thoracic n.
    articular n.
    axillary n.
    Bell n.
    descending cervical n.
    transverse cervical n.
    circumflex n.
    cluneal n's, inferior
    cluneal n's, middle
    cluneal n's, superior
    common fibular n.
    common peroneal n.
    crural interosseous n.
    cubital n.
    cutaneous n.
    deep fibular n.

nerve *(continued)*

deep peroneal n.
digital n's, radial dorsal
digital n's, ulnar dorsal
digital n's of foot, dorsal
digital n's of lateral plantar
n., common plantar
digital n's of lateral plantar
n., proper plantar
digital n's of lateral surface
of great toe and of medial
surface of second toe,
dorsal
digital n's of medial plantar
n., common plantar
digital n's of medial plantar
n., proper plantar
digital n's of median n.,
common palmar
digital n's of median n.,
proper palmar
digital n's of radial n., dorsal
digital n's of ulnar n., collateral palmar
digital n's of ulnar n., common palmar
digital n's of ulnar n., dorsal
digital n's of ulnar n.,
proper palmar
dorsal n. of scapula, dorsal
scapular n.
femoral n.
femoral cutaneous n.
superficial fibular n.
furcal n.
fusimotor n's
genitofemoral n.
gluteal n's
gluteal n., inferior
gluteal n's, middle
gluteal n., superior
hypoglossal n.
iliohypogastric n.
ilioinguinal n.
iliopubic n.
intercostal n's
intercostobrachial n's
interdigital n.

nerve *(continued)*

inferior laryngeal n.
intermediate dorsal cuta-
neous n.
intermetatarsal n.
interosseous n. of forearm,
anterior
interosseous n. of forearm,
posterior
interosseous n. of leg
ischiadic n.
n. of Kunzel
Latarjet n.
lumbar n's
lumboinguinal n.
mandibular n.
medial articular n.
medial brachial n.
median n.
mixed n., n. of mixed fibers
motor n.
musculocutaneous n.
musculocutaneous n. of
foot
musculocutaneous n. of leg
musculospiral n.
myelinated n.
obturator n.
obturator n., accessory
obturator n., internal
n. to pectineus
pectoral n., lateral
pectoral n., medial
peripheral n.
peroneal n., accessory
deep
peroneal n., common
peroneal n., deep
peroneal n., superficial
phrenic n.
piriform n., n. to piriformis
plantar n., lateral
plantar n., medial
popliteal n., external
popliteal n., internal
popliteal n., lateral
popliteal n., medial
n. to quadratus femoris
n. to quadratus femoris
and gemellus inferior

nerve *(continued)*
  posterior interosseous n.
  radial n.
  radial n., deep
  radial n., superficial
  radial digital n.
  radial sensory n.
  recurrent laryngeal n.
  regeneration of n.
  n. root
  sacral n.
  saphenous n.
  n. to sartorius
  scapular n., dorsal
  sciatic n.
  sciatic n., small
  sensory n.
  sinuvertebral n.
  spinal accessory n.
  spinal n's
  subclavian n.
  n. to subclavius
  subcostal n.
  subscapular n's
  superficial peroneal n.
  superior gluteal n.
  superior laryngeal n.
  supraclavicular n's
  supraclavicular n's, anterior
  supraclavicular n's, intermediate
  supraclavicular n's, lateral
  supraclavicular n's, medial
  supraclavicular n's, middle
  supraclavicular n's, posterior
  suprascapular n.
  sural n.
  sural cutaneous n., lateral
  sural cutaneous n., medial
  sympathetic n.
  thoracic n's
  thoracic n., long
  thoracodorsal n.
  tibial n.
  transverse n. of neck
  ulnar n.
  vagus n.
  vertebral n.

nerve *(continued)*
  n. of Willis
  Wrisberg n.

nerve block
  digital n. b.
  median n. b.
  musculocutaneous n. b.
  peripheral n. b.
  recurrent median n. b.
  ulnar n. b.

nervus
  n. accessorius
  n. anococcygeus
  n. articularis
  n. axillaris
  nervi cervicales
  nervi clunium inferiores
  nervi clunium medii
  nervi clunium superiores
  n. coccygeus
  nervi digitales dorsales hallucis lateralis et digiti secundi medialis
  nervi digitales dorsales nervi radialis
  nervi digitales dorsales nervi ulnaris
  nervi digitales dorsales pedis
  nervi digitales palmares communes nervi mediani
  nervi digitales palmares communes nervi ulnaris
  nervi digitales palmares proprii nervi mediani
  nervi digitales palmares proprii nervi ulnaris
  nervi digitales plantares communes nervi plantaris lateralis
  nervi digitales plantares communes nervi plantaris medialis
  nervi digitales plantares proprii nervi plantaris lateralis
  nervi digitales plantares proprii nervi plantaris medialis

nervus *(continued)*
- n. dorsalis scapulae
- n. femoralis
- n. fibularis communis
- n. fibularis profundus
- n. fibularis superficialis
- n. genitofemoralis
- n. gluteus inferior
- n. gluteus superior
- n. iliohypogastricus
- n. ilioinguinalis
- n. iliopubicus
- nervi intercostales
- nervi intercostobrachiales
- n. interosseus antebrachii anterior
- n. interosseus antebrachii posterior
- n. interosseus cruris
- n. ischiadicus
- nervi lumbales, nervi lumbares
- n. lumboinguinalis
- n. medianus
- n. mixtus
- n. motorius
- n. musculi obturatorii interni
- n. musculi piriformis
- n. musculi quadrati femoris
- n. obturatorius
- n. obturatorius accessorius
- n. obturatorius internus
- n. pectoralis lateralis
- n. pectoralis medialis
- n. peroneus communis
- n. peroneus profundus
- n. peroneus profundus accessorius
- n. peroneus superficialis
- n. quadratus femoris
- n. radialis
- nervi sacrales
- nervi sacrales et n. coccygeus
- n. saphenus
- n. sciaticus
- n. sensorius
- nervi spinales

nervus *(continued)*
- n. subclavius
- n. subcostalis
- nervi subscapulares
- nervi supraclaviculares
- nervi supraclaviculares intermedii
- nervi supraclaviculares laterales
- nervi supraclaviculares mediales
- nervi supraclaviculares posteriores
- n. suprascapularis
- n. suralis
- nervi thoracici
- n. thoracicus longus
- n. thoracodorsalis
- n. tibialis
- n. transversus cervicalis
- n. ulnaris
- n. vagus
- n. vertebralis

network
- achilleocalcaneal vascular n.

Neufeld
- N. cast
- N. dynamic method
- N. nail
- N. pin
- N. plate
- N. screw
- N. traction

NeuFlex metacarpophalangeal joint implant

Neurairtome drill

neural
- n. foramen
- n. foraminotomy
- n. nevus
- n. tissue

neuralgia
- genicular n.
- geniculate n.
- glossopharyngeal n.
- intercostal n.

neuralgia *(continued)*
    trigeminal n.
    vagoglossopharyngeal n.
    vidian n.

neurapraxia

neurarthropathy

neuraxial compression

neurectomy
    adductor tenotomy and ob-
      turator n.
    obturator n.
    Phelps n.
    ulnar motor n.

neuroarthropathic foot

neurofibromatosis

neurofunctional subluxation

neurogenic
    n. arthrogryposis
    n. fracture
    n. motor-evoked potential

neurolysis
    distal n.
    external n.
    Morton neuroma n.

neuroma
    amputation stump n.
    incisional n.
    n.-in-continuity
    interdigital n.
    Morton n.
    Morton interdigital n.
    sural n.
    traumatic n.

neuromuscular
    n. gait pattern change
    n. scoliosis

neuromyotonia

neuron
    motor n.

neuropathic
    n. ankle
    n. forefoot ulceration

neuropathic *(continued)*
    n. fracture
    n. hyperkyphoscoliosis
    n. midfoot deformity
    n. osteoarthropathy
    n. tarsal-metatarsal joint

neuropathy
    compressive n.
    epineurial-perineurial n.
    fascicular n.
    hereditary sensory mo-
      tor n.
    periepineurial n.
    peripheral n.
    peroneal n.
    porphyritic n.
    spontaenous median n.
    sural n.
    ulnar n.

neurorrhaphy

neuroskeletal

neuroskeleton

neurotendinous

Neu-Visc

Neviaser
    N. acromioclavicular tech-
      nique
    N. classification of frozen
      shoulder

nevus
    neural n.

Newington
    N. brace
    N. orthosis

Newman-Keuls procedure

Newport MC hip orthosis

Newton ankle prosthesis

newtonian body

NexGen
    N. complete knee system
    N. component
    N. knee implant

NexGen *(continued)*
  N. offset stem extension

Nextep knee brace

Nicola
  N. forceps
  N. shoulder procedure

Nicoll
  N. cancellous bone graft
  N. extractor
  N. fracture operation
  N. fracture repair proce-
    dure
  N. plate
  N. tendon prosthesis

nidus
  radiolucent n.

Niebauer
  N. implant
  N. metacarpophalangeal
    joint prosthesis
  N. trapeziometacarpal ar-
    throplasty

Nightimer carpal tunnel support

nightstick fracture

nipper
  English anvil nail n.

Niro
  N. bone cutting forceps
  N. wire-twisting forceps

nitro-paracetamol

nociception

node
  Bouchard n's
  gouty n.
  Haygarth n.
  Heberden n's
  Osler n.
  Parrot n.
  Schmorl n.
  syphilitic n.

nodule
  Jeanselme n's
  juxta-articular n's
  Lisch n.
  Lutz-Jeanselme n's
  rheumatoid n's

Noiles fully constrained tricompartmental knee prosthesis

noise
  endplate n.

No-Lok
  N.-L. bolt
  N.-L. screw

nonarticular distal radial fracture

nonbeaded guidepin

noncemented total hip arthroplasty

noncontiguous fracture

nonfenestrated stem

nonlamellated bone

nonphyseal fracture

nonporous-coated endoprosthesis

nonreamed nail

nonrotational burst fracture

nontraumatic idiopathic osteonecrosis

nonunion
  n. of acromion
  avascular n.
  fracture n.
  metaphyseal-articular n.
  oligotrophic fracture n.
  scaphoid n.
  supracondylar n.
  talar body n.

nonvalgus

Norco

Norian SRS cement

Norton ball reamer

notalgia

notch
    A-frame n.
    acetabular n.
    clavicular n. of sternum
    condylar n.
    coracoid n.
    costal n's of sternum
    cotyloid n.
    fibular n.
    fibular n. of tibia
    greater n. of ischium
    interclavicular n.
    intercondylar n. of femur
    interpeduncular n.
    intervertebral n.
    ischiadic n., greater
    ischiadic n., lesser
    ischial n., greater
    ischial n., lesser
    jugular n. of manubrium of
      sternum
    jugular n. of sternum
    lesser n. of ischium
    popliteal n.
    presternal n.
    radial n.
    radial n. of ulna
    sacrosciatic n., greater
    sacrosciatic n., lesser
    scapular n.

notch *(continued)*
    sciatic n.
    sciatic n., greater
    sciatic n., lesser
    semilunar n. of scapula
    spinoglenoid n.
    sternal n.
    suprascapular n.
    suprasternal n.
    trochlear n. of ulna
    ulnar n.
    ulnar n. of radius
    vertebral n., inferior
    vertebral n., superior

notchplasty

Novus LC

Noyes flexion rotation drawer
   test

nucha

nuchae
    ligamentum n.

nuchal ligament

nucleus *pl.* nuclei
    n. gelatinosus
    n. pulposus
    n. pulposus disci interver-
      tebralis
    periaqueductal n.
    pulpy n. of intervertebral
      disk

NuKo knee orthosis

O

OA
osteoarthritis

OASIS
osteotomy analysis simulation software

Oasis wound dressing

Ober
O. anterior transfer
O. incision
O. operation
O. release
O. sign
O. tendon technique
O. test

oblique
o. base-wedge osteotomy
o. displacement
o. facet wiring
o. fracture
o. meniscal tear
o. metaphyseal osteotomy
o. metatarsocuneiform joint
o. osteotomy with derotation
o. popliteal ligament
o. retinacular ligament
o. screw insertion
o. slide osteotomy

obliquity
pelvic o.
o. of pelvis

O'Brien pelvic halo operation

Obwegeser sagittal mandibular osteotomy

occipital
o.-axis joint
o. condyle fracture
o. fiber analysis

occipitoatlantal

occipitoatlantoaxial
o. fusion

occipitoatlantoaxial *(continued)*
o. joint

occlusal joint

occult
o. fracture
o. talar lesion

OCL
Orthopedic Casting Lab
OCL volar splint

Odland ankle prosthesis

O'Donoghue
O'D. ACL (anterior cruciate ligament) reconstruction
O'D. facetectomy

odontoid
o.-axial area
o. condyle
o. process osteosynthesis

odontoidectomy

odontoideum
os o.

ODQ
opponens digiti quinti

Odgen plate

Ogee acetabular component
olecranoid

Oklahoma ankle splint orthosis

olecranon
o. bursa
o. fossa
o. fracture

Olerud
O. pedicle fixation system
O. PSF screw

oligoarthritis

oligoarticular

oligotrophic fracture nonunion

olisthesis

olisthetic vertebra

olisthy

Ollier
O. arthrodesis approach
O. disease
lateral O. approach
O. law
O. layer
O. rake retractor
O.-Thiersch skin graft

omagra

omalgia

omarthritis

Ombrédanne mallet

Omega compression hip screw
system

Omer-Capen carpectomy

omitis

Ommaya reservoir device

Omnifit HA hip stem prosthesis

Omniflex hip prosthesis

Omni-Flexor device

Omni knee brace

Omnipaque contrast medium

OMNI pretibial buttress

omoclavicular

omodynia

omohyoid muscle

omosternum

omovertebral bone

onkinocele

onlay
o. bone graft
o. cancellous iliac graft

On-Q

Ontak

OnTrack knee brace system

onychectomy

Onychocare

onychogryphosis

onychomycosis

onychoosteodysplasia

onychotomy

OP-1
osteogenic protein 1

opaque synovium

open-book fracture

opening
o. in adductor magnus
muscle
o. of Hunter's canal, inferior
inferior o. of pelvis
inferior o. of sacral canal
saphenous o.
superior o. of pelvis
tendinous o.

opera-glass hand

operation
Abbe o.
Abbott-Lucas shoulder o.
Adams hip o.
Akin o.
Albee o.
Albee-Delbet o.
Albert o.
Alouette o.
Armistead ulnar lengthen-
ing o.
Baker patellar advance-
ment o.
Baker translocation o.
Bankart o.
Bankart-Putti-Platt o.
Barker o.
Barr tendon transfer o.
Barsky o.
Barton o.

operation *(continued)*
    Bauer-Tondra-Trusler o.
    Berger o.
    Bier o.
    Bristow o.
    Brooks-Gallie cervical o.
    Buck o.
    Bunnell posterior tibial tendon transfer o.
    Caldwell-Durham tendon o.
    Chopart o.
    Colonna o.
    Cotrel-Dubousset derotation o.
    Cracchiolo-Sculco implant o.
    Dupuytren o.
    DuVries modified McBride hallux valgus o.
    Eaton-Malerich fracture-dislocation o.
    Elmslie peroneal tendon o.
    Elmslie-Cholmely foot o.
    Elmslie-Trillat peroneal tendon o.
    flap o.
    French supracondylar fracture o.
    Galeazzi patellar o.
    Girdlestone o.
    Gritti o.
    Guyon o.
    Hancock o.
    Hey o.
    Hibbs o.
    Hoffa o.
    Hoffa-Lorenz o.
    Hoffmann metatarsal arch o.
    Hoke Achilles tendon lengthening o.
    Isseis-Aussies scoliosis o.
    Jaboulay o.
    Janecki-Nelson shoulder o.
    Jones cock-up toe o.
    Juvara foot o.
    Keller o.
    Keller hallux valgus o.
    Kessler posterior tibial tendon transfer o.

operation *(continued)*
    Kirk distal thigh o.
    Kocher o.
    Lambrinudi drop foot o.
    Lapidus o.
    Larrey o.
    Lisfranc o.
    Lorenz o.
    McBride o.
    MacNab o.
    Mayo hallux valgus modified o.
    Mikulicz o.
    Mitchell o.
    Miyakawa knee o.
    Moe scoliosis o.
    Nicoll fracture o.
    Ober o.
    O'Brien pelvic halo o.
    Paddu knee o.
    Péan o.
    Phelps o.
    Phemister o.
    resurfacing o.
    Schede o.
    Selig hip o.
    Silver o.
    Steindler o.
    Stokes o.
    Syme o.
    Teale o.
    tendon lengthening o.
    Vladimiroff o.
    Vulpius equinus deformity o.
    Whitman o.
    Zickel subtrochanteric fracture o.

opisthenar

Oppenheim
    O. brace
    O. gait
    O. reflex
    O. sign

Oppenheimer
    O. spring-wire splint
    O. wire

opponens
    o. bar
    o. digiti quinti (ODQ)
    o. splint
    o. transfer

opponensplasty
    Bunnell o.
    Goldmar o.
    Groves o.
    Huber o.
    Littler o.
    Manske-McCarroll o.
    Phalen-Miller o.
    Riordan finger o.

opposition
    o. contracture
    o. test
    thumb o.

OpSite wound dressing

Optetrak total knee replacement system

Opti-Fix
    O. femoral prosthesis
    O. hip stem
    O. total hip system

Oratek chisel

Orbeli
    O. effect
    O. phenomenon

order of activation

Orfit splint

Orfizip knee cast

organ
    Golgi tendon o.
    neurotendinous o.
    tendon o.

orgotein

ORIF
    open reduction and internal fixation

Oris pin

Orlando hip-knee-ankle-foot orthosis

ORLAU
    Orthotic Research and Locomotor Assessment Unit
        ORLAU swivel walker orthosis

Ormandy screw

Orozco plate

Orr
    O. method
    O. technique
    O. treatment
    O.-Buck traction

orthesis (*see* orthosis)

orthetic

orthetist

Ortho-Cel pad

Orthocomp cement

orthodactylous

orthodigita

Orthofix
    O. M-100 distractor
    O. pin
    O. screw

OrthoGen bone growth stimulator

Ortho-Glass

Ortho-Grip silicone rubber handle

orthokinetic exercise

Ortholav
    O. irrigation and suction device
    O. jet
    O. jet lavage

OrthoLogic

Orthomedics brace

Ortho-Mold
    O. spinal brace
    O. splint

orthopaedic (*variant of* orthopedic)

orthopaedics (*variant of* orthopedics)

OrthoPak bone growth stimulator system

orthopedic (*spelled also* orthopaedic)
    o. bed

orthopedics (*spelled also* orthopaedics)

orthopedist

Orthoplast
    O. fracture brace
    O. isoprene splint
    O. jacket
    O. slipper cast

orthopod

orthopraxis

orthopraxy

orthorrhachic

Orthoset cement

orthosis
    abduction hip o.
    accommodative o.
    airplane splint o.
    Alznner o.
    Amfit o.
    Amfit custom o.
    ankle o.
    ankle-foot o.
    Atlanta brace o.
    Atlanta–Scottish Rite abduction o.
    balanced forearm o.
    Bauerfeind Malleolic ankle o.
    Beaty lateral o.
    Beaufort seating o.
    Biothotic foot o.

orthosis (*continued*)
    Boston brace thoracolumbosacral o.
    cable-twister o.
    C-bar o.
    cervical o.
    cervicothoracolumbosacral o. (CTLSO)
    copolymer ankle-foot o.
    corrective o.
    Craig-Scott o.
    cruciform anterior spinal hyperextension o.
    CTLSO o.
    dynamic o.
    elbow o.
    elbow-wrist-hand o. (EWHO)
    Engen extension o.
    Engen palmar finger o.
    Fillauer bar foot o.
    flexion-extension control cervical o.
    flexor hinge o.
    flexor hinge hand o.
    functional o.
    floor-reaction ankle-foot o.
    Gillette joint o.
    halo o.
    hand o.
    hindfoot o.
    hip o.
    hip-knee-ankle-foot o.
    Hyperex o.
    hyperextension o.
    Hyperex thoracic o.
    Ilfeld splint o.
    ischial weight-bearing o.
    J-24 cervical o.
    J-45 contraflexion o.
    Jewett-Benjamin cervical o.
    Jewett contraflexion o.
    Jewett hyperextension o.
    Jewett postfusion o.
    Jewett thoracolumbosacral o.
    knee o.
    knee-ankle-foot o.
    knee extension o.

orthosis *(continued)*
    L.A. cervical o.
    Legg-Perthes disease o.
    Lenox Hill knee o.
    Ligamentus ankle o.
    L'Nard Multi-Podus o.
    long leg o.
    lumbosacral o.
    Lynco foot o.
    Malibu cervical o.
    Malleotec ankle o.
    MCF shoulder o.
    metal hybrid o.
    metatarsocuneiform joint o.
    Milwaukee scoliosis o.
    Minerva o.
    molded ankle-foot o.
      (MAFO)
    neoprene wrist o.
    Newington o.
    Newport MC hip o.
    NuKo knee o.
    Oklahoma ankle splint o.
    Orlando hip-knee-ankle-
      foot o.
    ORLAU swivel walker o.
    opponens o.
    parapodium o.
    patellar tendon-bearing o.
    Phelps o.
    Plastizote cervical collar o.
    pneumatic o.
    Polydor o.
    polypropylene glycol ankle-
      foot o.
    poster o.
    PowerStep o.
    prehension o.
    Pro-glide o.
    PSA thermoplastic o.
    PTB (patellar tendon–bear-
      ing) plastic o.
    Pucci rehab knee o.
    reciprocating gait o. (RGO)
    resting o.
    rib belt o.
    SACH (solid ankle, cush-
      ioned heel) o.
    sacroiliac o.

orthosis *(continued)*
    SAWA shoulder o.
    Scottish Rite hip o.
    serial stretch o.
    soft collar cervical o.
    SOMI o.
    spinal o.
    spring-loaded lock o.
    standing o.
    static o.
    supramalleolar o.
    therapeutic o.
    Thomas collar cervical o.
    thoracolumbosacral o.
      (TLSO)
    tone-reducing ankle-foot o.
      (TRAFO)
    Toronto Legg-Perthes o.
    total contact o.
    TRAFO o.
    turnbuckle wrist o.
    UCB foot o.
    Universal plantar fasci-
      itis o.
    Vari-Duct hip and knee o.
    Visclas o.
    von Rosen split hip o.
    Williams o.
    wrist-driven flexor hinge o.
    wrist-hand o.
    XPE foot o.
    Zinco ankle o.

OrthoSorb
    O. absorbable pin
    O. pin nail

orthotherapy

orthotic

orthotics

orthotist

orthotome resector

orthotripsy

Ortolani
    O. click
    O. maneuver
    O. sign

oryzoid bodies

os *pl.* ossa
- o. acetabuli
- o. acromiale
- o. calcis
- o. capitatum
- o. carpale distale primum
- o. carpale distale quartum
- o. carpale distale secundum
- o. carpale distale tertium
- ossa carpalia
- ossa carpalia accessoria
- ossa carpi
- o. centrale
- o. centrale tarsi
- o. coccygis
- o. costae
- o. costale
- o. coxae
- o. cuboideum
- o. cuneiforme intermedium
- o. cuneiforme laterale
- o. cuneiforme mediale
- o. cuneiforme primum
- o. cuneiforme secundum
- o. cuneiforme tertium
- ossa digitorum manus
- ossa digitorum pedis
- o. femorale
- o. femoris
- o. hamatum
- o. iliacum
- o. ilii
- o. ilium
- o. innominatum
- o. intercuneiforme
- o. intermedium
- o. intermetatarseum
- o. ischii
- o. lunatum
- o. magnum
- ossa manus
- ossa membri inferioris
- ossa membri superioris
- ossa metacarpalia
- o. metacarpale tertium

os *(continued)*
- ossa metacarpi
- o. metacarpi tertium
- ossa metatarsalia
- ossa metatarsi
- o. multangulum majus
- o. multangulum minus
- o. naviculare
- o. naviculare manus
- o. naviculare pedis
- o. naviculare pedis retardatum
- o. odontoideum
- ossa pedis
- o. pelvicum
- o. peroneum
- o. pisiforme
- o. pubis
- o. radiale
- o. sacrale
- o. sacrum
- o. scaphoideum
- o. sedentarium
- ossa sesamoidea manus
- ossa sesamoidea pedis
- o. subtibiale
- ossa suprasternalia
- ossa tarsalia
- o. tarsale distale primum
- o. tarsale distale quartum
- o. tarsale distale secundum
- o. tarsale distale tertium
- ossa tarsi
- o. tarsi fibulare
- o. tarsi tibiale
- ossa thoracis
- o. tibiale externum
- o. trapezium
- o. trapezoideum
- o. trigonum
- o. triquetrum
- o. vesalianum pedis

Osada saw

Osborne
- O. plate
- O. posterior approach

OSCAR bone cement

oscillating gouge

oscillation

Osgood
  O. rotational osteotomy
  O.-Schlatter disease
  O.-Schlatter lesion

Osher irrigating implant hook

OSI
  Orthopedic Systems, Inc.
    OSI arthroscopic leg
      holder
    OSI extremity elevator

Osler node

Os-5/Plus 2 knee brace

ossa (*plural of* os)

OssaTron orthopedic extracorporeal shock wave system

ossein

osseoaponeurotic

osseocartilaginous

osseofascial compartment

osseofibrous

osseointegrated

osseointegration

osseous
  o. attachment
  o. defect
  o. drift
  o. equinus
  o. foraminal encroachment
  o. homeostasis
  o. patellae outgrowth
  o. ring of Lacroix
  o. tissue

ossicle
  accessory o.
  episternal o's

ossidesmosis

ossiferous

ossific

ossification
  bilateral heterotrophic o.
  cartilaginous o.
  ectopic o.
  enchondral o.
  endochondral o.
  endplate o.
  heterotopic o.
  iliac crest o.
  intramembranous o.
  membranous o.
  pelvitrochanteric heterotopic o.
  periarticular heterotopic o.
  perichondral o.
  periosteal o.
  pisiform o.
  trapezium o.
  trapezoid o.
  triquetrum o.

ossifluence

ossifying

Ossigel

Ossotome bur

ostalgia

ostarthritis

ostealgia

osteanabrosis

osteanagenesis

osteanaphysis

ostearthritis

ostearthrotomy

ostectomy
  fibular o.

osteectomy

osteectopia

osteectopy

ostein

osteite

osteitis
    acute o.
    o. albuminosa
    carious o.
    o. carnosa
    caseous o.
    central o.
    chronic o.
    chronic nonsuppurative o.
    o. condensans
    o. condensans generalisata
    o. condensans ilii
    condensing o.
    cortical o.
    o. deformans
    o. fibrosa cystica
    o. fibrosa cystica generalis-
        ata
    o. fibrosa disseminata
    o. fibrosa localisata
    o. fibrosa osteoplastica
    formative o.
    o. fragilitans
    o. fungosa
    Garré o.
    o. granulosa
    gummatous o.
    necrotic o.
    o. ossificans
    parathyroid o.
    productive o.
    o. pubis
    rarefying o.
    sclerosing o.
    secondary hyperplastic o.
    vascular o.

ostempyesis

osteoanagenesis

osteoanesthesia

osteoaneurysm

osteoarthritic

OsteoArthritic knee brace

osteoarthritis (OA)
    o. deformans
    o. deformans endemica
    degenerative o.
    endemic o.
    hyperplastic o.
    interphalangeal o.
    midtarsal o.
    tarsometatarsal o.

osteoarthropathy
    familial o. of fingers
    hypertrophic pulmonary o.
    idiopathic hypertrophic o.
    neuropathic o.
    primary hypertrophic o.
    pulmonary o.
    secondary hypertrophic o.

osteoarthrosis
    o. juvenilis

osteoarthrotomy

osteoarticular
    o. allograft implantation
    o. defect
    o. graft

osteoblast

osteoblastic
    o. bone regeneration

osteoblastoma
    spinal o.

Osteobond copolymer bone cement

osteobunionectomy

osteocachectic

osteocachexia

osteocalcin

osteocampsia

osteocampsis

OsteoCap hip prosthesis

osteocartilaginous
  o. exostosis
  o. loose body

osteochondral
  o. allograft
  o. autograft transfer system
  o. prominence

osteochondritis
  calcaneal o.
  o. deformans juvenilis
  o. deformans juvenilis
    dorsi
  o. dissecans
  epiphyseal o.
  juvenile deforming metatar-
    sophalangeal o.
  o. juvenilis
  o. necroticans
  o. ossis metacarpi et meta-
    tarsi
  patellar o. dissecans

osteochondrodesmodysplasia

osteochondrodystrophy

osteochondrofibroma

osteochondrolysis

osteochondroma
  epiphyseal o.
  fibrosing o.
  intra-articular o.

osteochondromatosis
  multiple o.
  synovial o.

osteochondromyxoma

osteochondropathy

osteochondrosarcoma

osteochondrosis
  o. deformans tibiae
  o. of metatarsal

osteochondrous

osteoclasis
  Moore osteotomy-o.

osteoclast

osteoclastic
  o. erosion

osteoclastoma

osteoconduction

osteocope

osteocutaneous free flap

osteocystoma

osteocyte

osteodesmosis

osteodiastasis

osteodynia

osteodysplasty
  o. of Melnick and Needles

osteodystrophia
  o. cystica
  o. fibrosa

osteodystrophy
  Albright o.
  azotemic o.

osteoectasia
  familial o.

osteoenchondroma

osteoepiphysis

osteofascial compartment

osteofibromatosis
  cystic o.

OsteoGen bone growth stimulator

osteogenesis
  distraction o.
  o. imperfecta
  o. imperfecta congenita
  o. imperfecta cystica
  o. imperfecta tarda

osteogenic
  o. protein 1 (OP-1)

osteogenous

osteogeny

OsteoGram 2000
   Automated O. 2000

osteography

Osteoguide

osteohalisteresis

osteoid
   calcified o.

osteoinduction

osteolipochondroma

Osteolock Omnifit-HA component

osteologia

osteologist

osteology

osteolysis
   acetabular o.
   femoral o.

osteolytic

osteoma
   cavalryman's o.
   compact o.
   o. durum
   o. eburneum
   giant osteoid o.
   intra-articular osteoid o.
   intracapsular osteoid o.
   ivory o.
   o. medullare
   osteoid o.
   parosteal o.
   o. spongiosum
   spongy o.
   trabecular o.

osteomalacia
   antacid-induced o.
   anticonvulsant o.
   familial hypophosphat-
      emic o.

osteomalacia *(continued)*
   hepatic o.
   nutritional o.
   oncogenic o.
   oncogenous o.
   senile o.

osteomalacosis

Osteomark

osteomatoid

osteomatosis

Osteomed screw

osteomere

osteometry

osteomiosis

osteomusculocutaneous flap

osteomyelitic
   o. sinus

osteomyelitis
   acute hematogenous o.
   anaerobic o.
   blastomycotic o.
   chronic pyogenic o.
   diffuse sclerosing o.
   femoral o.
   Gaenslen o.
   Garré o.
   Garré sclerosing o.
   iatrogenic o.
   pedal o.
   pin-track o.
   postfracture o.
   salmonella o.
   sclerosing o.
   sclerosing nonsuppura-
      tive o.
   spinal o.
   supparative o.
   vertebral o.

osteomyelodysplasia

osteomyxochondroma

osteon

osteonal lamellar bone

osteonecrosis
dysbaric o.
idiopathic o.
steroid-induced o.

osteonectin

osteoneuralgia

Osteonics
O. acetabular dome hole
plug
O. jig
O. Omnifit-C
O. Scorpio insert

osteonosus

osteo-onychodysplasia
hereditary o.-o.

Osteopatch

osteopathia
o. condensans
o. condensans disseminata
o. condensans generalisata
o. hyperostotica congenita
o. hyperostotica multiplex
infantilis
o. striata

osteopathic

osteopathology

osteopathy
disseminated condensing o.
myelogenic o.

osteopecilia

osteopenia

osteopenic

osteoperiosteal

osteoperiostitis

osteopetrosis

osteophage

osteophlebitis

osteophyma

osteophyte
beaklike o.
bony o.
o. elevator
o. formation

osteophytosis

osteoplaque

osteoplast

osteoplastic
o. laminectomy
o. reconstruction

osteoplastica

osteoplasty
Maquet anteromedial o.

osteopoikilosis

osteopoikilotic

osteopontin

osteoporosis
o. of disuse
femoral o.
idiopathic juvenile o.
idiopathic transient o.
involutional o.
posttraumatic o.
senile o.
transient o.

osteoporotic
o. bone
o. spine

osteopsathyrosis idiopathica

osteorrhagia

osteorrhaphy

osteosarcoma
chondroblastic o.
classical o.
extraosseous o.
fibroblastic o.
gnathic o.
high-grade surface o.
intracortical o.

osteosarcoma *(continued)*
  intraosseous low-grade o.
  o. of jaw
  juxtacortical o.
  multicentric o.
  osteoblastic o.
  parosteal o.
  periosteal o.
  small-cell o.
  telangiectatic o.

osteosarcomatosis

osteosarcomatous

osteosclerosis
  o. fragilis
  o. fragilis generalisata
  o. myelofibrosis

osteosclerotic

Osteoset bone graft substitute

osteosis
  o. eburnisans monomelica
  parathyroid o.

Osteo-Stim implantable bone
  growth stimulator

osteosynovitis

osteosynthesis
  anterior column o.
  odontoid process o.
  plate-screw o.
  vertebral o.

osteothrombophlebitis

osteothrombosis

osteotome
  Acufex o.
  Albee o.
  Anderson-Neivert o.
  Army o.
  arthroscopic o.
  Aufranc o.
  backcutting o.
  Blount o.
  Bowen o.
  box o.
  Carroll-Legg o.
  Carroll-Smith-Petersen o.

osteotome *(continued)*
  chevron osteotomy
  chevron-Akin double oste-
    otomy
  chevron osteotomy with
    rigid screw fixation
  Cinelli o.
  Cloward spinal fusion o.
  Compere o.
  Cottle o.
  curved o.
  Dautrey o.
  Dawson-Yuhl o.
  Hendel guided o.
  Hibbs o.
  Hibbs curved o.
  Hibbs straight o.
  Hoke o.
  Lambotte o.
  Leinbach o.
  Lexer o.
  Meyerding curved o.
  Meyerding straight o.
  MGH o.
  Micro-Aire o.
  Moberg o.
  Moe o.
  Parkes o.
  Peck o.
  Rhoton o.
  rotary o.
  Silver o.
  Smith-Petersen curved o.
  Smith-Petersen straight o.
  Stille o.
  Weck o.
  West o.

osteotomize

osteotomy
  Abbott-Gill o.
  abduction o.
  adduction o.
  Agliette supracondylar o.
  Aiken o.
  Akin proximal phalange-
    al o.
  Amspacher-Messenbaugh
    closing wedge o.
  Amstutz-Wilson o.

osteotomy *(continued)*
  Anderson-Fowler anterior calcaneal o.
  Anderson-Fowler calcaneal displacement o.
  angulation o.
  anterior calcaneal o.
  arcuate o.
  Austin o.
  Axer lateral opening wedge o.
  Bailey-Dubow o.
  Baker-Hill o.
  Balacescu closing wedge o.
  Barouk microscrew with shortening o.
  basal o.
  base wedge o.
  basilar crescentic o.
  basilar metatarsal o.
  Bellemore-Barrett closing wedge o.
  Berman-Gartland metatarsal o.
  bicorrectional Austin o.
  bifurcation o.
  block o.
  Blount displacement o.
  Blundell-Jones hip o.
  Bonney-Kessel dorsiflexionary tilt-up o.
  Borden-Spence-Herman o.
  Brackett o.
  Brett-Campbell tibial o.
  o./bunionectomy
  calcaneal L o.
  Campbell tibial o.
  Canale o.
  chevron o.
  Chiari innominate o.
  Chiari-Salter-Steel pelvic o.
  closed-wedge o.
  closing abductory-wedge o. (CAWO)
  Coventry proximal tibial o.
  Crego femoral o.
  crescentic base wedge o.
  crescentic calcaneal o.
  cuneiform o.

osteotomy *(continued)*
  cup-and-ball o.
  decompressive o.
  Dega pelvic o.
  derotational o.
  diaphyseal o.
  Dimon o.
  Dimon-Hughston intertrochanteric o.
  displacement o.
  distal Akin phalangeal o.
  dome o.
  dorsal closing wedge o.
  dorsal-V o.
  dorsiflexory wedge o.
  Dunn-Hess trochanteric o.
  Emmon o.
  epiphyseal-metaphyseal o.
  Estersohn o. for tailor's bunion
  Evans calcaneal o.
  eversion o.
  extension o.
  failed femoral o.
  femoral derotation o.
  fibular o.
  Fish cuneiform o.
  Fulkerson o.
  flexion o.
  Gant o.
  Gerbert o.
  Giannestras metatarsal oblique o.
  Gibson-Piggott o.
  Gigli saw o.
  Gleich o.
  glenoid o.
  Green-Reverdin o.
  Gudas scarf Z-plasty o.
  Haas o.
  Haber-Kraft o.
  Haddad o.
  Haddad metatarsal o.
  high tibial o. (HTO)
  Hirayama o.
  Hohmann o.
  horizontal o.
  iliac o.
  innominate o.
  intertrochanteric varus o.

osteotomy *(continued)*
  intraarticular o.
  intracapsular o.
  intraepiphyseal o.
  Japas o.
  Kalish o.
  Kawamura dome o.
  Kawamura pelvic o.
  Keck and Kelly o.
  Kelikian modified Z o.
  Kelly-Keck o.
  Kempf-Grosse-Abalo
    Z-step o.
  Lambrinudi o.
  Lindgren oblique o.
  linear o.
  Lorenz o.
  Lucas-Cottrell o.
  Macewen-Shands o.
  malleolar o.
  mandibular o.
  Maquet dome o.
  Mau o.
  metacarpal o.
  metaphyseal o.
  metatarsal head o.
  metatarsal oblique o.
  metatarsal Reverdin o.
  metatarsal V-shaped o.
  Mitchell step-down o.
  Molesworth o.
  Moore o.-osteoclasis
  Müller intertrochanteric va-
    rus o.
  Müller transposition o.
  Obwegeser sagittal mandi-
    bular o.
  oblique o.
  oblique base-wedge o.
  oblique o. with derotation
  oblique metaphyseal o.
  oblique slide o.
  os calcis o.
  Osgood rotational o.
  Pauwels proximal o.
  Pauwels valgus o.
  Pauwels Y-o.
  Peimer reduction o.
  pelvic o.

osteotomy *(continued)*
  Pemberton pericapsular o.
  percutaneous o.
  pericapsular o.
  phalangeal o.
  Platou o.
  Pol Le Coueur o.
  Potts eversion o.
  Rappaport o.
  Reverdin o.
  Reverdin-Green o.
  reverse wedge o.
  Root-Siegal varus derota-
    tional o.
  sagittal-Z o.
  Sakoff o.
  Salter innominate o.
  Salter pelvic o.
  Samilson crescentic calca-
    neal o.
  Sarmiento intertrochanter-
    ic o.
  Schanz o.
  Schanz angulation o.
  Schanz femoral o.
  Schede hip o.
  Schwartz dorsiflexory o.
  Siffert intraepiphyseal o.
  Simmonds-Menelaus meta-
    tarsal o.
  Simmonds-Menelaus proxi-
    mal phalangeal o.
  Smith-Petersen o.
  Sofield o.
  spike o.
  spinal o.
  Sponsel oblique o.
  Stamm metatarsal o.
  step-cut o.
  step-down o.
  subcapital o.
  subcondylar o.
  subtrochaneteric o.
  tarsal wedge o.
  Thompson telescoping V o.
  tibial tuberosity o.
  tilt-up o.
  Trethowan metatarsal o.
  Trillat o.

osteotomy *(continued)*
    U-o.
    V-o.
    valgus extension o.
    varus derotational o.
    varus rotational o. (VRO)
    V-shaped o.
    Wagdy double-Y o.
    Waterman o.
    Weber humeral o.
    wedge-shaped o.
    Wiltse ankle o.
    Wiltse varus supramalleo-
        lar o.
    Yancey o.

Osteotone stimulator for bone
    union

OsteoView

ostitis

ostium *pl.* ostia

ostosis

ostracosis

Ostrum-Furst syndrome

Otto
    O. Bock 3R45 modular knee
        joint
    O. disease
    O. pelvis
    O. pelvis dislocation

Outerbridge ridge

outlet
    pelvic o.

Overdyke hip prosthesis

Overholt clip-applying forceps

overpronation

Overto dowel graft

Owestry staple

oxycinesia

Paas disease

PaBa anchor

pachydactylia

pachydactyly

pachydermoperiostosis

pachyperiostitis

pack
  Bodylce cold p.
  cold p.
  dry p.
  DynaHeat hot p.
  full p.
  Glacier P.
  half p.
  hot p.
  Hydrocollator p.
  ice p.
  one sheet p.
  partial p.
  salt p.
  Thera-Med cold p.
  Thermaphore heat p.
  three-quarters p.
  wet p.
  wet-sheet p.

pad
  Achilles heel p.
  Airex balance p.
  AirLITE support p.
  Aliplast p.
  Arthropor cup p.
  calcaneal fat p.
  Decubinex p.
  dinner p.
  foveal fat p.
  heating p.
  Hydrocollator p.
  infrapatellar fat p.
  Kerlix cast p.
  Mikulicz p.
  Ortho-Cel p.
  patellar orthosis p.
  Pelite p.

pad *(continued)*
  reticulated polyurethane p.
  retropatellar fat p.
  Roho heel p.
  scalene fat p.
  Silipos digital p.
  spur p.
  T-foam p.
  Zimfoam p.

Paddu knee operation

Paget
  P. disease
  P. disease of bone
  P. quiet necrosis

pagetic

pagetoid bone

pain
  Achilles tendon p.
  back p.
  band-like p.
  causalgic p.
  deafferentation p.
  dermatomal p.
  diskogenic p.
  epicritic p.
  fibromyalgic p.
  functional back p.
  glenohumeral p.
  gouty p.
  impingement p.
  joint line p.
  jumping p.
  lancinating p.
  osteocopic p.
  patellofemoral p.
  perimalleolar p.
  periscapulitis shoulder p.
  phantom p.
  radicular p.
  recalcitrant p.
  referred neuritic p.
  scapulothoracic p.
  sclerosomal p.
  sclerotomal p.
  splint-like p.

pain *(continued)*
    static foot p.

paired
    p. scintigraphy
    p. *t*-test

Pais fracture

PAL
    posterior axillary line

Palacos
    P. cement adhesive
    P. radiopaque bone cement

Paladon
    P. implant material
    P. prosthesis

Palex expansion screw

palmar
    p. advancement flap
    p. aponeurosis
    p. arch
    p. carpometacarpal ligaments
    p. cock-up splint
    p. crease
    p. fasciotomy
    p. flexion
    p. intercarpal ligaments
    p. interosseous muscle
    p. luxation
    p. metacarpal ligaments
    p. radiocarpal ligament
    p. synovectomy
    p. ulnocarpal ligament

palmare
    ligamentum radiocarpale p.
    ligamentum ulnocarpale p.

palmaris
    p. longus
    p. longus muscle
    p. longus tendon

Palmer
    P. bone nail
    P. method
    P. screw

Palmer *(continued)*
    P. transscaphoid perilunar dislocation
    P.-Dobyns-Linscheid ligament repair
    P.-Widen shoulder technique

palsy
    brachial plexus p.
    Erb p.
    Erb-Duchenne p.
    Hoke procedure for tibial p.
    Klumpke p.
    median nerve p.
    peripheral nerve p.
    peroneal nerve p.
    radial nerve p.
    sciatic nerve p.
    thenar p.
    tourniquet p.
    ulnar nerve p.

Palumbo
    P. ankle stabilizer
    P. dynamic patellar brace
    P. knee brace

Panalok absorbable anchor

panarthritis

panastragaloid arthrodesis

panclavicular dislocation

Pancoast syndrome

Panje prosthesis

Panner disease

panosteitis

panostitis

Panoview arthroscope

pan splint

pantalar
    p. arthrodesis
    p. fusion

pantalocrural arthritis

pantaloon spica cast

pants-over-vest
    p.-o.-v. capsulorrhaphy
    p.-o.-v. technique

Papavasiliou olecranon fracture
    classification

Papineau graft

papule
    Gottron p.
    painful piezogenic pedal
        p's
    piezogenic p's

paracoxalgia

paradox
    Weber p.

paraesthesia (*variant of* pares-
    thesia)

parallagma

paralysis
    p. agitans
    Chaves-Rapp p.
    Dewar-Harris p.
    flaccid p.
    Haas p.
    intrinsic p.
    Klumpke p.
    myopathic p.
    pseudohypertrophic mus-
        cular p.
    tourniquet p.
    Volkmann ischemic p.
    Whitman p.

ParaMax ACL guide system

parameniscitis

parameniscus

paraparesis

parapatellar
    p. arthrotomy
    p. plica
    p. synovitis

paraplegia
    Pott p.
    spastic p.
    traumatic p.

parapodium orthosis

parapophysis

parasacral

parasagittal groove

parascapular

parasternal heave

parasynovitis

paratarsium

paratenon

parathenar incision

paratrooper fracture

paravertebral
    p. musculature

Paré reduction of elbow dislo-
    cation

paresthesia (*spelled also* par-
    aesthesia)
    intermittent p's

paresthetica
    cheiralgia p.
    meralgia p.

Parham-Martin fracture appa-
    ratus

Parkes osteotome

parkinsonian gait

Parona space

paronychia
    p. bur
    p. tendinosa

parosteal
    p. osteoma

parosteitis

parosteosis

parostosis

Parrish-Mann hammertoe technique

Parrot node

parry fracture

pars
- p. abdominalis musculi pectoralis majoris
- p. anularis vaginae fibrosae digitorum manus
- p. anularis vaginae fibrosae digitorum pedis
- p. calcaneocuboidea ligamenti bifurcati
- p. calcaneonavicularis ligamenti bifurcati
- p. cartilaginea systematis skeletalis
- p. clavicularis musculi pectoralis majoris
- p. cruciformis vaginae fibrosae digitorum manus
- p. cruciformis vaginae fibrosae digitorum pedis
- p. iliaca lineae terminalis
- p. interarticularis
- p. lateralis arcus pedis longitudinalis
- p. lateralis musculorum intertransversariorum posteriorum cervicis
- p. lateralis ossis sacri
- p. libera membri inferioris
- p. libera membri superioris
- p. medialis arcus pedis longitudinalis
- p. medialis musculorum intertransversariorum posteriorum cervicis
- p. ossea systematis skeletalis
- p. sacralis lineae terminalis
- p. sternocostalis musculi pectoralis majoris

pars *(continued)*
- p. tibiocalcanea ligamenti collateralis medialis
- p. tibionavicularis ligamenti collateralis medialis
- p. tibiotalaris anterior ligamenti collateralis medialis
- p. tibiotalaris posterior ligamenti collateralis medialis

part
- annular p. of fibrous sheaths of fingers
- annular p. of fibrous sheaths of toes
- broad p. of anterior annular ligament of leg
- cruciate p. of fibrous sheaths of fingers
- cruciate p. of fibrous sheaths of toes
- lambdoidal p. of anterior annular ligament of leg
- lower p. of anterior annular ligament of leg
- superior p. of anterior annular ligament of leg
- third p. of quadriceps femoris muscle
- transverse p. of anterior annular ligament of leg

particulate
- p. cancellous bone graft
- p. synovitis

Partsch
- P. chisel
- P. gouge

PASA
- proximal articular set angle

passer
- Batzdorf cervical wire p.
- wire p.

passive
- p. exercise

Passow chisel

paste
 bone p.
 Coe-pak p.
 Unna p.

patella *pl.* patellae
 absent p.
 p. alta
 p. baja
 p. bipartita
 bipartite p.
 chondromalacia patellae
 p. cubiti
 floating p.
 high-riding p.
 p. infera
 low-riding p.
 maltracking p.
 p. minima
 multipartite p.
 p. partita
 prosthetic p.
 slipping p.
 subluxing p.
 p. tripartita
 tripartite p.

patellapexy

patellaplasty

patellar
 p. alignment
 p. apprehension test
 p. bone-tendon-bone autograft
 p. bursitis
 p. cement clamp
 p. clonus
 p. glide
 p. groove
 p. intraarticular dislocation
 p. jerk
 p. malalignment syndrome
 p. osteochondritis dissecans
 p. realignment
 p. reamer guide
 p. reamer shaft
 p. reduction clamp

patellar *(continued)*
 p. retinacular release
 p. retinaculum
 p. retinaculum release
 p. retraction test
 p. rotation
 p. sleeve
 p. sleeve fracture
 p. subluxation
 p. tap test
 p. tendinitis
 p. tendon–bearing below-
   knee prosthesis
 p. tendon graft
 p. tendon transfer
 p. tracking
 p. transplant

patellectomy
 Westin-Soto-Hall p.

patellofemoral
 p. articulation
 p. congruence
 p. crepitation
 p. dysarthrosis
 p. dysplasia
 p. groove
 p. ligament

patellomeniscal ligament

patelloquadriceps
 p. tendon

patellotibial ligament

Patel medial meniscectomy

pathological plica

pathologic spondylolisthesis

Patrick
 P. fabere test
 P. test

Patten-Bottom-Perthes brace

pattern
 cloverleaf p.
 dermatomal p.
 facilitation p.
 full interference p.
 gait p.

pattern *(continued)*
  interference p.
  intermediate interference p.
  lamellar p.
  recruitment p.
  reduced interference p.
  storiform p.
  whorled p.

pauciarticular
  p. arthritis

Paulson knee retractor

Paulus plate

Pauly point

Pauwels
  P. angle
  P. proximal osteotomy
  P. valgus osteotomy
  P. Y-osteotomy

Pavlik
  P. harness splint
  P. sling

Payr sign

PCA
  patient-controlled analgesia
  porous-coated anatomic
    PCA cutting guide
    PCA hip stem
    PCA medullary guide
    PCA primary total knee system
    PCA prosthesis
    PCA total hip replacement
    PCA unconstrained tricompartmental prosthesis
    PCA unicompartmental knee prosthesis
    PCA Universal total knee instrument system

PCL
  posterior cruciate ligament

pDEXA
  peripheral dual-energy x-ray absorptiometry

PDN
  prosthetic disk nucleus
    PDN device

PDS knot

PEAK
  PEAK anterior compression plate system
  PEAK channeled plate system
  PEAK fixation system

Péan
  P. clamp
  P. operation

pear bur

Pease bone drill

PEC
  PEC modular total knee system
  PEC total hip system

pechyagra

Peck osteotome

pecten
  p. ossis pubis

pectineal

pectoralgia

pectus
  p. carinatum
  p. excavatum
  p. gallinatum
  p. recurvatum

pedal
  p. hypophalangism
  p. osteomyelitis

pedarthrocace

pedes

pedialgia

pedicle
    p. axis angle
    p. bone graft
    p. clamp
    p. cortex disruption
    p. fat graft
    p. fixation
    p. localization
    p. method
    p. plate
    p. screw
    p. screw construct
    p. screw fixation
    p. screw insertion
    p. screw plating
    p. screw system
    p. sounding probe
    p. of vertebral arch

pediculus
    p. arcus vertebrae

pedionalgia

pediphalanx

pedobarograph

pedobarography

pedodynamometer

pedograph

pedometer

pedorthic

pedorthist

peg
    Beath bone intermedullary p.
    bone p.
    p.-in-hole prosthesis

pegged tibial prosthesis

Peimer reduction osteotomy

Pelite pad

Pellegrini
    P. disease

Pellegrini *(continued)*
    P.-Stieda disease
    P.-Stieda syndrome

pelvic
    p. angle
    p. avulsion fracture
    p. discontinuity
    p. flexion contracture
    p. hyperextension traction
    p. obliquity
    p. osteotomy
    p. ring fracture
    p. rotation
    p. splint
    p. straddle fracture

pelvifemoral

pelvis
    assimilation p.
    beaked p.
    bony p.
    coxalgic p.
    dwarf p.
    false p.
    flat p.
    greater p.
    high-assimilation p.
    kyphoscoliotic p.
    large p.
    lesser p.
    lordotic p.
    low-assimilation p.
    p. major
    p. minor
    p. nana
    p. ossea
    osteomalacic p.
    Otto p.
    p. plana
    Prague p.
    pseudo-osteomalacic p.
    rachitic p.
    Rokitansky p.
    scoliotic p.
    small p.
    p. spinosa
    spondylolisthetic p.
    p. spuria

pelvis *(continued)*
    true p.

pelvisacrum

pelvisternum

pelvitrochanteric heterotopic
    ossification

pelvivertebral angle

pelvospondylitis
    p. ossificans

PelvX

Pemberton
    P. acetabuloplasty
    P. pericapsular osteotomy
    P. spur-crushing clamp

Penfield periosteal elevator

Pennig dynamic wrist fixator

Pennsaid

PENS
    percutaneous electrical
      nerve stimulation

pentadactyl

PepGen P-15

PEP syndrome

P-ER
    pronation–external rota-
      tion

perarticulation

percussor

percutaneous
    p. autogenous dowel bone
      graft
    p. heel cord lengthening
    p. lumbar diskectomy
    p. osteotomy
    p. pin insertion
    p. stapling
    p. tenotomy

perforans
    p. manus

perforation
    attritional p.
    cortical p.
    femoral cortical p.

periarthritis
    p. of shoulder

periarthrosis humeri

periarticular
    p. fracture
    p. heterotopic ossification

pericapsular osteotomy

perichondral

perichondritis

perichondroma

pericoxitis

peridesmic

peridesmitis

peridesmium

periepineurial neuropathy

perihamate injury

perilunate
    p. carpal dislocation
    p. transscaphoid disloca-
      tion

perimysial

perimysiitis

perimysitis

perimysium
    external p.
    p. externum
    internal p.
    p. internum

Perio-Glas

periost

periosteal
    p. chondroma

periosteal elevator
  Adson p. e.
  Alexander p. e.
  Aufranc p. e.
  Bethune p. e.
  Bristow p. e.
  Brophy p. e.
  Buck p. e.
  Cameron-Haight p. e.
  Campbell p. e.
  Carroll-Legg p. e.
  Cheyne p. e.
  Coryllos-Doyen p. e.
  Darrach p. e.
  Doyen p. e.
  Farabeuf p. e.
  Fomon p. e.
  Freer p. e.
  Hoen p. e.
  J-p. e.
  Kahre-Williger p. e.
  Langenbeck p. e.
  Lempert p. e.
  Molt p. e.
  Penfield p. e.
  Sebileau p. e.
  Sédillot p. e.
  von Langenbeck p. e.
  Wiberg p. e.
  Willauer-Gibbon p. e.
  Willliger p. e.
  Yankauer p. e.

periosteitis

periosteodema

periosteoedema

periosteoma

periosteomedullitis

periosteomyelitis

periosteophyte

periosteosis

periosteotome
  Alexander costal p.
  Alexander-Farabeuf p.
  Ballenger p.

periosteotome *(continued)*
  elevator-p.
  Fomon p.

periosteotomy

periosteum

periostitis
  p. albuminosa
  albuminous p.
  diffuse p.
  hemorrhagic p.
  p. hyperplastica
  p. ossificans
  precocious p.
  supparative p.

periostoma

periostomedullitis

periostosis

periostosteitis

periostotome

periostotomy

peripatellar

peripisiform injury

periprosthetic
  p. fracture
  p. membrane

periscapulitis shoulder pain

perisclerium

perispondylic

perispondylitis
  Gibney p.

perisynovial

peritendineum

peritendinitis
  Achilles p.
  p. calcarea
  p. crepitans
  p. serosa

peritendinous

peritenon

peritenonitis

peritrochanteric fracture

Perman cartilage forceps

peronarthrosis

perone

peroneal
p. compartment syndrome
p. dislocation
p. nerve
p. subluxation
p. tendinitis
p. tendon sheath

peroneum
os p.

peroneus
p. brevis
p. brevis elongation
p. brevis graft
p. brevis muscle
p. longus
p. longus muscle
p. longus tendon
p. tertius muscle
p. tertius tendon

Perrin-Ferraton disease

Perry
P. extensile anterior approach
P.-Nickel cranial halo
P.-Nickel technique
P.-O'Brien-Hodgson triple tenodesis
P.-Robinson cervical technique

Per-Q-Graft

Perthes
P. disease
P. epiphysis
P. lesion
P. reamer
P.-Bankart lesion

pes
p. abductus

pes *(continued)*
p. adductus
p. anserinus
p. calcaneocavus
p. cavovalgus
p. cavovarus
p. cavus
p. equinovalgus
p. equinovarus
p. equinovarus adductus
p. equinus
p. gigas
p. planovalgus
p. planovalgus adductus
p. planus
p. valgus
p. valgus, congenital convex
p. varus

Petit triangle

Petrie spica cast

pétrissage

petroclinoid ligament

Pfannenstiel transverse approach

PGP flexible nail system

PGR cemented modular system

phalangeal
p. condylectomy
p. diaphyseal fracture
p. dislocation
p. fracture fixation
p. malunion correction
p. osteotomy

phalangectomy

phalangette
drop p.

phalangitis

phalangization

phalangophalangeal

phalanx *pl.* phalanges
accessory p.

phalanx *(continued)*
    delta p.
    phalanges digitorum manus
    phalanges digitorum pedis
    p. distalis digitorum manus
    p. distalis digitorum pedis
    phalanges of fingers
    p. media digitorum manus
    p. media digitorum pedis
    p. prima digitorum manus
    p. prima digitorum pedis
    p. proximalis digitorum manus
    p. proximalis digitorum pedis
    p. secunda digitorum manus
    p. secunda digitorum pedis
    p. tertia digitorum manus
    p. tertia digitorum pedis
    phalanges of toes
    proximal p.
    ungual p. of fingers
    ungual p. of toes

Phalen
    P. maneuver
    reverse P. test
    P.-Miller opponensplasty

phase
    granulation p.
    motofacient p.
    nonmotofacient p.
    reparative p.
    reversal p.
    stance p.
    swing p.

Phelps
    P. neurectomy
    P. operation
    P. orthosis
    P. scapulectomy
    P. splint

Phemister
    P. acromioclavicular pin fixation
    P. biopsy trephine
    P. elevator

Phemister *(continued)*
    P. graft
    P. onlay bone graft
    P. operation

phenomenon
    brake p.
    combined-flexion p.
    give-way p.
    Gowers p.
    halisteresis p.
    Herendeen p.
    Kohnstamm p.
    Kühne muscular p.
    Orbeli p.
    pivot shift p.
    Porret p.
    referred trigger point p.
    Rieger p.
    Rust p.

Philadelphia collar

Phillips muscle

phocomelic dwarfism

phonomyoclonus

phonomyogram

phonomyography

photon densitometry

photoplethysmography
    digital p.

physeal
    p. cartilage
    p. distraction

physiatrics

physiatrist

physiatry

Physio-Stim Lite

physiotherapist

physiotherapy

physis *pl.* physes

physique
    ectomesomorphic p.

physique *(continued)*
    ectomorphic p.

Phytodolor

Picot incision

Pidcock pin

Piedmont fracture

Piffard curet

pilaster
    p. of Broca

pillar
    articular p's

Pillet hand prosthesis

pillion

pillow
    abduction p.
    Bio-Gel decubitus p.
    Capello slim-line abduction p.
    cervical sleep p.
    crescent p.
    Flip-Flop p.
    Frejka p.
    Neck-Hugger cervical support p.
    Pillo-Wedge p.
    shoulder abduction p.

Pillo-Wedge pillow

pilon fracture

pin
    absorbable polyparadioxanone p.
    Acufex distractor p.
    Allofix cortical bone p.
    Arthrex zebra p.
    ARUM Colles fixation p.
    ASIF screw p.
    Asnis p.
    Austin Moore p.
    Barr p.
    beaded hip p.
    Beath p.
    bevel-point Rush p.
    Biofix system p.

pin *(continued)*
    Böhler p.
    Böhler-Knowles hip p.
    Bohlman p.
    calcaneal p.
    calibrated p.
    Canakis beaded hip p.
    cancellous p.
    Charnley p.
    cloverleaf p.
    Compere threaded p.
    Compton clavicle p.
    Conley p.
    cortical p.
    Crego-McCarroll p.
    DePuy p.
    Deyerle II p.
    distraction p.
    distractor p.
    Fahey-Compere p.
    femoral guide p.
    FIN p.
    fixation p.
    guide p. *(see* guidepin)
    Hagie hip p.
    Hegge p.
    hexhead p.
    Hoffmann apex fixation p.
    Hoffmann transfixion p.
    Intraflex intramedullary p.
    intramedullary p.
    Jones compression p.
    Kirschner wire p.
    Küntscher p.
    Lottes p.
    medullary p.
    Moore fixation p.
    Moule screw p.
    Neufeld p.
    Oris p.
    Orthofix p.
    OrthoSorb absorbable p.
    osseous p.
    osteotomy p.
    Pidcock p.
    Pugh hip p.
    resorbable polydioxanone p.
    Rhinelander p.
    Risser-Stille p.

pin *(continued)*
 Rush intramedullary fixa-
   tion p.
 Safir p.
 Scand p.
 Schweitzer p.
 self-broaching p.
 self-tapering p.
 Smillie p.
 SMo (stainless steel and
   molybdenum) Moore p.
 Steinmann p.
 Steinmann p. with Crowe
   pilot point
 Steinmann fixation p.
 strut-type p.
 Tachdjian p.
 tapered p.
 titanium half p.
 transarticular p.
 transcapitellar p.
 transfixion p.
 Triad p.
 trochanteric p.
 Tutofix p.
 union broach retention p.
 Varney p.
 Venable-Stuck fracture p.
 Watanabe p.
 Z p.
 Zimfoam p.
 Zimmer p.
Pinn ACL (anterior cruciate lig-
 ament) guide system
pinning
 Asnis p.
 Sofield p.
Pinto distractor
PIP
 proximal interphalangeal
   PIP articulation
   PIP flexion creaking
   PIP joint
PIPJ
 proximal interphalangeal
   joint

Pirie bone

Pirogoff amputation

pisiform
 p. bone
 p. bursa
 p. metacarpal ligament
 p. ossification

pisohamate ligament

pisometacarpal ligament

pisotriquetral
 p. arthritis
 p. joint

pivot
 Accu-Line dual p.
 p.-shift test

placement
 variable screw p. (VSP)

plafond
 p. fracture
 tibial p.

plana
 coxa p.

plane
 anatomic p.
 axial p.
 auricular p. of sacral bone
 coronal p.
 facet p.
 flexion-extension p.
 Hensen p.
 Hodge p.
 Ludwig p.
 median sagittal p.
 mesiodistal p.
 midsagittal p.
 popliteal p. of femur
 sagittal p.
 sternal p.
 sternoxiphoid p.
 subcostal p.
 suprasternal p.
 thoracic p.

plate   257

plane *(continued)*
    transverse p.
    varus-valgus p.
    vertical p.

planovalgus
    p. deformity
    talipes p.

planta
    p. pedis

plantalgia

plantar
    p. aponeurosis
    p. Babinski response
    p. bromhidrosis
    p. calcaneocuboid ligament
    p. calcaneonavicular ligament
    p. capsuloligamentous complex
    p. condylectomy
    p. cuboideonavicular ligament
    p. cuneocuboid ligament
    p. cuneonavicular ligament
    p. fasciitis
    p. fasciotomy
    p. flexion
    p. flexion-inversion deformity
    p.-hindfoot-midfoot-bony mass
    p. intercuneiform ligaments
    p.-lateral release
    p. ligaments of tarsus
    p.-medial release
    p. tarsometatarsal ligaments
    p. tendopathy

plantarflex

plantaris
    arcus p.
    p. muscle
    p. tendon
    verruca p.

plantarward

plantigrade
    p. foot

planum
    p. popliteum femoris
    p. sternale

plaque
    attachment p's

plast
    Putti bone p.

plaster
    p.-of-Paris disease
    x-ray in p. (XIP)

Plastizote
    P. cervical collar orthosis
    P. foam

plastron

plate
    90-90 p.
    acetabular reconstruction p.
    AcroMed VSP p.
    anchor p.
    anterior cervical p.
    antiglide p.
    AO-ASIF compression p.
    AO blade p.
    AO condylar blade p.
    AO dynamic compression p.
    Armstrong p.
    ASIF right-angle blade p.
    autocompression p.
    Badgley p.
    Bagby angled compression p.
    Batchelor p.
    Belos compression p.
    p. bender
    BioSorbFX SR p. and screw
    blade p.
    Blair talar body fusion blade p.
    Blair tibiotalar arthrodesis blade p.

plate *(continued)*
    bone p.
    bone flap fixation p.
    Bosworth spine p.
    buttress-type p.
    calcaneal Y p.
    coaptation p.
    compression p.
    condylar p.
    contoured anterior spinal p. (CASP)
    cortical p.
    craniocervical p.
    cribriform p.
    cruciform tibial base p.
    C-Tek anterior cervical p.
    DePuy p.
    Deyerle p.
    Driessen hinged p.
    Duopress p.
    Dwyer-Hall p.
    eccentric dynamic compression p. (EDCP)
    Eggers p.
    Eggers bone p.
    epiphyseal p.
    epiphyseal growth p.
    ferromagnetic metal p.
    fibrocartilaginous p.
    five-hole p.
    fixed angle blade p.
    flexor p.
    force p.
    four-hole side p.
    gait p.
    Gallenaugh p.
    growth p.
    Hagie sliding nail p.
    Harris p.
    Hoen skull p.
    p.-holding forceps
    I-p.
    interfragmentary p.
    intertrochanteric p.
    Jergeson tapered p.
    Jewett nail overlay p.
    Kessel p.
    Laing p.
    Lane p's

plate *(continued)*
    Leibinger titanium p.
    Letournel p.
    limited-contact dynamic compression p.
    Luque II p.
    Massie p.
    May p.
    May anatomical bone p.
    McBride p.
    Medoff sliding p.
    Milch p.
    Moe p.
    Moe intertrochanteric p.
    Moore sliding nail p.
    Moreira p.
    Morscher p.
    Müller compression blade p.
    narrow AO dynamic compression p.
    Neufeld p.
    Nicoll p.
    occipitocervical p.
    Odgen p.
    Orozco p.
    orthotic p.
    Osborne p.
    palmar p.
    Paulus p.
    pedicle p.
    peg-base p.
    plain pattern p.
    pterygoid p.
    Pugh p.
    pylon attachment p.
    quadrangular positioning p.
    Richards-Hirschorn p.
    Rohadur gait p.
    round-hole compression p.
    Roy-Camille p.
    RSDCP p.
    Schweitzer spring p.
    p.-screw
    p. and screw
    p.-screw fixation
    p.-screw osteosynthesis
    semitubular blade p.

plate *(continued)*
    Senn p.
    seven-hole p.
    Sherman p.
    six-hole p.
    slotted femur p.
    Smith-Petersen intertro-
        chanteric p.
    SMO (supramalleolar or-
        thosis) p.
    spinous process p.
    static compression p.
    Steffee pedicle p.
    Steffee screw p.
    strut p.
    subchondral p.
    supracondylar p.
    Synthes pie p.
    Tacoma sacral p.
    tarsal p.
    T buttress p.
    tendon band p.
    thoracolumbosacral p.
    Thornton nail p.
    three-hole p.
    tibial base p.
    titanium p.
    toe p.
    Townley tibial plateau p.
    T-shaped AO p.
    TSRH p.
    two-hole p.
    UCBL (University of Califor-
        nia–Berkeley laboratory)
        foot p.
    Universal bone p.
    Uslenghi p.
    variable screw p.
    V blade p.
    Venable p.
    Vitallium p.
    V nail p.
    volar p.
    VSP (variable screw place-
        ment) p.
    Wainwright p.
    Wenger p.
    wing p.
    Würzburg p.

plate *(continued)*
    X p.
    X-shaped p.
    Y bone p.
    Y-shaped p.
    Zimmer femoral condyle
        blade p.

plateau
    bicondylar tibial p.
    proximal tibial p.
    tibial p.

platform
    force p.
    Kistler force p.
    plantigrade p.

plating
    anterior spinal p.
    diaphyseal p.
    pedicle screw p.
    posterior spinal p.
    tension band p.
    variable spinal p.

Platou osteotomy

platybasia

platycnemia

platyhieric

platyknemia

platymeria

platymeric

platypodia

platyspondylia

platyspondylisis

pleonosteosis
    Léri p.

plethysmography
    digital p.

pleuralgia

pleurapophysis

pleurocentrum

pleurodynia

Plexiglas jig

plexus
> brachial p.
> sacral p.

plica *pl.* plicae
> plicae alares
> bucket-handle p.
> infrapatellar p.
> mediopatellar p.
> parapatellar p.
> pathological p.
> suprapatellar p.
> symptomatic synovial p.
> synovial p.
> p. synovialis
> p. synovialis infrapatellaris
> p. synovialis mediopatel-
> laris
> p. synovialis suprapatel-
> laris

plicectomy

plinth

PLL
> posterior longitudinal liga-
> ment

plug
> bone femoral p.
> Exeter intramedullary bo-
> ne p.
> Osteonics acetabular dome
> hole p.
> polyethylene femoral
> buck p.

PMMA
> polymethyl methacrylate
> PMMA bone cement

pneumatic compression boot

Pneu-trac cervical collar

podagra

podagral

podagric

podagrous

podalgia

podarthritis

pododynia

podogram

podograph

POEMS syndrome

Pogrun lateral approach

point
> anchoring p.
> Crowe pilot p.
> Crutchfield drill p.
> electrodesiccated
> bleeding p.
> Erb p.
> glenoid p.
> inflexion p.
> isometric p.
> Krackow p.
> motor p.
> myofascial drill p.
> ossification p.
> ossification p., primary
> ossification p., secondary
> Pauly p.
> Raney-Crutchfield drill p.
> Steinmann pin with Crowe
> pilot p.
> supraclavicular p.
> Universal drill p.
> Ziemssen motor p.

pointer
> hip p.
> shoulder p.

Poirier
> space of P.

poison
> fatigue p.

Poisson ratio

POL
> posterior oblique ligament

Polarus
> P. humeral rod

Polarus *(continued)*
    P. Plus humeral fixation
    system

Polk finger goniometer

Pol Le Coueur osteotomy

pollex
    p. adductus
    p. extensus
    p. flexus
    p. valgus
    p. varus

pollical

pollicization
    Gillies p.

polyarteritis
    p. nodosa

polyarthric

polyarthritis
    chronic secondary p.
    chronic villous p.
    p. destruens
    peripheral p.
    tuberculous p.

polyarthropathy

polyarticular

polyaxial cervical screw

polychondritis
    relapsing p.

Polydor orthosis

polydysspondylism

polyether implant material

Polyform splint

polymer
    self-curing p.

polymerization of bone cement

polymetacarpia

polymetatarsalia

polymetatarsia

polymethyl methacrylate
    (PMMA)
    antibiotic-impregnated
    p. m.
    p. m. bone cement

polymyalgia
    p. arteritica
    p. rheumatica

polymyopathy

polymyositis

polyneuromyositis

polyostotic

polyperiostitis
    p. hyperesthetica

polyphasic action potential

polyradiculopathy

polysynovitis

polytendinitis

polytendinobursitis

polytenosynovitis

polytetrafluoroethylene (PTFE)
    p. graft

PolyWic dressing

Poncet
    P. disease
    P. rheumatism

Ponseti splint

Pontenza arthrodesis

ponesiatrics

ponograph

poples

popliteal
    p. fossa
    p. ligament
    p. pterygium syndrome
    p. tendon

popliteomeniscal fascicle

Popoff suture

Porak-Durante syndrome

Porocoat
    P. noncemented prosthesis
    P. porous coating
    P. prosthetic material

porosis

porotic

Porret phenomenon

port
    S-D-p.

portal
    anterocentral p.
    Caspari arthroscopic p.
    midpatellar p.

Porter-Richardson-Vainio syn-
    ovectomy

Portmann drill

portmanteau procedure

Porzett splint

posaconazole

Posadas fracture

Posey bed cradle

position
    90-90 p.
    angular p.
    "arch and slouch" p.
    beach chair p.
    Bonner p.
    Brickner p.
    figure-of-four p.
    Jones p.

positioner
    Allen arthroscopic elbow p.
    Allen arthroscopic knee p.
    Allen arthroscopic wrist p.
    Mark II Stulberg leg p.
    Wixson hip p.

postaxial

postbrachial

postcubital

postglenoid

postischial

Posture Pump

posturography

potential
    action p.
    after-p.
    bioelectric p.
    bizarre high-frequency p.
    compound action p.
    compound muscle action p.
    demarcation p.
    dermatosensory evoked p.
    evoked p.
    fasciculation p.
    fibrillation p.
    injury p.
    motor unit p.
    motor unit action p.
    muscle action p.
    muscle fiber action p.
    myotonic p.
    negative after-p.
    neurogenic motor-
        evoked p.
    polyphasic action p.
    positive after-p.
    satellite p.
    serrated action p.
    somatosensory evoked p.
        (SEP, SSEP)
    spike p.

potentiation
    posttetanic p.

Pott
    P. abscess
    P. curvature
    P. disease
    P. fracture
    P. paraplegia

Potts
    P. eversion osteotomy

Potts *(continued)*
    P. splint

pouce
    p. flottant

poultice

Poupart ligament

PowerStep
    P. orthosis

Prague pelvis

Pratt open reduction

preaxial

Preclude Spinal Membrane

precostal

prediction
    Anderson-Green growth p.

prehallux

Preiser disease

Premalok
    Weber P.

Presbyterian Hospital staphy-
    lorrhaphy elevator

prescapula

prescapular

prespondylolisthesis

Press-Fit
    P.-F. condylar knee arthro-
      plasty
    P.-F. femoral component
    P.-F. fixation

pressure
    intradiscal p.

prezygapophysis

Pridie ankle arthrodesis

probe
    Bunnell dissecting p.
    pedicle sounding p.
    reverse-cutting meniscal p.

procallus

procedure
    Adams p.
    Axer-Clark p.
    Bandi p.
    Baxter-D'Astous p.
    Bickel-Moe p.
    Bilhaut-Cloquet p.
    bone block p.
    Brantigan-Voshell p.
    Bristow p.
    Bristow-Helfet p.
    Bristow-May p.
    Campbell ankle p.
    Campbell-Goldthwaite p.
    Chrisman-Snook p.
    Darrach p.
    Fulkerson p.
    femorodistal bypass p.
    forage p.
    Ghormley shelf p.
    Hass p.
    Hauser heel cord p.
    Hoke p. for tibial palsy
    Jansey p.
    Job-Glousman capsular
      shift p.
    Juvara p.
    Kelikian-McFarland p.
    Lindeman p.
    Maquet p.
    Müller knee p.
    Neer capsular shift p.
    Newman-Keuls p.
    Putti-Platt shoulder p.
    Nicola shoulder p.
    Nicoll fracture repair p.
    Regnauld p.
    Reverdin-Green foot p.
    reverse Putti-Platt p.
    Skoog p. for release of Du-
      puytren contracture
    Souter hip p.
    Stamm p. for intraarticular
      hip fusion
    Vulpius-Stoffel p.
    Wallenberg p.
    Watson-Cheyne-
      Burghard p.

procedure *(continued)*
    Whitman-Thompson p.
    Yoke transposition p.
    Youngswick-Austin p.
    Yount p.
    Zancolli-Losso p.
    Zarins-Rowe p.

process
    accessory p. of sacrum, spurious
    acromial p.
    acromion p.
    alar p. of sacrum
    anconeal p. of ulna
    anterior articular p. of axis
    ascending p. of vertebra
    calcaneal p. of cuboid bone
    calcanean p. of cuboid bone
    capitular p.
    condyloid p. of vertebra, inferior
    condyloid p. of vertebra, superior
    conoid p.
    coracoid p.
    coronoid p.
    costal p.
    cubital p. of humerus
    dentoid p. of axis
    descending p. of vertebra
    ensiform p. of sternum
    epiphyseal p.
    falciform p. of rectus abdominis muscle
    false articular p. of coccyx
    hamular p. of unciform bone
    inframalleolar p. of calcaneus
    intercondylar p. of tibia
    internal p. of humerus
    lateral p. of calcaneus
    mammillary p. of lumbar vertebra
    mammillary p. of sacrum, oblique
    oblique p. of vertebra, inferior

process *(continued)*
    oblique p. of vertebra, superior
    odontoid p. of axis
    olecranon p. of ulna
    spinous p. of sacrum, spurious
    spinous p. of tibia
    spurious articular p. of sacrum
    Stieda p.
    styloid p. of fibula
    synovial p.
    transverse p. of sacrum
    transverse p. of vertebrae, accessory
    trochlear p. of calcaneus
    unciform p. of scapula
    uncinate p. of cervical vertebra
    uncinate p. of unciform bone
    ungual p. of third phalanx of foot
    spinous p. of vertebra
    xiphoid p.

processus
    p. accessorius
    p. accessorii spurii
    p. articularis inferior vertebrae
    p. articularis superior ossis sacri
    p. articularis superior vertebrae
    p. calcaneus ossis cuboidei
    p. coracoideus scapulae
    p. coronoideus ulnae
    p. costalis vertebrae
    p. costiformis
    p. falciformis ligamenti sacrotuberalis
    p. lateralis tali
    p. lateralis tuberis calcanei
    p. mammillaris
    p. medialis tuberis calcanei
    p. posterior tali
    p. spinosus vertebrae

processus *(continued)*
  p. styloideus fibulae
  p. styloideus ossis meta-
    carpalis III
  p. styloideus ossis meta-
    carpi III
  p. styloideus radii
  p. styloideus ulnae
  p. supracondylaris humeri
  p. supracondyloideus hu-
    meri
  p. transversus vertebrae
  p. trochlearis calcanei
  p. xiphoideus

prochondral

procurvation

Profix porous femoral component

Profore
  P. boot
  P. four-layer bandaging sys-
    tem

profunda femoris

Pro-glide
  P. orthosis
  P. splint

program
  ABAQUS modeling p.

progressive
  p. resistance exercise
  p. resistive exercise

projection
  axial calcaneal p.
  axial sesamoid p.

prominence
  osteochondral p.

promontorium
  p. ossis sacri

promontory
  sacral p.

pronation
  p.-abduction fracture
  p.-eversion fracture
  p.–external rotation (P-ER)

pronation *(continued)*
  p.–external rotation frac-
    ture
  p. of the foot

pronatoflexor

pronator

pronometer

Pro Osteon
  P. O. granules
  P. O. 200 implant
  P. O. 200R implant
  P. O. 500 implant
  P. O. 500R implant

Propel cannulated interference
  screw

proprioceptive neuromuscular
  facilitation method

PROSTALAC
  prosthetic antibiotic-
    loaded acrylic cement
      PROSTALAC prosthe-
        sis

prosternation

prosthesis
  acetabular p.
  AcuMatch femoral hip p.
  Aesculap-PM noncemented
    femoral p.
  AFI total hip replace-
    ment p.
  Allen-Brown p.
  Amstutz cemented hip p.
  Anametric total knee p.
  Arthropor cup p.
  Attenborough total knee p.
  Aufranc cobra hip p.
  Aufranc-Turner cemented
    hip p.
  Austin Moore p.
  Autophor ceramic total
    hip p.
  Autophor femoral p.
  Bechtol hip p.
  Beck-Steffee total ankle p.
  bicentric p.

prosthesis *(continued)*
bicondylar knee p.
Bi-Metric hip p.
BioFit Press-Fit acetabu-
lar p.
Biometric p.
Bombelli-Mathys-Morscher
hip p.
Brigham p.
Buchholz p.
Byars mandibular p.
Callender technique hip p.
Calman-Nicolle finger p.
capitellocondylar uncon-
strained elbow p.
Cathcart Orthocentric
hip p.
Centralign precoat hip p.
Charnley p.
Charnley acetabular cup p.
Charnley cemented p.
Charnley-Hastings p.
Charnley-Müller hip p.
Chatzidakis hinged Vital-
lium implant p.
Christiansen hip p.
Cintor knee p.
cobalt-chromium alloy p.
Cofield shoulder p.
Conaxial ankle p.
d'Aubigné femoral p.
DeBakey p.
de la Caffinière trapezio-
metacarpal p.
DeLaura knee p.
DePalma hip p.
duocondylar knee p.
Dynaplex knee p.
Eaton trapezium finger
joint replacement p.
Eicher femoral p.
Eicher hip p.
Engh porous metal hip p.
ePTFE (expanded polytet-
rafluoroethylene) graft p.
Exeter cemented hip p.
femoral p.
Finney-Flexirod p.

prosthesis *(continued)*
four-bar Polycentric
knee p.
Galante hip p.
Gerard p.
Gillies p.
Gore-Tex knee p.
Greissinger foot p.
Hanslik patellar p.
heat-cured acrylic femoral
head p.
hip p.
HPS II total hip p.
humeral p.
implant metal p.
Intermedics Natural-Knee
knee p.
ischial weight-bearing p.
Jaffe-Capello-Averill hip p.
Jobst p.
Jonas p.
knee p.
Küntscher humeral p.
Landers-Foulks p.
LAPOC p.
LaPorte total toe p.
Lewis expandable adjusta-
ble p. (LEAP)
Lippman hip p.
McBride-Moore p.
McGehee elbow p.
McKeever-MacIntosh tibial
plateau p.
Macrofit hip p.
Mallory-Head hip p.
Mediloy implant metal p.
medullary p.
Metasul metal-on-metal
hip p.
Michael Reese articula-
ted p.
Microloc knee p.
Moore femoral neck p.
Müller-Charnley hip p.
Müller dual-lock hip p.
Müller total hip replace-
ment p.
Natural-Hip p.

prosthesis *(continued)*
    Natural-Lok acetabular cup p.
    NEB (New England Baptist) total hip p.
    Newton ankle p.
    Nicoll tendon p.
    Niebauer metacarpophalangeal joint p.
    Odland ankle p.
    Omnifit HA hip stem p.
    Omniflex hip p.
    Opti-Fix femoral p.
    OsteoCap hip p.
    Overdyke hip p.
    Paladon p.
    Panje p.
    patellar tendon–bearing below-knee p.
    PCA (porous-coated anatomic) p.
    PCA (porous-coated anatomic) unconstrained tricompartmental p.
    PCA (porous-coated anatomic) unicompartmental knee p.
    pegged tibial p.
    peg-in-hole p.
    Pillet hand p.
    Porocoat noncemented p.
    PROSTALAC p.
    Rastelli p.
    Richards Zirconia femoral head p.
    Ring knee p.
    Ring total hip p.
    Rosenfeld hip p.
    Sampson p.
    Sarmiento hip p.
    Sauerbruch p.
    Savastano hemi-knee p.
    Sbarbaro hip p.
    Sbarbaro tibial plateau p.
    Schlein trisurface ankle p.
    self-centering Universal hip p.
    Silastic ball spacer p.
    Silastic radial head p.

prosthesis *(continued)*
    Silflex intramedullary p.
    silicone trapezium p.
    SKI knee p.
    Sportono hip p.
    S-ROM hip p.
    STD hip p.
    stemmed tibial p.
    Stenzel rod p.
    Synatomic total knee p.
    Thompson p.
    total hip p.
    total knee p.
    Triad p.
    Universal femoral head p.
    Universal hip p.
    trapeziometacarpal p.
    unicompartmental knee p.
    unicondylar p.
    Valls hip p.
    Vanghetti limb p.
    Varikopf hip p.
    Villadot p.
    Vinertia implant metal p.
    Vitallium humeral replacement p.
    Vitallium implant metal p.
    Vitalock talon locking-cup hip p.
    Wadsworth unconstrained elbow p.
    Walldius Vitallium mechanical knee p.
    Warsaw hip p.
    Waugh knee p.
    Waugh total ankle replacement p.
    Weller total hip joint p.
    well-seated p.
    Wilson-Burstein hip internal p.
    Xenophor femoral p.
    Young hinged knee p.
    Young Vitallium hinged p.
    Zimalite implant metal p.
    Zimaloy implant metal p.
    Zimmer Centralign Precoat hip p.

prosthetic
  p. antibiotic-loaded acrylic cement (PROSTALAC)

Protector meniscus suturing system

protein
  bone morphogenetic p.
  fusion p.
  Ne-Osteo bone morphogenetic p.
  osteogenic p. 1 (OP-1)

protochondral

protochondrium

protocol
  Evans-Burkhalter p.

Protoplast cement

ProTrac

protrusio
  p. acetabuli

protrusion
  disk p.
  intrapelvic p.

proximal
  p. interphalangeal joint (PIPJ)
  p. tibiofibular joint

prozonal

pseudankylosis

pseudarthrosis
  extraarticular p.
  fibular p.

pseudoankylosis

pseudoantagonist

pseudoarthrosis

pseudocoxalgia

pseudodiabetes
  uremic p. mellitus

pseudoepiphysis

pseudogout

pseudoluxation

pseudo-osteomalacia

psoas

psoitis

psoriasis
  arthritic p.
  p. arthropathica
  p. arthopica

PTB
  patellar tendon–bearing
    PTB plastic orthosis

pternalgia

PTFE
  polytetrafluoroethylene
    PTFE graft

pubococcygeal

pubococcygeus

pubofemoral

pubotibial

Pucci
  P. rehab knee orthosis
  P. splint

Pugh
  P. hip pin
  P. plate
  P. sliding nail

Puka chisel

pull

pulley
  C1–C3 cruciate p.

pulp
  digital p.

pump
  Posture P.

punch
  Hirsch hypophyseal p.
  Kerrison p.

punctum
    p. ossificationis
    p. ossificationis primarium
    p. ossificationis secundar-
      ium

purchase
    bony p.

purpura
    Schönlein p.

Push-Ease Quad cuff

Puth abduction splint

Putti
    P. knee arthrodesis
    P. posterior approach
    P.-Platt arthroplasty
    P.-Platt instrumentation
    reverse P.-Platt procedure

Putti *(continued)*
    P.-Platt shoulder procedure

putty
    AlloMatrix injectable p.
    Grafton p.

pyarthrosis

pyknodysostosis

Pyle disease

pylon
    AirStance p.
    metal p.

Pylon intramedullary nail sys-
    tem

pyoarthrosis

pyramidale

pyriform bursa

Q

Q
  quadriceps
    Q angle

Q disk

QuadraCut ACL shaver system

quadrangular cartilage

quadrate ligament

quadratipronator

quadratus
  q. femoris
  q. femoris fascia

quadriceps
  q. (Q) angle

quadricepsplasty
  Coonse-Adams q.
  Judet q.

quadriplegic
  q. standing frame

Quain
  triangular fascia of Q.

quartisternal

Queckenstedt sign

Quengel apparatus

Quervain
  Q. disease
  Q. fracture

Questus leading edge grasper-
  cutter

Quick Tack fixation system

quinti
  abductor digiti q. (ADQ)
  extensor digiti q.
  opponens digiti q. (ODQ)

rabbetting

rachial

rachialgia

rachidial

rachidian

rachigraph

rachilysis

rachiocampsis

rachiocyphosis

rachiodynia

rachiokyphosis

rachiometer

rachiopathy

rachioscoliosis

rachiotome

rachiotomy
Capener lateral r.
decompression r.

rachis

rachischisis
r. partialis
r. posterior
r. totalis

rachitic

rachitome

rachitomy

radial
r.-based flap
r. bursa
r. carpal collateral ligament
r. collateral ligament
r. deviation
r. digital nerve
r. epicondylalgia
r. head anlage
r. head dislocation
r. head fracture

radial (continued)
r. head of humerus
r. head subluxation
r. hemimelia
r. laminectomy
r. malalignment
r. meniscal tear
r. metacarpal ligament
r. nerve injury
r. pseudarthrosis
r. sensory nerve entrapment syndrome
r. slab splint
r. styloid fracture
r. tuberosity
r. wedge osteotomy
r. wrist extensor tendinitis

radiale
ligamentum collaterale r.
ligamentum collaterale carpi r.

radialis
r. brevis
flexor carpi r.

radiatum
ligamentum capitis costae r.
ligamentum carpi r.

radicotomy

radiculectomy

radiculitis
cervical r.

radiculopathy

radii (plural of radius)

radiobicipital

radiocapitate ligament

radiocapitellar
r. articulation
r. joint

radiocarpal
r. arthritis

271

radiocarpal *(continued)*
    r. arthrodesis
    r. arthroscopy
    r. articulation
    r. joint
    r. ligament

radiocarpus

radiodigital

radiohumeral

RadioLucent wrist fixation system

radiolunate fusion

radiopraxis

radioscaphocapitate (RSC)

radioscaphoid
    r. fusion

radioscapholunate

radiotriquetral ligament

radioulnar

radius *pl.* radii
    r. of angulation
    annular ligament of r.
    r. curvus
    Kapandji fracture of r.
    ligamentum anulare radii
    proximal r.
    tuber of r.

radix
    r. arcus vertebrae

Ragnell retractor

Raimondi hemostatic forceps

raising
    straight leg r. (SLR)

Ralks bone drill

raloxifene hydrochloride

Ralston-Thompson pseudarthrosis technique

ramus *pl.* rami
    dorsal r.

ramus *(continued)*
    gray r. communicans
    r. inferior ossis ischii
    r. inferior ossis pubis
    dorsal r.
    ischial r.
    ischiopubic r.
    r. ischiopubicus
    r. of ischium
    r. ossis ischii
    r. ossis pubis
    pubic r., inferior
    pubic r., superior
    r. of pubis
    r. of pubis, ascending
    r. of pubis, descending
    r. superior ossis ischii
    r. superior ossis pubis

Ranawat classification

Raney
    R. bone drill
    R. perforator drill
    R.-Crutchfield drill point

range
    active r. of movement
    r. of excursion
    r. of movement

range of motion (ROM)
    active r. o. m.
    active-assisted r. o. m.
    active ankle joint complex
      r. o. m. (AAROM)
    active integral r. o. m.
      (AIROM)
    active and passive r. o. m.
    back r. o. m. (BROM)
    r. o. m. exercise
    passive r. o. m.

raphe
    anterolateral r.
    median r.

Rappaport osteotomy

rasp
    Aufricht glabellar r.
    carbon-tungsten r.

rasp *(continued)*
    Coryllos r.
    Doyen costal r.
    Farabeuf-Collin r.
    femoral r.
    Gallagher r.
    Langenbeck r.
    ulnar r.

Rastelli prosthesis

ratio
    abductor/adductor
      (AB/AD) r.
    ankle/brachial pressure r.
    Blackburne-Peel r.
    external/internal rotation r.
    Insall-Salvati r.
    metaphyseal to diaphyseal
      width r.
    Poisson r.
    vastus medialis obliquus/
      vastus lateralis r.

Rauchfuss sling

ravuconazole

Ray
    R. screw
    R. TFC (threaded fusion
      cage)

ray
    r. amputation
    long axis r.
    metatarsal r.
    pollical r.
    pollicized r.

RC
    rotator cuff

REACT muscle stimulator

reaction
    r. of degeneration
    r. of exhaustion
    implant r.
    Jolly r.
    lengthening r.
    myasthenic r.
    neurotonic r.
    shortening r.

reaction *(continued)*
    vagal r.

Read gouge

realignment
    Galeazzi r.
    Genutrain PE patellar r.
    patellar r.

reamer
    acetabular r.
    acorn r.
    Anspach r.
    Arthrex coring r.
    Aufranc r.
    Austin Moore r.
    ball r.
    blunt tapered T-handled r.
    bone r.
    brace-type r.
    calcar r.
    cannulated Henderson r.
    Caparosa r.
    chamfer r.
    Charnley r.
    Charnley deepening r.
    Charnley trochanter r.
    concave-surface r.
    conical r.
    deepening r.
    DePuy r.
    expanding r.
    fenestrated r.
    flexible medullary r.
    Hall Versipower r.
    hollow mill r.
    humeral r.
    Intracone intramedullary r.
    Küntscher r.
    medullary canal r.
    Norton ball r.
    Perthes r.
    Rush rod awl r.
    Smith-Petersen r.
    spiral cortical r.
    spiral trochanteric r.
    step-cut r.
    T-handled r.
    trochanteric r.
    Wagner acetabular r.

rearfoot

recalcitrant
   r. pain
   r. plantar fasciitis

receptor
   epicritic r.
   nociceptive r.
   paciniform r's

recess
   accessory r. of elbow
   acetabular r.
   annular periradial r.
   Flatt r.
   lateral r.
   popliteal r.
   sacciform r. of articulation
      of elbow

recessus
   r. sacciformis articulationis
      cubiti
   r. sacciformis articulationis
      radioulnaris distalis
   r. subpopliteus

reciprocal
   r. innervation
   r. relaxation

reciprocating gait orthosis
   (RGO)

Recklinghausen
   R. disease
   R. disease of bone

Recon
   R. nail
   R. proximal drill guide bolt

reconstruction
   ACL (anterior cruciate liga-
      ment) r.
   Andrews iliotibial band r.
   anterior capsulolabral r.
      (ACLR)
   arthroscopically-assisted
      anterior cruciate liga-
      ment r.

reconstruction *(continued)*
   Bankart r.
   Brown knee joint r.
   capsular-shift r.
   Chrisman-Snook r. of ankle
      ligament
   Clancy cruciate ligament r.
   cruciate ligament r.
   d'Aubigné femoral r.
   d'Aubigné resection r.
   Ellison lateral knee r.
   Elmslie r.
   endoscopic anterior cruci-
      ate ligament r.
   Eriksson cruciate liga-
      ment r.
   Evans lateral ankle r.
   extraarticular r.
   Goldner r.
   Harmon hip r.
   Hughston-Degenhardt r.
   Hughston lateral compart-
      ment r.
   index metacarpophalangeal
      joint r.
   Insall anterior cruciate liga-
      ment r.
   intra-articular r.
   joint r.
   Jones-Ellison ACL (anterior
      cruciate ligament) r.
   juxtacubital r.
   Krukenberg hand r.
   Kugelberg r.
   Lange Achilles tendon r.
   Larson ligament r.
   lateral compartment r.
   Lee r.
   L'Episcopo hip r.
   Neer posterior shoulder r.
   O'Donoghue ACL (anterior
      cruciate ligament) r.
   osteoplastic r.
   sternoclavicular joint r.
   sural island flap for foot
      and hand r.
   tenoplastic r.
   Torg knee r.

reconstruction *(continued)*
    two-stage tendon graft r.
    Verdan osteoplastic
      thumb r.
    Vulpius Achilles tendon r.
    Watson-Jones r.
    Whitman femoral neck r.
    Zancolli r.

rectus
    r. abdominis
    r. femoris

recurrent
    r. hyperextension
    r. median nerve block
    r. patellar dislocation
    r. synovitis

recurvatum deformity

Redi-Trac traction apparatus

reduction
    Ace bandage r.
    Agee force-couple splint r.
    Allen open r. of calcaneal
      fracture
    Becton open r.
    calcaneal fracture r.
    closed r.
    concentric r.
    Cotton r. of elbow disloca-
      tion
    Crego hip r.
    delayed open r.
    Eaton closed r.
    Eaton-Malerich r.
    Essex-Lopresti open r.
    femoral neck fracture r.
    Ferguson hip r.
    r./fixation
    Flynn femoral neck frac-
      ture r.
    fracture r.
    r. of fracture
    fracture-dislocation r.
    hip r.
    incomplete r.
    internal fixation, closed r.
    Kaplan open r.

reduction *(continued)*
    King open r.
    Lange hip r.
    Lavine r.
    McBride hallux abductoval-
      gus r.
    McBride hallux valgus r.
    Moberg-Gedda open r.
    Neer open r.
    open r.
    open r. and internal fixa-
      tion (ORIF)
    r. osteotomy
    Paré r. of elbow dislocation
    Pratt open r.
    radial fracture r.
    Ridlon hip r.
    shoulder r.
    Speed-Boyd open r.
    spondylolisthesis r.
    sternoclavicular joint r.
    surgical r.
    swan-neck deformity r.
    r. syndactyly
    trial r.
    Weber-Brunner-Freuler
      open r.

reefing
    capsular r.
    median retinaculum r.

reflex
    accommodation r.
    Achilles tendon r.
    adductor r.
    ankle r.
    antigravity r.
    r. arc
    asymmetric incurvatum r.
    asymmetric tonic neck r.
    axon r.
    Babinski r.
    Bekhterev-Mendel r.
    biceps r.
    bulbocavernosus r.
    crossed extensor r.
    deep tendon r. (DTR)
    delayed r.

reflex *(continued)*
depressed r.
dorsal r.
elbow r.
extensor thrust r.
flexor withdrawal r.
Gordon r.
r. hammer
Hirschberg r.
Hoffmann r.
hyperactive deep tendon r.
hypoactive deep tendon r.
incurvatum r.
jaw opening r. (JOR)
knee jerk r.
Liddell and Sherrington r.
Mendel-Bekhterev r.
muscle stretch r.
muscular r.
myotatic r.
Oppenheim r.
patellar r.
patelloadductor r.
pectoral r.
plantar r.
quadriceps r.
radial r.
Remak r.
righting r.
scapular r.
scapulohumeral r.
somatosomatic r.
stretch r.
suprapatellar r.
tendon r.
tonic neck r.
triceps surae r.
ulnar r.
vertical suspension r.
viscerosomatic r.
von Bekhterev r.

Refobacin Palacos cement

regeneration of nerve

Regen flexion exercise

regio *pl.* regiones
r. antebrachialis
r. antebrachialis anterior

regio *(continued)*
r. antebrachialis posterior
r. antebrachii anterior
r. antebrachii posterior
r. brachialis anterior
r. brachialis posterior
r. brachii anterior
r. brachii posterior
r. calcanea
r. carpalis
r. carpalis anterior
r. carpalis posterior
r. cervicalis posterior
r. coxae
r. cruralis anterior
r. cruralis posterior
r. cruris
r. cruris anterior
r. cruris posterior
r. cubitalis
r. cubitalis anterior
r. cubitalis posterior
r. dorsalis manus
r. dorsalis pedis
r. femoralis
r. femoralis anterior
r. femoralis posterior
r. femoris
r. femoris anterior
r. femoris posterior
r. genualis anterior
r. genualis posterior
r. genus
r. genus anterior
r. genus posterior
r. manus
regiones membri inferioris
regiones membri superioris
r. metacarpalis
r. metatarsalis
r. nuchalis
r. palmaris
r. pedis
r. plantaris
r. retromalleolaris lateralis
r. retromalleolaris medialis
r. surae
r. suralis
r. talocruralis anterior

regio *(continued)*
    r. talocruralis posterior
    r. tarsalis

region
    ankle r.
    ankle r., anterior
    ankle r., posterior
    antebrachial r.
    anterior r. of arm
    anterior r. of forearm
    anterior r. of knee
    anterior r. of leg
    anterior r. of wrist
    calcaneal r.
    carpal r.
    carpal r., anterior
    carpal r., posterior
    crural r., anterior
    crural r., posterior
    cubital r.
    cubital r., anterior
    cubital r., posterior
    deltoid r.
    dorsal r. of foot
    extrapolar r.
    femoral r.
    foot r.
    hand r.
    heel r.
    hip r.
    knee r.
    metacarpal r.
    metatarsal r.
    metazonal r.
    r. of nape
    nuchal r.
    palmar r.
    physeal r.
    posterior r. of arm
    posterior r. of forearm
    posterior r. of knee
    posterior r. of leg
    posterior oblique fiber r.
    posterior r. of wrist
    posteromedial r.
    retromalleolar r., lateral
    retromalleolar r., medial
    superomedial r.
    sural r.

region *(continued)*
    talocrural r., anterior
    talocrural r., posterior
    true acetabular r.

Regnauld
    R. degeneration of MTP (metatarsophalangeal) joint
    R. enclavement
    R. modification of Keller arthroplasty
    R. procedure

Reichel syndrome

Reichert-Mundinger stereotactic device

Reinert acetabular extensile approach

relaxation
    reciprocal r.

release
    adductor tendon and lateral capsular r.
    anterior hip r.
    anterior shoulder r.
    alterolateral r.
    Beaty lateral r.
    brevis r.
    capsular r.
    carpal tunnel r.
    circumferential periosteal r.
    complete subtalar r.
    Dupuytren contracture r.
    Eberle contracture r.
    ectopic carpal tunnel r. (ECTR)
    endoscopic carpal tunnel r.
    Endotrac endoscopic carpal tunnel r.
    extensile r.
    fascial r.
    Ferkel bipolar r.
    flexor–hallucis longus tendon r.
    flexor-pronator origin r.
    Guyon tunnel r.

release *(continued)*
    hamstring r.
    joint r.
    key r.
    lateral r.
    leg compartment r.
    ligamentous r.
    myofascial r.
    Ober r.
    patellar retinacular r.
    patellar retinaculum r.
    plantar-lateral r.
    plantar-medial r.
    plantar plate r.
    posterolateral r.
    posteromedial r.
    pronator teres r.
    quadriceps r.
    radical flexor r.
    retinacular r.
    retrogeniculate hamstring r.
    tarsal tunnel r.
    tendon r.
    triceps surae r.
    trigger finger r.
    trigger thumb r.
    Turco r.
    ulnar nerve r.
    unipolar r.
    Williams-Haddad r.
    Z-plasty r.

reluxation

Remak reflex

removal
    Winograd nail plate r.

Renografin contrast medium

repair
    ACL (anterior cruciate ligament) r.
    acromioclavicular joint r.
    Bankart shoulder r.
    Becker tendon r.
    bone graft r.
    Bosworth tendo calcaneus r.
    brachial plexus r.
    Bunnell tendon r.

repair *(continued)*
    Caspari r.
    dural r.
    DuVries hammertoe r.
    Ecker-Lotke-Glazer patellar tendon r.
    end-to-end tendon r.
    end-to-side r.
    epineurial r.
    extensor tendon r.
    fascicular r.
    five-in-one knee ligament r.
    flexor tendon r.
    Froimson-Oh r.
    glenohumeral dislocation r.
    group fascicular r.
    Jones first-toe r.
    Kelikian-Riashi-Gleason patellar tendon r.
    Kleinert r.
    Lindholm tendo calcaneus r.
    MacNab shoulder r.
    Ma-Griffith ruptured Achilles tendon r.
    Ma-Griffith tendo calcaneus r.
    Mandelbaum-Nartolozzi-Carney patellar tendon r.
    medial r.
    meniscal r.
    Palmer-Dobyns-Linscheid ligament r.
    patellar tendon r.
    pseudarthrosis r.
    rotator cuff r.
    shoulder r.
    Scuderi r.
    Speed sternoclavicular r.
    Strickland tendon r.
    suture r.
    tendo calcaneus r.
    tendon r.
    TEPP r.
    triad knee r.
    Turco r. of talipes equinovarus
    Turco-Spinella tendo calcaneus r.
    volar plate r.

repair *(continued)*
    Watson-Jones fracture r.

replacement
    allograft ligament r.
    Amstutz total hip r.
    calcar r.
    Charnley total hip r.
    Contour DF-80 total hip r.
    Ewald total elbow r.
    facet r.
    failed joint r.
    hip r.
    Howse total hip r.
    hybrid total hip r.
    intercalary segmental r.
    PCA (porous-coated anatomic) total hip r.
    SAF (self-articulating femoral) hip r.
    Stanmore r.
    total articular r.
    total elbow r.
    total hip r. (THR)
    total joint r.
    total knee r. (TKR)
    total ossicular r. (TORP)
    total shoulder r.
    total wrist r.

resection
    r. arthrodesis
    r. arthroplasty
    Badgley r. of iliac wing
    bony bridge r.
    calcaneal r.
    calcaneonavicular r.
    caudal lamina r.
    Darrach r.
    en bloc r.
    Enneking r.-arthrodesis
    epiphyseal bar r.
    femoral r.
    first rib r.
    Girdlestone r.
    iliac wing r.
    innominate bone r.
    intercalary r.
    Janecki-Nelson shoulder girdle r.
    Mankin r.

resection *(continued)*
    marginal r.
    medial eminence r.
    medial malleolus r.
    r. of the meniscus
    proximal femoral r.
    r.-realignment
    wedge r.

resector
    Accu-Line femoral r.
    Accu-Line tibial r.
    full-radius r.
    orthotome r.

resistance
    isometric r.
    strength against r.

resonator
    Jacobson r.

resorption
    bone r.
    osteoclastic r.

response
    average evoked r.
    decremental r.
    decrementing r.
    delayed r.
    evoked r.
    galvanic skin r.
    incremental r.
    paired r.
    plantar Babinski r.
    sensory r.
    visual evoked r.

resurfacing
    bone r.
    r. operation
    patellar r.
    Salzer r.

reticulum *pl.* reticula
    endoplasmic r.
    sarcoplasmic r.

retinaculum *pl.* retinacula
    r. of arcuate ligament
    r. capsulae articularis coxae
    caudal r.

retinaculum *(continued)*
    r. costae ultimae
    extensor r. of foot
    extensor r. of hand
    r. extensorum manus
    flexor r.
    flexor r. of foot
    flexor r. of hand
    r. flexorum manus
    inferior extensor r. of foot
    inferior peroneal r.
    lateral patellar r.
    r. ligamenti arcuati
    medial patellar r.
    r. musculorum extensorum
      inferius pedis
    r. musculorum extensorum
      manus
    r. musculorum extensorum
      pedis inferius
    r. musculorum extensorum
      pedis superius
    r. musculorum extensorum
      superius pedis
    r. musculorum fibularium
      inferius
    r. musculorum fibularium
      superius
    r. musculorum flexorum
      manus
    r. musculorum flexorum
      pedis
    r. musculorum peroneorum
      inferius
    r. musculorum peroneorum
      superius
    r. patellae laterale
    r. patellae mediale
    patellar r.
    superior extensor r. of foot
    superior peroneal r.
    r. tendinum
    r. tendinum musculorum
      extensorum
    r. tendinum musculorum
      extensorum inferius
    r. tendinum musculorum
      extensorum superius
    r. tendinum musculorum
      flexorum

retinaculum *(continued)*
    Weitbrecht r.

retraction

retractor
    Adson hemilaminectomy r.
    Allport r.
    amputation r.
    Army-Navy r.
    Aufranc cobra r.
    Badgley laminectomy r.
    Balfour self-retaining r.
    Ballantine hemilaminecto-
      my r.
    Beckman r.
    Bertin hip r.
    Blount knee r.
    Bodner r.
    Busenkell posterior hip r.
    Carroll-Bennett r.
    Chandler knee r.
    Charnley pin r.
    Charnley self-retaining r.
    Cloward blade r.
    Collis r.
    Collis-Taylor r.
    Crego r.
    Cushing r.
    Darrach r.
    Deaver r.
    D'Errico r.
    Downey hemilaminecto-
      my r.
    Finochietto rib r.
    Freebody-Steinmann r.
    Fukuda humeral head r.
    Gelpi r.
    hand-held r.
    Hayes r.
    Hedblom rib r.
    Henning meniscal r.
    Hibbs r.
    Hibbs-type r.
    hip r.
    Hoen r.
    Hohmann r.
    Holscher knee r.
    Homan r.
    humeral head r.
    Kasdan r.

retractor *(continued)*
 knee r.
 Kocher r.
 Lange bone r.
 Luongo hand r.
 McCullough r.
 Markham-Meyerding r.
 Mark II concave total
  knee r.
 Mark II lateral collateral ligament r.
 Mark II modular weight r.
 Mark II "S" total knee r.
 Mark II wide PCL knee r.
 Mayo-Collins r.
 Meyerding r.
 Myers knee r.
 Müller r.
 Ollier rake r.
 Paulson knee r.
 Ragnell r.
 rib r.
 Sauerbruch r.
 Schink metatarsal r.
 Scoville r.
 self-retaining r.
 Senn r.
 Sims r.
 Smillie r.
 Sofield r.
 Volkmann rake r.
 Wagner r.
 Watanabe r.
 Weit-Arner r.
 Weitlaner r.
 Wichman r.

retroacetabular lesion

retrocalcaneal
 r. bursitis
 r. exostosis

retrocollic

retrocollis

retrocrural

retroflexion

retrogeniculate hamstring release

retrolisthesis

retropatellar
 r. fat pad

retroperitoneal
 r. decompression

retropulsed

retropulsion of gait

retrospondylolisthesis

retrotorsion
 femoral r.
 tibial r.

retroversion
 femoral r.

revascularization
 endosteal r.

Revelation hip system

Reverdin
 R. bunionectomy
 R. osteotomy
 R.-Green foot procedure
 R.-Green osteotomy
 R.-Laird bunionectomy
 R.-McBride bunionectomy

reverse
 r. Colles fracture
 r.-cutting meniscal probe
 r. Hill-Sachs lesion
 r. Lasègue test
 r. Monteggia fracture
 r. Phalen test
 r. pivot shift
 r. Putti-Platt procedure
 r. threaded screw
 r. wedge osteotomy

ReVision nail

Revo knot

Rezaian external fixation apparatus

RGO
 reciprocating gait orthosis

rhabdomyolysis
 exertional r.

rhabdomyoma

rhaebocrania

rhaeboscelia

rhaebosis

rheobase

rheostosis

rheumatalgia

rheumatic

rheumatism
  articular r., chronic
  Besnier r.
  Heberden r.
  muscular r.
  palindromic r.
  Poncet r.
  subacute r.
  tuberculous r.

Rhinelander pin

rhizomelic

rhizomesomelic bone dysplasia

rhizotomy
  intradural dorsal spinal
    root r.
  posterior r.

rhomboideus
  r. major muscle
  r. minor muscle

rhomboid flap

Rhoton
  R. elevator
  R. osteotome

rib
  abdominal r's
  asternal r's
  bicipital r.
  r. cage
  cervical r.
  false r's
  floating r's
  slipping r.

rib *(continued)*
  spurious r's
  sternal r's
  Stiller r.
  true r's
  vertebral r's
  vertebrocostal r's
  vertebrosternal r's

Rica
  R. bone drill
  R. wire guidepin

Ricard amputation

Richards
  R. angle guide
  R. arthrodesis
  R. bone clamp
  R. classic compression hip
    screw
  R. drill guide
  R. hip endoprosthesis sys-
    tem
  R. lag screw
  R. locking rod
  R. modular hip system
  R. modular stem
  R. pistol-grip drill
  R. sideplate
  R. Zirconia femoral head
    prosthesis
  R.-Colles external fixator
  R.-Hirschorn plate

Richmond subarachnoid screw

Richter bone drill

rickets
  adult r.
  anticonvulsant r.
  autosomal dominant vita-
    min D–resistant r.
  familial hypophosphate-
    mic r.
  florid r.
  hepatic r.
  hereditary hypophospha-
    temic r. with hypercalci-
    uria
  hypophosphatemic r.

rickets *(continued)*
    oncogenous r.
    pseudodeficiency r.
    pseudovitamin D–deficiency r.
    refractory r.
    vitamin D–dependent r., type I
    vitamin D–dependent r., type II
    vitamin D–refractory r.
    vitamin D–resistant r.

ridge
    bicipital r., anterior
    bicipital r., external
    bicipital r., internal
    bicipital r., outer
    bicipital r., posterior
    deltoid r.
    epicondylic r., lateral
    epicondylic r., medial
    gastrocnemial r.
    gluteal r. of femur
    r. of humerus
    interarticular r. of head of rib
    interosseous r. of fibula
    interosseous r. of radius
    interosseous r. of tibia
    interosseous r. of ulna
    intertrochanteric r.
    middle r. of femur
    r. of neck of rib
    oblique r's of scapula
    osteochondral r.
    Outerbridge r.
    pectoral r.
    radial r. of wrist
    rough r. of femur
    supinator r.
    supracondylar r. of humerus, lateral
    supracondylar r. of humerus, medial
    supraepicondylar r. of humerus, lateral
    supraepicondylar r. of humerus, medial
    transverse r's of sacrum

ridge *(continued)*
    trapezoid r.
    tubercular r. of sacrum
    ulnar r. of wrist
    vastus lateralis r.

Ridlon hip reduction

Rieger phenomenon

righting reflex

rim
    acetabular r.
    alar r.
    glenoid r.
    sclerotic marginal r.
    tibial r.

Ring
    R. knee prosthesis
    R. total hip prosthesis

ring
    r. block anesthesia
    epiphyseal r.
    fibroosseous r. of Lacroix
    fibrous r. of intervertebral disk
    fibrous r. of Lacroix
    r. fracture
    interpubic fibrous r.
    Ilizarov r.
    ischial weightbearing r.
    orthosis drop-back r.
    osseous r. of Lacroix
    pelvic r.
    perichondral r.
    periosteal bone r.
    protrusio r.
    proximal-to-distal r.
    reduction r.
    r. sublimus aponeuroplasty
    V1 halo r.

Riordan finger opponensplasty

Risser
    R. jacket
    R. turnbuckle cast
    R.-Stille pin

Robert Jones splint

Robert ligament

Rochester
    R. lamina elevator
    R. recipient bone cutter

rocker-bottom
    r.-b. deformity
    r.-b. flatfoot
    r.-b. foot

Rockwood anterior acromio-
    plasty

rod
    Acufex TAG r.
    alignment guide r.
    Alta CFX reconstruction r.
    Alta tibial-humeral r.
    autoreinforced polyglyco-
        lide r.
    Bailey-Dubow r.
    Bickel intramedullary r.
    Biofix absorbable r's and
        screws
    compression r.
    compressive r.
    Cotrel-Dubousset r.
    Dacron-impregnated sili-
        cone r.
    distraction r.
    Ender r.
    Enneking r.
    Fixateur Interne r.
    Harrington r.
    Harrington compression r.
    hinge r.
    Hunter Silastic r.
    impacter r.
    intramedullary alignment r.
    Isola spinal implant system
        eye r.
    Kaneda r.
    Knodt r.
    Luque r.
    Moe modified Harrington r.
    Moe square-end r.
    Mouradian r.
    muscle r.
    Polarus humeral r.
    Richards locking r.
    Rush r.
    Sage r.

rod (continued)
    Schneider r.
    screw alignment r.
    Serrato forearm r.
    silicone-Dacron tendon r.
    spinal fixation r.
    Stenzel r.
    telescopic r.
    tendon r.
    threaded r.
    V-A alignment r.
    Wiltse system spinal r.
    Wissinger r.
    Zickel r.
    Zielke r.

rod bender
    DePuy r. b.
    Luque r. b.

roentgenogram
    biplane r.
    lateral r.

roentgenography
    preoperative r.
    intraoperative r.

Roger Anderson splint

Rogozinski
    R. screw system
    R. spinal fixation
    R. spinal fixation system

Rohadur
    R. gait plate

Roho
    R. bed
    R. heel pad

Rokitansky pelvis

Rolando fracture

Rollett secondary substance

Rolyan
    R. arm elevator
    R. tibial fracture brace

ROM
    range of motion
        ROM knee brace

Romberg test

Rome criteria for rheumatoid
arthritis

rongeur
Adson r.
angular bone r.
Bacon bone r.
Baer bone r.
Bane bone r.
Bane-Hartmann bone r.
basket r.
Beyer r.
Beyer-Stille r.
Beyer-Stille bone r.
Blumenthal bone r.
Bruening-Citelli r.
Campbell r.
Cicherelli bone r.
Cleveland bone r.
Cloward r.
Colclough laminectomy r.
Corbett bone r.
Cushing r.
Defourmental r.
downbiting r.
duckbill r.
Echlin duckbill r.
Ferris Smith r.
Ferris Smith–Spurling
disk r.
flat-bottomed Kerrison r.
r. forceps
Friedman bone r.
Guleke bone r.
Hartmann bone r.
Hein r.
Hoen r.
Jackson intervertebral
disk r.
Kerrison downbiting r.
Kleinert-Kutz synovecto-
my r.
Lebsche r.
Leksell r.
Lempert r.
Liston-Littauer r.
Luer bone r.
Markwalder bone r.
McIndoe bone r.
Montenovesi r.

rongeur *(continued)*
Ruskin r.
Schleisinger cervical r.
Smith-Petersen r.
Spurling r.
Stille r.
Stille-Luer bone r.
Super Cut laminectomy r.
upbiting r.
upcut r.

Rood method

Roos
R. approach
R. rib cutter

root
r. of arch of vertebra
cervical r.
r. infiltration
nerve r.

Root-Siegal varus derotational
osteotomy

Rorabeck fasciotomy

Rosenfeld hip prosthesis

Rosen splint

Rossiter System *(stretching program)*

Rotablator rotating bur

rotation
Borggreve limb r.
cervical r. in extension
external r. in extension
(ERE)
external r. in flexion (ERF)
r. fracture
Hermodsson internal r.
hip r.
knee r.
patellar r.
pelvic r.
pronation–external r.
(P-ER)
supination–external r.
van Ness r.

rotationplasty
Kotz-Salzer r.

rotationplasty *(continued)*
  tibial hindfoot osteomusculocutaneous r.
  van Ness r.
  Winkelmann r.

rotator
  r. cuff tear
  r. cuff tendinitis
  Howmedica monotube external r.

rotatory
  r. atlantoaxial subluxation
  r. torque
  r.-variable-differential transducer

Rotorloc

rouleaux formation

Rousek extender

Roux-duToit staple capsulorrhaphy

Roy-Camille plate

RSC
  radioscaphocapitate

RSDCP plate

rubra vera

Ruedi fracture

rugby knee

ruler
  Berndt hip r.

rupture
  Achilles tendon r. (ATR)

rupture *(continued)*
  adductor longus muscle r.
  buttonhole r.
  flexor tendon r.

ruptured disk

Rush
  bevel-point R. pin
  R. bone clamp
  R. flexible medullary nail
  R. intramedullary fixation pin
  R. pin reamer awl
  R. rod
  R. rod awl reamer

Ruskin
  R. rongeur
  R.-Liston bone cutting forceps

Russe bone graft

Russell
  R. fibular head autograft
  R. splint
  R. traction
  R.-Silver dwarfism

Rust
  R. disease
  R. phenomenon
  R. sign
  R. syndrome

Rydell nail

Ryerson
  R. bone graft
  R. triple arthrodesis

saber-cut incision

Sabolich socket system

sac
  bursal s.
  thecal s.

SACH
  solid ankle, cushioned heel
    SACH foot
    SACH foot adaptor
    SACH orthopedic heel

sacral
  s. agenesis
  s. ala
  s. alar screw
  s. arcuate line
  s. base angle
  s. horizontal plane line
  s. nerve root sparing
  s. pedicle screw fixation
  s. plexus
  s. promontory
  s. spine decompression
  s. spine fixation
  s. spine modular instru-
    mentation
  s. tilt
  s. triangle

sacralgia

sacralization

sacrarthrogenic

sacrectomy

sacrococcygeal

sacrococcyx

sacrocoxalgia

sacrocoxitis

sacrodynia

sacrofemoral angle

sacrohorizontal angle

sacroiliac
  s. disarticulation

sacroiliac *(continued)*
  s. extension fixation
  s. flexion fixation
  s. joint
  s. joint arthroplasty
  s. orthosis
  s. subluxation

sacroiliitis

sacrolisthesis

sacrolumbar

sacropromontory

sacrosciatic

sacrospinal

sacrospinous

sacrotomy

sacrotuberale
  ligamentum s.

sacrotuberous ligament

sacrovertebral
  s. angle

sacrum
  assimilation s.
  s. fusion screw fixation
  scimitar s.
  tilted s.

SAF
  self-articulating femoral
    SAF hip replacement

SAFHS
  Sonic Accelerated Fracture
    Healing System
    SAFSH 2000

Safir pin

Sage
  S. cheilectomy
  S. forearm nail
  S. rod
  S. tibial nail
  S.-Clark cheilectomy

sagittal
  s. kyphosis
  s. pedicle angle
  s. plane
  s.-Z osteotomy

Sakoff osteotomy

Salenius meniscus knife

salicylate
  sodium s.

salt
  bone s's
  gold s.

saltans
  coxa s.

Salter
  S. epiphyseal fracture
  S. fracture
  S. innominate osteotomy
  S. pelvic osteotomy
  S.-Harris fracture

Salzer resurfacing

Samilson crescentic calcaneal
  osteotomy

Sampson
  S. medullary nail
  S. prosthesis

Samuels forceps

sanguineous

Sapphire View arthroscope

sarcoenchondroma

sarcogenic

sarcolemma

sarcolemmic

sarcolemmous

sarcoma
  bicompartmental soft-tis-
    sue s.
  chondroblastic s.

sarcoma *(continued)*
  Ewing s.
  extracompartmental soft-
    tissue s.
  fibroblastic s.
  giant cell s.
  high-grade surface osteo-
    genic s.
  intracortical osteogenic s.
  Kaposi s.
  multicentric osteogenic s.
  multipotential primary s. of
    bone
  osteoblastic s.
  osteogenic s.
  parosteal s.
  synovial s.

sarcomere

sarcopenia

sarcoplasm

sarcoplasmic

sarcoplast

sarcopoietic

sarcostyle

sarcotubules

sarcous

Sarmiento
  S. fracture brace
  S. hip prosthesis
  S. intertrochanteric osteot-
    omy
  S. nail

sartorius
  s. muscle
  s. tendon

SAS
  Shoulder Arm System
    SAS II brace

Satterlee bone saw

Saturn splint

saucerization

Sauerbruch
S. prosthesis
S. retractor
S. rib elevator
S. rib forceps

Sauvé-Kapandji arthroplasty

SAVANT
Surgical Anatomy Visualization and Navigation Tools

Savastano
S. hemiknee
S. hemiknee prosthesis

saw
Adams s.
Aesculap s.
air-driven oscillating s.
amputating s.
bone s.
Butcher s.
Charriere s.
Charriere bone s.
Cottle s.
crescentic s.
end-cutting reciprocating s.
Engel plaster s.
Gigli s.
Hall Versipower oscillating s.
Henschke-Mauch s.
Hey s.
Horsley bone s.
humeral s.
Langenbeck bone s.
Lebsche wire s.
Luck-Bishop bone s.
Miltex bone s.
Mitek bone s.
Osada s.
reciprocating motor s.
Satterlee bone s.
Shrady s.
Sklar bone s.
subcutaneous s.
Tuke s.
Zimmer oscillating s.

Sawa shoulder brace

Sayre
S. apparatus
S. elevator
S. splint

Sbarbaro
S. hip prosthesis
S. spica cast
S. tibial plateau prosthesis

scaffold
collagen s.
VITOSS s.

scale
Arthritis Impact Measurement S. (AIMS)

scalene
s. block
s. fascia
s. maneuver

scalenectomy

scalenotomy

scalenus
s. anticus muscle
s. anticus syndrome

scalpel
Bard-Parker s.

scan
adenosine thallium s.
DEXA (dual-energy x-ray absorption) s.

Scand pin

scaphocapitate
s. fusion

scaphocapitolunate (SCL) arthrodesis

scaphoid
bipartite s.
s. bone
carpal s.
s. fracture

scaphoid *(continued)*
  s. nonunion

scaphoiditis
  tarsal s.

scaphoid-lunate *(see* scapholunate)

scapholunate *(also* scaphoid-lunate)
  s. angle
  s. dissociation
  s. interosseous ligament

scaphotrapeziotrapezoid arthrodesis

scaphotrapezoid-trapezial

scapula *pl.* scapulae
  alar s.
  s. alata
  elevated s.
  Graves s.
  scaphoid s.
  winged s.

scapulalgia

scapular
  s. approximation test
  s. ligament
  s. notch

scapulectomy
  Das Gupta s.
  Phelps s.

scapuloclavicular
  s. articulation

scapulodynia

scapulohumeral

scapuloperoneal

scapulopexy

scapulothoracic
  s. arthrodesis
  s. fusion
  s. muscle

scapulovertebral border

Scarpa
  ligament of S.

SCD
  sequential compression device

scelalgia

Schäfer
  dumbbells of S.

Schanz
  S. angulation osteotomy
  S. collar
  S. collar brace
  S. disease
  S. femoral osteotomy
  S. osteotomy
  S. screw
  S. syndrome

Schatzker tibial plateau fracture

Schauwecker
  S. patellar tension band wire
  S. patellar wiring

Schede
  S. bone curet
  S. hip osteotomy
  S. operation

Schepens hollow silicone hemisphere implant material

Scheuermann
  S. disease
  S. dystrophic spondylosis
  S. kyphosis

Schink metatarsal retractor

schistorachis

schizotonia

Schlatter
  S. disease
  S. sprain
  S.-Osgood disease

Schlein
  S. elbow arthroplasty

Schlein *(continued)*
S. trisurface ankle prosthesis

Schleisinger cervical rongeur

Schlemm ligaments

Schmid metaphyseal dyostosis

Schmorl
S. body
S. disease
S. node

Schneider
S. extractor
S. rod

Schnute wedge resection technique

Schönlein
S. disease
S. purpura

Schrudde rotational flap

Schwann cell

Schwartz
S. clip-applying forceps
S. dorsiflexory osteotomy

Schwartze chisel

Schwediauer *(variant of* Swediaur)

Schweitzer
S. pin
S. spring plate

sciatic
s. foramen
s. leg block
s. nerve injury
s. notch

sciatica

scintigraphy
bone s.
paired s.

scissors
meniscal s.

scissors *(continued)*
Sistron s.
Sistrunk s.
Smillie meniscal s.

SCIWORA
spinal cord injury without
radiographic abnormality
SCIWORA syndrome

SCL
scaphocapitolunate
SCL arthrodesis

sclerosing
s. osteomyelitis

sclerosis *pl.* scleroses
amyotrophic lateral s.
anterolateral s.
diaphyseal s.
endplate s.
Mönckeberg s.
systemic s.

sclerotic

sclerotomal pain

sclerozone

Scoffert triple arthrodesis

SCOI
Southern California Ortho-
pedic Institute
SCOI stitch

scoliokyphosis

scoliorachitic

scoliosiometry

scoliosis
adolescent s.
adolescent idiopathic s.
(AIS)
Aussies-Isseis unstable s.
s. brace
Brissaud s.
cicatricial s.
congenital s.
Cotrel s.
coxitic s.

scoliosis *(continued)*
- dextrorotary s.
- empyematic s.
- fracture with s.
- functional s.
- Galen s.
- habit s.
- idiopathic s.
- inflammatory s.
- ischiatic s.
- King-Moe s.
- kyphosing s.
- levorotary s.
- levoscoliosis
- myopathic s.
- neuromuscular s.
- ocular s.
- ophthalmic s.
- osteopathic s.
- paralytic s.
- rachitic s.
- rheumatic s.
- rotational s.
- sciatic s.
- static s.
- thoracolumbar spine s.

scoliotic

scoliotone

scolopsia

score
- Fries s. for rheumatoid arthritis
- Glasgow coma s. (GCS)
- Merle-d'Aubigné hip s.

Scorpio total knee system

Scott humeral splint

Scottish Rite
- S. R. brace
- S. R. hip orthosis
- S. R. splint

Scoville
- angled S. curet
- S. curet
- S. retractor

screw
- AcroMed s.
- alar s.
- Alta s.
- Alta cancellous s.
- Alta cortical s.
- Alta cross-locking s.
- Alta lag s.
- Alta transverse s.
- AMBI compression hip s.
- AMBI hip s.
- anchor s.
- AO-ASIF s.
- AO cancellous s.
- AO spongiosa s.
- Arthrex sheathed interference s.
- arthrodesis s.
- ASIF s.
- Asnis cannulated cancellous s.
- Aten olecranon s.
- axial compression s.
- Barouk cannulated bone s.
- Basile hip s.
- Bechtol s.
- bicortical s.
- Biofix absorbable rods and s's
- Bionix absorbable cannulated s.
- BioRCI bioabsorbable s.
- BioSorbFX SR plate and s.
- Bone Mulch s.
- Bosworth coracoclavicular s.
- buttress thread s.
- Campbell cannulated s.
- cancellous bone s.
- CAPIS s.
- Carrell-Girard s.
- cervical s.
- cervical s. insertion
- compression hip s.
- Concise compression hip s.
- CorIS interference s.
- cortical cancellous s.
- Cotrel pedicle s.

screw *(continued)*
- Coventry s.
- Cubbins s.
- DeMuth hip s.
- DePuy interference s.
- Deyerle s.
- distal locking s.
- Duo-Drive s.
- Dynamic condylar s.
- Eggers s.
- Fabian s.
- Fixateur Interne s.
- Glasgow s.
- Glass-Bessen transfixion s.
- glenoid fixation s.
- Guardian femoral s.
- Heck s.
- Herbert scaphoid s.
- hex s.
- Howmedica ICS s.
- Ilizarov s.
- interfragmentary lag s.
- Isola vertebral s.
- Johannson lag s.
- lag s.
- Lane bone s.
- Leinbach olecranon s.
- Leone expansion s.
- Lorenzo s.
- Luhr s.
- lumbar pedicle s.
- Luque pedicle s.
- McLaughlin carpal scaphoid s.
- malleolar s.
- maxillofacial bone s.
- Medoff axial compression s.
- mille pattes s.
- Moberg s.
- Mouradian s.
- Neufeld s.
- No-Lok s.
- Olerud PSF s.
- Ormandy s.
- Orthofix s.
- Osteomed s.
- Palex expansion s.

screw *(continued)*
- Palmer s.
- pedicle s.
- plate-s.
- plate and s.
- polyaxial cervical s.
- Propel cannulated interference s.
- Ray s.
- reverse threaded s.
- Richards classic compression hip s.
- Richards lag s.
- Richmond subarachnoid s.
- sacral alar s.
- Schanz s.
- Scuderi s.
- self-tapping bone s.
- Sharpey s.
- Simmons-Martin s.
- spongiosa s.
- Spontak pedicle s.
- Steffee s.
- Stryker lag s.
- syndesmotic s.
- Synthes compression hip s.
- threaded cancellous s.
- titanium s.
- Tivanium cancellous bone s.
- traction tongs s.
- transarticular s.
- transfixion s.
- triangulated pedicle s.
- TSRH pedicle s.
- Venable s.
- Vitallium s.
- VLC compression s.
- Wagner-Schanz s.
- Weise jack s.
- Woodruff s.
- Yuan s.
- Zimmer compression s.
- Zimmer compresssion hip s.
- Zuelzer s.

screwdriver
- Allen head s.
- Cardan s.

screwdriver *(continued)*
Lane s.

screw-plate
Calandruccio impaction s.-p.
Zimmer impaction s.-p.

SCS
spinal canal stenosis

SCSP
supracondylar-suprapatel-
lar

Scuderi
S. repair
S. screw
S. technique

scutum
s. pectoris

S-D-port

S-D-sorb
S. E-Z Tac system
S. meniscal stapler

SDBT
segmentally demineralized
bone technology

seal-fin deformity

seam
osteoid s.

seat belt fracture

Seattle foot

Sebileau
S. muscle
S. periosteal elevator

Sedan goniometer

Seddon
S. dorsal spine costotrans-
versectomy
S. modification

Sédillot periosteal elevator

segmentally demineralized
bone

Segmented Orthopaedic System
(S.O.S.)

Segond fracture

Seidel bone-holding clamp

self-articulating
s.-a. femoral (SAF) hip replacement

self-broaching

self-centering Universal hip
prosthesis

self-curing polymer

self-locking nail

self-sealing cannula

self-tapping bone screw

Selig hip operation

Selverstone rongeur forceps

semicanal of humerus

semilaminotomy

semilunar
s. bone
s. cartilage of knee joint
s. cartilage knife

semimembranous

semiopen sliding tenotomy

semipenniform

semitendinosus
s.-gracilis graft
s. graft
s. tendon transfer
s. tenodesis

semitendinous graft

Senegas hip approach

Senn
S. plate
S. retractor

sense
joint position s. (JPS)

SEP
somatosensory evoked po-
tential

separation
  AC joint s.
  acromioclavicular s.
  lamellar s.
  shoulder s.
  transepiphyseal s.

septum
  Bigelow s.
  s. of Cloquet
  crural s.
  femoral s.
  s. femorale
  s. femorale [Cloqueti]
  intermuscular s., anterior crural
  intermuscular s., posterior crural
  intermuscular s. of arm, external
  intermuscular s. of arm, internal
  intermuscular s. of arm, lateral
  intermuscular s. of arm, medial
  intermuscular s. of leg, anterior
  intermuscular s. of leg, posterior
  intermuscular s. of thigh, external
  intermuscular s. of thigh, lateral
  intermuscular s. of thigh, medial
  s. intermusculare anterius cruris
  s. intermusculare brachii laterale
  s. intermusculare brachii mediale
  s. intermusculare cruris anterius
  s. intermusculare cruris posterius
  s. intermusculare femoris laterale
  s. intermusculare femoris mediale

septum (continued)
  s. intermusculare humeri laterale
  s. intermusculare humeri mediale
  s. intermusculare posterius cruris

sequester

sequestral

sequestration
  disk s.

sequestrectomy

sequestrotomy

sequestrum
  avascular s.
  primary s.
  secondary s.
  tertiary s.

Seradge hand exercises

Series II humeral head

serosynovitis

Serrato forearm rod

service
  EpicelSM s.

sesamoid
  accessory s.
  bipartite tibial s.
  s. bone
  fibular s.
  hallucal s.
  s. ligament
  tibial s.

sesamoidectomy
  fibular s.

sesamoideum

sesamoidometatarsal joint

sesamophalangeal ligament

set
  acetabular trial s.
  Bankart shoulder repair s.
  Brown-Mueller T-fastener s.

set *(continued)*
    phalangeal s.
    Stille bone drill s.

Seton hip brace

Sever disease

sexdigitate

shaft
    s. of femur
    s. of fibula
    s. of humerus
    s. of metacarpal bone
    s. of metatarsal bone
    ministem s.
    patellar reamer s.
    s. of phalanx of hand
    s. of phalanx of foot
    s. of radius
    s. of rib
    s. of tibia
    s. of ulna

shank
    calcar trimmer with Zim-
      mer-Hudson s.

Sharp acetabular angle

Sharpey
    S. fiber
    S. screw

SharpShooter

shaver
    arthroscopic s.
    Dyonics s.
    Kuda s.
    Microsect s.
    synovial s.

shaving
    femoral condylar s.

shear
    s. fracture
    s. maneuver
    s. testing
    vertical s.

shears
    Bethune-Coryllos rib s.

shears *(continued)*
    Brunn plaster s.
    Stille plaster s.

sheath
    arthroscope s.
    common s. of tendons of
      fibular muscles
    common s. of tendons of
      peroneal muscles
    fibroosseous s.
    fibrous s's of fingers
    fibrous s. of tendon
    fibrous s's of toes
    intertubercular mucous s.
    intertubercular synovial s.
    muscle s.
    mucous s's
    mucous s. of tendon
    mucous s's of tendons of
      fingers
    mucous s's of tendons of
      toes
    peroneal tendon s.
    plantar tendinous s. of long
      fibular muscle
    plantar tendinous s. of long
      peroneal muscle
    s. of plantar tendon of long
      fibular muscle
    s. of plantar tendon of long
      peroneal muscle
    rectus s.
    synovial s. of bicipital
      groove
    synovial s. of intertubercu-
      lar groove
    synovial s. of tendon
    synovial s. of tendons of
      foot
    tendinous s's of flexor mus-
      cles of fingers
    tendinous s's of flexor mus-
      cles of toes
    tendinous s. of leg
    tendon s.
    tendon s. of anterior tibial
      muscle
    tendon s's of long extensor
      muscles of toes

sheath *(continued)*
    tendon s's of long flexor
       muscles of toes
    tendon s. of posterior tibial
       muscle
    tenosynovial s.

Shepherd fracture

Sherrington law

Sherman plate

Shiatsu massage

shift
    reverse pivot s.

shin
    cucumber s.
    saber s.
    s. splints

SHIP-Shaw rod hammertoe im-
    plant

shoe
    Ambulator s's

shortening
    femoral diaphyseal s.
    femoral metaphyseal s.
    Winquist-Hansen-Pearson
       closed femoral diaphy-
       seal s.

shoulder
    s. ankylosis
    s. brace
    s. disarticulation
    drop s.
    frozen s.
    knocked-down s.
    loose s.
    s. reduction
    s. subluxation inhibitor
    stubbed s.

shoulderblade

Shrady saw

shunt
    Sundt s.

Shy-Magee syndrome

Sibson
    S. aponeurosis
    S. fascia
    S. groove

sideplate
    Richards s.

Sielke instrumentation

Siffert
    S. intraepiphyseal osteot-
       omy
    S.-Forster-Nachamie ar-
       throdesis

sign
    Achilles bulge s.
    Adson s.
    Allen s.
    Allis s.
    Amoss s.
    Anghelescu s.
    anterior drawer s.
    Apley s.
    apprehension s.
    Babinski s.
    Barlow s.
    Bassett s.
    Battle s.
    bayonet s.
    Bryant s.
    Burton s.
    Cantelli s.
    Chaddock s.
    Chvostek s.
    Cleeman s.
    click s.
    Codman s.
    cogwheel s.
    Comolli s.
    contralateral s.
    Coopernail s.
    dancing patella s.
    Darier s.
    Dawbarn s.
    Desault s.
    drawer s's
    Dugas s.
    Dupuytren s.

sign *(continued)*
  Egawa s.
  Ely s.
  Erichsen s.
  fabere s.
  fadir s.
  Fairbanks s.
  Forestier bowstring s.
  Froment paper s.
  Gaenslen s.
  Gage s.
  Galeazzi s.
  Goldthwait s.
  Gottron s.
  Gowers s.
  Guilland s.
  halo s.
  Hamman s.
  Hawkins s.
  Hawkins impingement s.
  Heberden s's
  heel varus s.
  Helbing s.
  Hill-Sachs s.
  Homans s.
  Hoover s.
  Hueter s.
  iliac apophysis s.
  impingement s.
  Jenet s.
  jerk s.
  Kanavel s.
  Keen s.
  Kehr s.
  Kernig s.
  Lachman s.
  Langoria s.
  Lasègue s.
  Laugier s.
  Léri s.
  L'hermitte s.
  Linder s.
  long tract s.
  Lorenz s.
  Ludington s.
  Ludloff s.
  Macewen s.
  McMurray s.
  Maisonneuve s.

sign *(continued)*
  Martel s.
  Matev s.
  Mendel-Bekhterev s.
  Mennell s.
  Minor s.
  Morquio s.
  Mudder s.
  Mulder s.
  Nelson s.
  Ober s.
  ocular s.
  Oppenheim s.
  Ortolani s.
  pathognomic s.
  Patrick s.
  Payr s.
  piriformis s.
  pivot shift s.
  positive impingement s.
  posterior drawer s.
  Queckenstedt s.
  Rust s.
  sciatic tension s.
  soft click s.
  soft pivot shift s.
  Soto-Hall s.
  Strümpell s.
  Strunsky s.
  sulcus s.
  thermoregulatory s.
  Thomas s.
  Thompson s.
  tibialis s.
  Tinel s.
  Trendelenburg s.
  trepidation s.
  Turyn s.
  vacant glenoid s.
  Vanzetti s.
  Voshell s.
  Waddell s.
  Wartenberg s.
  Wilson s.
  Winberger s.
  Yergason s.

Silastic
  S. ball spacer prosthesis

Silastic *(continued)*
    S. finger joint
    S. gel dressing
    S. joint
    S. lunate arthroplasty
    S. radial head prosthesis

silence
    electrical s.

Silflex intramedullary prosthesis

Silfverskiöld syndrome

silicone
    s. arthritis
    s.-Dacron tendon rod
    s. gel socket insert
    s. rubber arthroplasty
    s. synovitis
    s. thermoplastic splint
    s. trapezium prosthesis
    s. wrist arthroplasty

Silipos
    S. digital pad
    S. mesh cap

Silver
    S. bunionectomy
    S. operation
    S. osteotome

silver
    s. fork deformity
    s. fork fracture

Silverman syndrome

Simal cervical stabilization system

Simmerlin dystrophy

Simmonds
    S.-Menelaus metatarsal osteotomy
    S.-Menelaus proximal phalangeal osteotomy

Simmons-Martin screw

Simplex P bone cement

Simpson sugar-tong splint

Sims retractor

Sinding-Larsen
    S.-L. disease
    S.-L.–Johansson disease

sinew
    weeping s.

single
    s.-axis
    s. photon emisssion computed tomography (SPECT)
    s.-stage
    s.-stemmed silicone hemiprosthesis

sinus
    anterior s. of atlas
    articular s. of atlas
    articular s. of atlas, superior
    articular s. of axis, anterior
    articular s. of vertebrae, inferior
    s. condylorum femoris
    costal s's of sternum
    lunate s. of radius
    lunate s. of ulna
    middle s. of atlas
    osteomyelitic s.
    peroneal s. of tibia
    semilunar s. of tibia
    tarsal s.
    s. tarsi

Sisson fracture-reducing elevator

Sistron scissors

Sistrunk scissors

SITEtrac spinal surgery system

Sjögren syndrome

skelasthenia

skeleton
    appendicular s.
    s. appendiculare
    axial s.

skeleton *(continued)*
  s. axiale
  bony s.
  s. membri inferioris liberi
  s. membri superioris liberi
  thoracic s.
  s. thoracicus
  s. thoracis
  visceral s.

skewfoot

SKI knee prosthesis

Skillern fracture

Sklar
  S. bone saw
  S. pin cutter

Skoog
  S. fasciotomy
  S. procedure for release of
    Dupuytren contracture

SLAC
  scapholunate advanced
    collapse
      SLAC wrist

sleeve
  patellar s.

SLE-like syndrome

slide
  flexor pronator s.

sling
  arm elevator s.
  Glisson s.
  Haacker s.
  Harris Hemi-Arm s.
  hemiarm s.
  s. immobilization
  Kodel knee s.
  Legg-Perthes s.
  Mersilene s.
  Pavlik s.
  pouch-type s.
  Rauchfuss s.
  soft tissue coaptation s.
  stockinette s.
  Thomas Kodel s.

sling *(continued)*
  triangle s.
  Uni-Versatil s.
  Velpeau s.
  Vogue arm s.
  Weil pelvic s.

slipped disk

Slocum
  S. anterior rotary drawer
    test
  S. fusion technique
  S. lateral pivot-shift test
  S. maneuver
  S. meniscal clamp
  S. nail
  S. pes anserinus transplant
  S. test

SLR
  straight leg raising

slurry
  bone marrow s.
  bony s.
  matrix–bone marrow s.

Smart-Magnetix prosthetic device for amputees

SmartScrew

Smedberg
  S. brace
  S. hand drill

Smedley dynamometer

Smillie
  S. cartilage chisel
  S. cartilage knife
  S. meniscal knife
  S. meniscal scissors
  S. meniscectomy chisel
  S. nail
  S. pin
  S. retractor
  S.-Beaver blade
  S.-Beaver knife

Smith
  S. cartilage knife
  S. dislocation

Smith *(continued)*
S. fracture
S.-Petersen cup arthro-
plasty
S.-Petersen curved gouge
S.-Petersen curved osteo-
tome
S.-Petersen hemiarthro-
plasty
S.-Petersen impactor
S.-Petersen intertrochan-
teric plate
S.-Petersen nail
S.-Petersen osteotomy
S.-Petersen reamer
S.-Petersen rongeur
S.-Petersen sacroiliac joint
fusion
S.-Petersen straight osteo-
tome
S.-Petersen synovectomy
S.-Petersen-Cave-Van Gor-
der anterolateral ap-
proach
S.-Richards instrumentation

SMO
supramalleolar orthosis
SMO plate

SMo
stainless steel and molybdenum
SMo Moore pin

Snap Lock wire/pin extractor

snapping hip

socket
variable circumference suprapatellar s. (VCSPS)

Socon spinal system

sodium
s. aurothiomalate
s. salicylate

Sofield
S. femoral deficiency tech-
nique
S. osteotomy

Sofield *(continued)*
S. pinning
S. retractor

software
Image-I analysis s.
osteotomy analysis simulation s. (OASIS)

soleus
s. complex
s. gastrocnemius

somatization

somatosensory
s. evoked potential (SEP,
SSEP)

Somerville anterior approach

SOMI
sternal-occipital-mandibu-
lar immobilization
SOMI brace
SOMI orthosis

Songer cable

Sonic Accelerated Fracture
Healing System (SAFHS)

Sonopuls

Sonotron

Sorbie-Questor total elbow system

Soren
S. ankle fusion
S. arthrodesis

S.O.S.
Segmented Orthopaedic
System

Soto-Hall
S.-H. bone graft
S.-H. maneuver
S.-H. sign

Soudre autogene

sounder
pedicle s.

sourcil in acetabulum

Souter
   S. hip procedure
   S. Strathclyde total elbow
      system
Southwick
   S. lateral slip angle
   S. screw extractor
   S.-Robinson anterior cervi-
      cal approach
space
   Barouk button s. for hallux
      valgus deformity
   costoclavicular s.
   disk s.
   epidural s.
   first web s.
   haversian s.
   hypoplastic disk s.
   increased lateral joint s.
   intercondylar s.
   intercostal s.
   intermetatarsal s.
   interosseous s's of meta-
      carpus
   interosseous s's of metatar-
      sus
   lateral joint s.
   marrow s.
   medullary s.
   midpalmar s.
   palmar s.
   Parona s.
   periaxial s.
   s. of Poirier
   popliteal s.
   prevertebral s.
   properitoneal s.
   retroperitoneal s.
   retropharyngeal s.
   subacromial s.
   subcoracoid s.
   suprasternal s.
   thenar s.
   tibiofibular s.
   web s.
spacer
   acetabular s.

spacer *(continued)*
   Telescopic Plate S. (TPS)
spanner gauge
spanning external fixator
sparing
   sacral nerve root s.
   Spartan jaw wire cutter
spasm
   carpal pedal s.
   muscle s.
   paravertebral muscle s.
   peroneal muscle s.
   retrocollic s.
   rotatory s.
   tetanic s.
   tonic s.
spatium *pl.* spatia
   s. intercostale
   spatia interossea metacarpi
   spatia interossea metatarsi
SPECT
   single photon emisssion
      computed tomography
Speed
   S. sternoclavicular repair
   S.-Boyd open reduction
Spence rongeur forceps
Spencer tendon lengthening
sphenoidal fossa
sphenopalatine ganglion block
spica cast
spicule
spike
   ball-tip s.
   endplate s.
   Glissane s.
   metaphyseal s.
   s. osteotomy
   supracollicular s. of corti-
      cal bone
spina
   s. bifida

spina *(continued)*
- s. bifida anterior
- s. bifida aperta
- s. bifida cystica
- s. bifida manifesta
- s. bifida occulta
- s. bifida posterior
- s. iliaca anterior inferior
- s. iliaca anterior superior
- s. iliaca posterior inferior
- s. iliaca posterior superior
- s. intercondyloidea
- s. ischiadica
- s. ischialis
- s. scapulae
- s. tibiae

spinal
- s. accessory nerve injury
- s. anesthesia
- s. arthrodesis
- s. axial load
- s. brace
- s. canal stenosis
- s. cord block
- s. cord compression
- s. cord–meningeal complex
- s. coronal plane deformity
- s. distraction
- s. dysarthria
- s. dysraphism
- s. evoked potential
- s. fixation
- s. fusion technique
- s. instrumentation
- s. manipulative therapy
- s. mobilization technique
- s. orthosis
- s. osteomyelitis
- s. osteotomy
- s. process apophysis
- s. rod cross-bracing
- s. stenosis
- s. transverse ligament

SpinaLogic

Spinal Technology bivalve
TLSO brace

spindle
- muscle s.

spindle *(continued)*
- neuromuscular s.
- neurotendinous s.
- s. cell
- tendon s.

spine
- anterior inferior iliac s.
- anterior occipitocervical s.
- anterior superior iliac s.
- bamboo s.
- cervical s.
- Charcot s.
- cleft s.
- coccygeal s.
- dorsal s.
- gibbous deformity of the s.
- s. of greater tubercle of humerus
- iliac s., anterior inferior
- iliac s., anterior superior
- iliac s., posterior inferior
- iliac s., posterior superior
- iliopectineal s.
- intercondyloid s.
- ischial s.
- s. of ischium
- kissing s's
- s. of lesser tubercle of humerus
- lumbar s.
- lumbosacral s.
- mandibular s.
- maxillary s.
- nasal s.
- neural s.
- obturator s.
- osteoporotic s.
- peroneal s. of calcaneus
- poker s.
- posterior-inferior s.
- s. of pubic bone
- s. of pubis
- rigid s.
- sacral s.
- sciatic s.
- s. of tibia
- thoracic s.
- thoracolumbar s.
- thoracolumbosacral s.
- tibial s.

spine *(continued)*
    trochanteric s., greater
    trochanteric s., lesser
    tuberculosis of s.
    typhoid s.
    s. of vertebra

SpineCATH intradiscal catheter

SpineVac

spinocerebellar

spinocostalis

spinoglenoid notch

splayfoot
    bunionette–hallux valgus–s.
    s. deformity

splenial

spleniserrate

splint
    Abbott s.
    Abouna s.
    acrylic cap s.
    acrylic template s.
    Adams s.
    Adjusta-Wrist s.
    Agnew s.
    Ainslie acrylic s.
    Airfoam s.
    airplane s.
    Air-Soft s.
    Alumafoam s.
    anchor s.
    Anderson s.
    ankle-foot orthotic s.
    anti-boutonnière s.
    anti–swan neck s.
    anti–ulnar deviation s.
    Asch s.
    Ashhurst leg s.
    Baldan fracture s.
    Balkan femoral s.
    banjo traction s.
    Bavarian s.
    Baylor metatarsal s.
    Bloom s.
    Blount s.
    Böhler-Braun s.

splint *(continued)*
    boutonnière s.
    Brady leg s.
    Brant aluminum s.
    Browne s.
    Buck extension s.
    Buck traction s.
    Budin hammer toe s.
    Bunnell finger extension s.
    Bunnell gutter s.
    Burnham finger s.
    Cabot leg s.
    Cabot posterior s.
    Campbell traction s.
    Capener coil s.
    Capener finger s.
    Capner s.
    Carter s.
    Clayton greenstick s.
    CMC (carpometacarpal) s.
    coaptation s's
    cock-up arm s.
    Colles s.
    compression sleeve shin s.
    Comprifix ankle s.
    counterrotational s.
    Cordon-Colles fracture s.
    countertraction s.
    Cramer s.
    cubital tunnel s.
    Culley ulnar s.
    Curry walking s.
    Davis metacarpal s.
    Denis Browne s.
    DePuy s.
    DonJoy wrist s.
    double-occlusal s.
    Dupuytren s.
    Dyna knee s.
    dynamic s.
    Easton cock-up s.
    Eggers contact s.
    elbow extension s.
    elbow flexion s.
    Engen palmar wrist s.
    Ezeform s.
    Fillauer night s.
    finger flexion s.
    flexor hinge hand s.

splint *(continued)*
>   flexor hinge s.
>   Formatray mandibular s.
>   Forrester s.
>   Fox clavicular s.
>   Frac-Sur s.
>   fracture s.
>   Framer s.
>   Freedom s.
>   Frejka pillow s.
>   Froimson s.
>   Fruehevald s.
>   functional s.
>   Funsten supination s.
>   Gagnon s.
>   Galveston s.
>   Ganley s.
>   Gibson s.
>   Gooch s.
>   Gunning s.
>   gutter s.
>   hallux valgus night s.
>   Hammond s.
>   Hexcelite s.
>   hand cock-up s.
>   hinged cylinder s.
>   Hodgen s.
>   humeral fracture abduction s.
>   Ilfeld s.
>   Isoprene plastic s.
>   Jacoby bunion s.
>   James s.
>   Jelanko s.
>   Jonell counteraction finger s.
>   Jonell thumb s.
>   Jones s.
>   Joseph s.
>   Kanavel cock-up s.
>   Kazanjian s.
>   Keller-Blake s.
>   Kirschner wire s.
>   Kleinert s.
>   knee brace s.
>   knee immobilizer s.
>   knuckle bender s.
>   Lambrinudi s.
>   Levis arm s.

splint *(continued)*
>   Liston s.
>   lively s.
>   LMB finger s.
>   long arm s.
>   long leg s.
>   McGee s.
>   McIntire s.
>   McLeod padded clavicular s.
>   magnet s.
>   Magnuson abduction humeral s.
>   malleable metal finger s.
>   mallet finger Abouna s.
>   Mason s.
>   Mayer s.
>   metal s.
>   Moberg s.
>   Mohr finger s.
>   Murphy s.
>   neutral position s.
>   occlusal s.
>   Oppenheimer spring-wire s.
>   OCL volar s.
>   open-air s.
>   opponens s.
>   Orfit s.
>   Ortho-Mold s.
>   Orthoplast isoprene s.
>   outrigger s.
>   padded aluminum s.
>   padded board s.
>   palmar cock-up s.
>   pan s.
>   Pavlik harness s.
>   pelvic s.
>   Phelps s.
>   plaster s.
>   plastic s.
>   Polyform s.
>   Ponseti s.
>   Porzett s.
>   posterior s.
>   Potts s.
>   Pro-glide s.
>   Pucci s.
>   Puth abduction s.
>   radial slab s.
>   radiolucent s.

splint *(continued)*
  resting s.
  Robert Jones s.
  Roger Anderson s.
  Rosen s.
  Russell s.
  Saturn s.
  Sayre s.
  Scott humeral s.
  Scottish Rite s.
  shin s's
  short arm s.
  shoulder spica s.
  silicone thermoplastic s.
  Simpson sugar-tong s.
  spica s.
  Stack s.
  Stader s.
  Stampelli s.
  static s.
  Stuart Gordon hand s.
  sugar-tong s.
  swan neck s.
  Swanson hand s.
  Synergy s.
  Taylor s.
  Teare arm s.
  tension night s.
  therapeutic s.
  Thomas s.
  Ticonium s.
  Toronto s.
  torsion bar s.
  traction s.
  U-s.
  ulnar deviation s.
  ulnar gutter s.
  Universal acromioclavicu-
    lar s.
  Universal gutter s.
  Urias air s.
  Urias arm s.
  Valentine s.
  Van Arsdale triangular s.
  Van Rosen s.
  Vesely-Street s.
  volar plaster s.
  Volkmann s.
  von Rosen abduction s.

splint *(continued)*
  Wanchik neutral position s.
  Weil s.
  Wertheim s.
  Wilson s.
  Winter s.
  wire s.
  wraparound s.
  wrist cock-up s.
  Zimmer airplane s.
  Zimmer clavicular cross s.
  Zollinger s.
  Zucker s.

splinted diaphragm

spondylalgia

spondylarthritis
  s. ankylopoietica

spondylarthrocace

spondylarthropathy

spondylectomy

spondylexarthrosis

spondylitic

spondylitis
  s. ankylopoietica
  s. ankylosans
  ankylosing s.
  Bekhterev (Bechterew) s.
  s. deformans
  hypertrophic s.
  s. infectiosa
  Kümmell s.
  Marie-Strümpell s.
  muscular s.
  post-traumatic s.
  rheumatoid s.
  rhizomelic s.
  traumatic s.
  s. tuberculosa
  tuberculous s.
  s. typhosa

spondylizema

spondyloarthropathy
  seronegative s's

spondylocace

spondylo construct

spondylodynia

spondyloepiphyseal dysplasia

spondylogenic

spondylolisthesis
    anteroinferior s.
    congenital s.
    degenerative s.
    dysplastic s.
    Gill-Manning-White s.
    high-grade s.
    isthmic s.
    lumbosacral s.
    pathologic s.
    postlaminectomy s.
    pathological s.
    sagittal roll s.
    slip angle s.
    symptomatic s.
    traumatic s.

spondylolisthetic

spondylolysis
    cervical s.
    contralateral s.

spondylomalacia
    s. traumatica

spondylopathy
    traumatic s.

spondyloptosis

spondylopyosis

spondyloschisis

spondylosis
    cervical s.
    s. chronica ankylopoietica
    degenerative s.
    lumbar s.
    rhizomelic s.
    Scheuermann dystrophic s.
    thoracolumbar s.
    s. uncovertebralis

spondylosyndesis

spondylotic

spondylotomy

spondylous

spongiosa
    s. screw

spongiosaplasty

Sponsel oblique osteotomy

Spontak pedicle screw

spoon
    meniscal s.

Sportono hip prosthesis

spot
    café au lait s.
    Carleton s's
    de Morgan s.

sprain
    inversion ankle s.
    rider's s.
    Schlatter s.
    syndesmotic s.
    talocrural s.
    talonavicular s.

spray
    low-pressure plasma s.
    (LPPS)

Spratt bone curet

spreader
    Beeson cast s.
    Bobechko s.
    Burford-Finochietto rib s.
    cast s.
    Harrington s.
    rib s.

Sprengel deformity

Springlite G foot component

sprinter's fracture

spur
    acromial s.
    bone s.

spur *(continued)*
    calcaneal s.
    cartilaginous s.
    chondroosseous s.
    fibrous s.
    Haglund s.
    heel s.
    occipital s.
    olecranon s.
    osteophytic s.
    spondylotic s.
    subacromial s.
    traction s.
    uncovertebral s.

Spurling
    S. maneuver
    S. rongeur
    S. test
    S.-Kerrison rongeur forceps

Spurway syndrome

square-shaped wrist test

squeeze dynamometer

S-ROM hip prosthesis

SRS injectable cement

SSEP
    somatosensory evoked potential

SSI
    segmental spinal instrumentation

stabilimeter

stability
    knee s.

stabilizer
    Palumbo ankle s.

stabilometry

Stableloc II external fixator system

Stack splint

Stader splint

Stamm
    S. metatarsal osteotomy

Stamm *(continued)*
    S. procedure for intraarticular hip fusion

Stampelli splint

stand
    Cherf cast s.

Stanmore replacement

staphylorrhaphy

staple
    Ellison fixation s.
    Howmedica Vitallium s.
    Nakayama s.
    Owestry s.

stapler
    GIA s.
    S-D-sorb meniscal s.
    Wiberg fracture s.

stapling
    Blount s.
    epiphyseal s.
    percutaneous s.

Statak anchor system

station
    gait and s.

Stauffer modification

Stayfuse

STD hip prosthesis

Stedman awl

Steffee
    S. pedicle plate
    S. plates and screws for lumbar fusion
    S. screw
    S. screw plate
    S. spinal instrumentation
    S. thumb arthroplasty

Steinbach mallet

Steinbrocker
    S. classification of rheumatoid arthritis
    S. syndrome

Steindler
- S. effect
- S. elbow arthrodesis
- S. flexorplasty
- S. matrixectomy
- S. operation

Steinhauser bone clamp

Steinmann
- S. extension nail
- S. fixation pin
- S. pin
- S. pin fixation
- S. pin with Crowe pilot point
- S. tendon forceps
- S. test
- S. traction

stellate
- s. fracture
- s. laceration

stem
- calcar replacement s.
- fenestrated s.
- Natural-Hip titanium hip s.
- nonfenestrated s.
- Opti-Fix hip s.
- PCA (porous-coated anatomic) hip s.
- Richards modular s.
- Synthes s.
- Ultima calcar s.

stemmed tibial prosthesis

stenosing tenosynovitis

stenosis
- anklyosing spinal s.
- foraminal s.
- lateral recess s.
- lateral recess spinal s.
- multisegmental spinal s.
- spinal s.
- spinal canal s. (SCS)

Stenzel
- S. rod
- S. rod prosthesis

stereotaxic anterior capsulotomy

sternal
- s. approximator
- s.-occipital-mandibular immobilization (SOMI)

sternalgia

sternen

sternoclavicular
- s. joint
- s. joint dislocation
- s. ligament

sternoclavicularis

sternocleidal

sternocleidomastoid
- s. muscle

sternocostal

sternodynia

sternohyoid muscle

sternomastoid muscle

sternoscapular

sternothyroid muscle

sternotrypesis

sternovertebral

sternoxiphoid plane

sternum

stethalgia

stethomyitis

stethomyositis

Stewart-Harley transmalleolar ankle arthrodesis

Stieda
- S. disease
- S. fracture
- S. process

Stiles-Bunnell technique

Still disease

Stille
- S. bone chisel
- S. bone drill set
- S. bone gouge
- S. brace
- S. bur
- S. osteotome
- S. plaster shears
- S. rongeur
- S.-Horsley rib forceps
- S.-Luer bone rongeur
- S.-Luer rongeur forceps

Stiller rib

Stimson
- S. anterior shoulder reduction technique
- S. method

StiM system

stimulation
- antidromic s.
- direct electrical nerve s.
- electrical surface s.
- functional electrical s.
- functional neuromuscular s.
- galvanic s.
- magnetic s.
- microamperage neural s.
- repetitive nerve s.
- transcutaneous electrical nerve s.

stimulator
- AME bone growth s.
- AMREX muscle s.
- bone growth s.
- electrical bone-growth s.
- galvanic electrode s.
- interferential s.
- Masterstim interferential s.
- OrthoGen bone growth s.
- OsteoGen bone growth s.
- Osteo-Stim implantable bone growth s.
- Osteotone s. for bone union

stimulator (continued)
- REACT muscle s.
- spinal fusion s.
- Synchrosonic s.
- Z-Stim s.

stimulus
- s. artifact
- conditioned s.
- electric s.
- liminal s.
- maximal s.
- mechanical s.
- paired s.
- subliminal s.
- subthreshold s.
- supraliminal s.
- supramaximal s.
- suprathreshold s.
- threshold s.

stinger

stippling

stirrup
- Aircast S.
- Böhler s.
- Finochietto s.
- traction s.

stitch
- SCOI (Southern California Orthopedic Institute) s.

STJ
- subtalar joint

stockings
- Jobst s.

Stokes
- S. amputation
- S. operation

Stone
- S. arthrodesis
- S. bunionectomy

stone
- chalk s.

Storz
- S. oblique arthroscope

Storz *(continued)*
    S. Microsystems plate cutter
    S. Microsystems plate-holding forceps

straight leg raising (SLR)

strain
    articular s.
    compression s.
    s. gauge
    high-jumper's s.
    postural s.
    shear s.

strait
    pelvic s., inferior
    pelvic s., superior

strap
    Levine patellar tendon s.

strapping
    adhesive s.
    Gibney s.

stratum
    s. fibrosum capsulae articularis
    s. fibrosum vaginae tendinis
    s. synoviale capsulae articularis
    s. synoviale vaginae tendinis

streblomicrodactyly

Streeter dysplasia

strength
    s. against resistance
    axial gripping s.
    cervical extension s.
    hand grasp s.
    instrinsic muscle s.
    muscle s.

strephenopodia

strephexopodia

strephopodia

streptomicrodactyly

stress
    adduction s. to finger
    laxity to varus s.
    s. test
    varus/valgus s. of the elbow

stria *pl.* striae
    striae of Amici

Strickland tendon repair

stripper
    Bunnell tendon s.
    tendon s.

Stromgren ankle brace

Strümpell
    S. sign
    S.-Marie disease

Strunsky sign

Struthers
    ligament of S.

strut plate

Stryker
    S. bed
    S. cartilage knife
    S. dermatome
    S. fracture frame
    S. lag screw
    S. power instrumentation
    S. viewing arthroscope

Stuart Gordon hand splint

stump
    conical s.
    s. edema

styloiditis

stylosteophyte

subacetabular

subacromial
    s. bursa
    s. decompression
    s. impingement syndrome
    s. space

subaponeurotic
s. abscess

subastragalar
s. dislocation
s. fusion

subaxial

subcapital

subcapsuloperiosteal

subchondral

subclavicular approach

subcoracoid
s. dislocation

subcostal plane

subglenoid
s. dislocation

subilium

subluxate

subluxation
atlantoaxial s.
atlantoaxial rotatory s.
atlantooccipital s.
calcaneocuboid (CC) s.
congenital hip s.
foraminal encroachment s.
glenohumeral joint s.
hip s.
neuroarticular s.
neurofunctional s.
patellar s.
peroneal s.
radial head s.
radioulnar s.
rotatory atlantoaxial s.
sacroiliac s.
shoulder s.
subaxial s.
tibiofibular s.
vertebral s.
Volkmann s.

subluxing patella

subpatellar

subperichondrial

subperiosteal
s. dissection
s. fracture

subperiosteocapsular

subspinous
s. dislocation

substance
compact s. of bones
cortical s. of bone
medullary s. of bone
medullary s. of bone, red
medullary s. of bone, yellow
Rollett secondary s.
sarcous s.
spongy s. of bone
trabecular s. of bone

substantia
s. compacta ossium
s. corticalis ossium
s. spongiosa ossium
s. trabecularis ossium

substitute
Osteoset bone graft s.

substitution
creeping s. of bone

subtalar
s. arthralgia
s. arthrodesis
s. arthrotomy
s. articulation
s. capsulectomy
s. instability
s. joint (STJ)

subtalo
luxatio pedis s.

subtarsal

subtrochanteric

subvertebral

Sudeck
S. atrophy
S. disease
S.-Leriche syndrome

sudomotor activity

sulcus *pl.* sulci
   s. arteriae subclaviae
   s. arteriae vertebralis atlantis
   bicipital s., lateral
   bicipital s., medial
   bicipital s., radial
   bicipital s., ulnar
   s. bicipitalis lateralis
   s. bicipitalis medialis
   s. bicipitalis radialis
   s. bicipitalis ulnaris
   calcaneal s.
   s. calcanei
   carpal s.
   s. carpi
   s. costae
   costal s.
   costal s., inferior
   cuboid s.
   interarticular s. of calcaneus
   interarticular s. of talus
   intertubercular s. of humerus
   s. intertubercularis humeri
   malleolar s. of fibula
   malleolar s. of tibia
   s. malleolaris fibulae
   s. malleolaris tibiae
   s. musculi flexoris hallucis longi calcanei
   s. musculi flexoris hallucis longi tali
   s. musculi peronei ossis cuboidei
   s. musculi subclavii
   s. nervi radialis
   s. nervi spinalis
   s. nervi ulnaris
   obturator s. of pubis
   s. obturatorius ossis pubis
   paraglenoid sulci of hip bone
   sulci paraglenoidales ossis coxae
   s. popliteus femoris
   radial s. of humerus

sulcus *(continued)*
   s. of radial nerve
   s. of semicanal of humerus
   semilunar s. of radius
   spiral s.
   spiral s. of humerus
   s. spiralis
   subclavian s.
   s. for subclavian artery
   s. for subclavian muscle
   s. for subclavian vein
   s. subclavius
   supra-acetabular s.
   s. supraacetabularis
   s. tali
   s. of talus
   s. tendinis musculi fibularis longi
   s. tendinis musculi flexoris hallucis longi calcanei
   s. tendinis musculi flexoris hallucis longi tali
   s. tendinis musculi peronei longi
   s. tendinum musculorum fibularium calcanei
   s. tendinum musculorum peroneorum calcanei
   s. for tendons of fibular muscles
   s. for tendon of flexor hallucis longus muscle of calcaneus
   s. for tendon of flexor hallucis longus muscle of talus
   s. for tendon of long fibular muscle
   s. for tendon of peroneus longus muscle
   s. for tendons of peroneus muscles
   s. for ulnar nerve
   s. venae subclaviae
   s. for vertebral artery of atlas
   s. of wrist

sulfasalazine

sulfinpyrazone

Sulzer fixation

Sundt shunt

superabduction

superacromial

Super Cut laminectomy rongeur

superextended

superextension

superflexion

supergenual

SuperSkin

supination
    s.-adduction fracture
    s.-eversion fracture
    s.–external rotation
    s. of the foot
    s.-inversion injury

supinator

support
    Accu-Back back s.
    Achillotrain active Achilles
      tendon s.
    Epitrain active elbow s.
    Nightimer carpal tunnel s.
    Valeo back s.

support hose
    Venosan s. h.

supra-acromial

supraclavicular

supracondylar

supracondyloid

supracostal

supracotyloid

supraepicondylar

supraepitrochlear

supraglenoid

supramalleolar

suprapatellar

suprascapular

supraspinal ligament

supraspinatus

supraspinous ligament

sural nerve

Suretac drill and guidewire

Surgical Simplex P bone cement

surface
    anterior s. of manubrium
      and gladiolus
    anterior s. of sacral bone
    anterior s. of scapula
    anterolateral s. of humerus
    anteromedial s. of humerus
    apposing articular s.
    articular s. of acetabulum
    articular s. of atlas, inferior
    articular s. of atlas, supe-
      rior
    articular s. of head of fibula
    articular s. of head of rib
    articular s. of sacral bone,
      lateral
    articular s. of tubercle of
      rib
    auricular s. of ilium
    auricular s. of sacrum
    condyloid s. of tibia
    costal s. of scapula
    dorsal s. of scapula
    extensor s.
    flexor s.
    pelvic s. of sacrum
    posterior s. of sacral bone
    posterior s. of scapula
    sacropelvic s. of ilium
    symphysial s. of pubic
      bone
    ventral s. of scapula

surgery
    ablative s.
    anterior cervical spine s.
    anterior cervicothoracic
      junction s.
    arthroscopic laser s.

surgery *(continued)*
    cineplastic s.
    orthopedic s.

Surgibone
    Boplant S.
    S. implant
    Unilab S.

Surgicel
    S. fibrillar hemostat
    S. implant

SurgiLav Plus Hydro débridement system

sustentaculum
    s. tali
    s. of talus

Sutter-CPM knee apparatus

suture
    braided s.
    bregmatomastoid s.
    Bunnell crisscross s.
    Bunnell wire pull-out s.
    caprolactam s.
    Czerny s.
    epitenon s.
    fishmouth end-to-end s.
    s. fixation
    lambdoid s.
    Le Dentu s.
    Le Fort s.
    mattress s.
    Popoff s.

suturing
    Johnson medial meniscal s.

swan-neck deformity

Swanson
    S. carpal scaphoid implant
    S. hand splint
    S. metatarsal broach
    S. scaphoid awl

swayback

Swediaur disease *(spelled also* Schwediauer)

Swedish
    S. gymnastics

Swedish *(continued)*
    S. massage
    S. movement

swelling
    blennorrhagic s.
    joint s.

Sygen (GM-1 ganglioside)

Syme
    S. amputation
    S. operation

sympathectomy
    cervical s.

symphalangia

symphalangism

symphyseal *(spelled also* symphysial)
    s. mobility

symphysial *(variant of* symphyseal)

symphysiorrhaphy

symphysis *pl.* symphyses
    s. intervertebralis
    s. manubriosternalis
    s. ossium pubis
    s. pubica
    s. pubis
    s. sacrococcygea
    sacrococcygeal s.
    sacroiliac s.

symptom
    Trendelenburg s.

synarthrodia

synarthrodial

synarthrophysis

synarthroses *(plural of* synarthrosis)

synarthrosis *pl.* synarthroses

Synatomic total knee prosthesis

synchondrosis
    costoclavicular s.
    s. manubriosternalis

synchondrosis *(continued)*
    neurocentral s.
    pubic s.
    s. pubis
    sacrococcygeal s.
    s. sternalis
    s. sternocostalis costae primae
    s. xiphisternalis

synchrondotomy

Synchrosonic stimulator

syndactylization

syndactyly
    burn s.
    complete s.
    complex s.
    Diamond-Gould reduction s.
    incomplete s.
    reduction s.

syndesis

syndesmitis
    s. metatarsea

syndesmology

syndesmoodontoid

syndesmopexy

syndesmosis
    s. radioulnaris
    s. tibiofibularis

syndrome
    acetabular rim s.
    Adair Dighton s.
    Albright s.
    Albright-McCune-Sternberg s.
    algodystrophy s.
    anterior compartment s.
    antiphospholipid-antibody s.
    Apert s.
    Arnold-Chiari s.
    Baastrup s.
    Babinski-Frohlich s.
    Bart-Pumphrey s.

syndrome *(continued)*
    Behçet s.
    benign hypermobility s.
    Bertolotti s.
    bilateral chronic radicular s.
    Brown-Séquard s.
    camptomelic s.
    carpal tunnel s. (CTS)
    cauda equina s.
    cervicogenic s.
    chronic back pain s. (CHPS)
    compartment s.
    Conradi s.
    Conradi-Hünermann s.
    Crow-Fukase s.
    Currarino-Silverman s.
    Cyriax s.
    de Barsy s.
    de Lange s.
    Eddowes s.
    Ekman s.
    Ekman-Lobstein s.
    entrapment s.
    facet joint s.
    failed back s. (FBS)
    failed back surgery s.
    Fanconi s.
    Felty s.
    fibromyalgia s.
    forearm compartment s.
    Fukuyama s.
    Gowers s.
    Grisel s.
    hand-shoulder s.
    Hench-Rosenberg s.
    Hoffmann s.
    Horner s.
    Horton s.
    hyperostosis s.
    hypothenar hammer s.
    idiopathic skeletal hyperostosis s.
    impingement s.
    intersection s.
    Jaccoud s.
    Kast s.
    Kearns-Sayre s.

syndrome *(continued)*
  Klippel-Feil s.
  König s.
  Kugelberg-Welander s.
  Larsen s.
  lateral patellar compres-
    sion s.
  Legg-Calvé-Perthes s.
  Leriche s.
  levator scapulae s.
  Leyden-Möbius s.
  Lobstein s.
  Looser-Milkman s.
  lumbago–mechanical insta-
    bility s.
  lupuslike s.
  McCune-Albright s.
  Maffucci s.
  Marie-Bamberger s.
  Martorell s.
  mechanical low back
    pain s.
  Melnick-Fraser s.
  metatarsal overload s.
  microgeodic s.
  Milkman s.
  Morton s.
  nail-patella s.
  osteoporosis pseudo-
    glioma s.
  os trigonum s.
  Ostrum-Furst s.
  overlap s.
  painful arc s.
  Pancoast s.
  patellar malalignment s.
  Pellegrini-Stieda s.
  PEP s.
  peroneal compartment s.
  pes anserinus s.
  plica s.
  POEMS s.
  popliteal pterygium s.
  Porak-Durante s.
  pronator teres s.
  Reichel s.
  Rust s.
  scalenus anticus s.
  scapulocostal s.

syndrome *(continued)*
  Schanz s.
  shoulder-hand s.
  Shy-Magee s.
  Silfverskiöld s.
  Silverman s.
  Sjögren s.
  skeletal hyperostosis s.
  SLE-like s.
  slipping rib s.
  Spurway s.
  Steinbrocker s.
  straight back s.
  subacromial impinge-
    ment s.
  Sudeck-Leriche s.
  supraspinatus s.
  Takayasu s.
  tensor fascia lata s.
  tethered cord s.
  Thiele s.
  Thiemann s.
  thoracic inlet s.
  thoracic outlet s.
  Touraine-Solente-Golé s.
  traumatic compartment s.
  Turner s.
  ulnar cubital tunnel s.
  ulnar nerve entrapment s.
  ulnocarpal abutment s.
  van Buchem s.
  van der Hoeve s.
  VATER s.
  Volkmann s.
  Wallenberg s.
  Weber s.
  Welander s.
  Wilkie s.
  Wohlfart-Kugelberg-Welan-
    der s.
  wrist pain s.

synergist

Synergy
  S. neurostimulation system
  S. splint
  S. system
  S. titanium posterior spinal
    system

synosteotic

synosteotomy

synostosis
  cervical s.
  congenital radiolunar s.
  fibula protibial s.
  radioulnar s.
  tarsal s.
  tibial-profibular s.

synostotic

synovectomy
  arthroscopic s.
  carpal s.
  palmar s.
  Porter-Richardson-Vainio s.
  radiation s.
  radioisotope s.
  Smith-Petersen s.
  volar s.
  Wilkinson s.

synovia

synovial
  s. cavity
  s. frond
  s. herniation
  s. joint
  s. membrane

synovialis

synovialoma

synovianalysis

synovin

synovioblast

synoviocyte

synovioma
  benign s.
  malignant s.

synoviorthesis

synoviosarcoma

synoviparous

synovitis
  bursal s.
  crystal-induced s.
  dendritic s.
  dry s.
  extraarticular pigmented
    villonodular s.
  florid s.
  fungous s.
  hypertrophic s.
  localized nodular s.
  monarticular s.
  parapatellar s.
  particulate s.
  pigmented villonodular s.
  proliferative s.
  purulent s.
  reactive s.
  recurrent s.
  serous s.
  s. sicca
  silicone s.
  simple s.
  tendinous s.
  vaginal s.
  vibration s.
  villonodular s.

synovium
  opaque s.

synphalangism

syntaxis

syntenosis

Synthes
  S. CerviFix system
  S. compression hip screw
  S. dorsal distal radius plate
    system
  S. Microsystem plate-hold-
    ing forceps
  S. Microsystem plate cutter
  S. pie plate
  S. Schuhli implant system
  S. stem
  S. USS (universal spinal
    system)
  S. wire guide

syntripsis

Synvisc

system
Accu-Flo ultrafiltration s.
Acculength arthroplasty
measuring s.
achilleocalcaneal plantar s.
Acufex MosaicPlasty com-
prehensive s.
Agee carpal tunnel re-
lease s.
Agee WristJack fracture re-
duction s.
Allo-Pro hip s.
Alta modular trauma s.
Amplatz anchor s.
Anametric total knee s.
Andersson hip status s.
anterior locking plate s.
(ALPS)
antimigration s. (AMS)
Apollo DXA bone densito-
metry s.
Apollo hip s.
Apollo knee s.
Arthro-Flo arthroscopic ir-
rigation s.
Arthro-Lok s.
articular ligamentous s.
Artisan cement s.
Asnis 3 cannulated screw s.
Axiom modular knee s.
AxyaWeld J-tip suture
welding s.
BacFix s.
BAK/C cervical interbody
fusion s.
BAK interbody fusion s.
Bassett electrical stimula-
tion s.
Becker orthopedic spinal s.
(BOSS)
BIAS total hip s.
Biomet Maxim knee s.
Biomet metal-on-metal ar-
ticulation hip s.
Boston Classification S.

system (continued)
Bridge hip s.
BTM hip s.
BWM (Bad Wildungen
Metz) spine s.
CAPIS bone plate s.
Cervi-Fix s.
Chiba spine s.
Chonstruct chondral re-
pair s.
Coblation-based spinal sur-
gery s.
ConstaVac autoreinfu-
sion s.
Contact SPH cup s.
Continuum knee s.
Coombs bone biopsy s.
cruciate condylar knee s.
C-Tek anterior cervical
plate s.
d'Aubigné hip status s.
Duracon total knee s.
Dyonics Access 15 arthro-
scopic fluid irrigation s.
EBI Xfix DynaFix S.
ElastaTrac home lumbar
traction s.
Endius Endoscopic
Access S.
Endotrac blade s.
E-series hip s.
Extend total hip s.
Fenlin total shoulder s.
Ficat-Marcus grading s.
Foundation total hip s.
Foundation total knee s.
Friatec manual arthrosco-
py s.
Global Fx shoulder frac-
ture s.
Hall modular acetabular
reamer s.
haversian s.
Hermes total knee s.
HJD total knee s.
Hock-Bowen cement re-
moval s.
Howmedica knee s.

system *(continued)*

   Howmedica microfixation s.
   Howmedica total ankle s.
   Indiana Tome s.
   In-Fast bone screw s.
   InFix interbody fusion s.
   In-Tac bone-anchoring s.
   Intermedics natural hip s.
   interstitial s.
   Isola fixation s.
   Isola spinal instrumenta-
      tion s.
   IsoMed infusion s.
   locomotor s.
   Malcolm-Lynn spinal re-
      traction s.
   Mallory-Head modular cal-
      car s.
   Mattrix spinal cord stimula-
      tion s.
   Maxim knee s.
   Medtronic spinal stimula-
      tion s.
   Moore hip endoprosthes-
      is s.
   Natural-Knee II s.
   Navitrack 3-D surgical guid-
      ance s.
   NC-stat nerve conduction
      monitoring s.
   NexGen complete knee s.
   Olerud pedicle fixation s.
   Omega compression hip
      screw s.
   OnTrack knee brace s.
   Optetrak total knee re-
      placement s.
   Opti-Fix total hip s.
   OrthoPak bone growth
      stimulator s.
   OssaTron orthopedic extra-
      corporeal shock wave s.
   osteochondral autograft
      transfer s.
   ParaMax ACL guide s.
   PCA (porous-coated ana-
      tomic) primary total
      knee s.

system *(continued)*

   PCA (porous-coated ana-
      tomic) Universal total
      knee instrument s.
   PEAK anterior compression
      plate s.
   PEAK channeled plate s.
   PEAK fixation s.
   PEC modular total knee s.
   PEC total hip s.
   pedicle screw s.
   PGP flexible nail s.
   PGR cemented modular s.
   Pinn ACL (anterior cruciate
      ligament) guide s.
   Polarus Plus humeral fixa-
      tion s.
   Profore four-layer bandag-
      ing s.
   Protector meniscus sutur-
      ing s.
   Pylon intramedullary nail s.
   QuadraCut ACL shaver s.
   Quick Tack fixation s.
   RadioLucent wrist fixa-
      tion s.
   Revelation hip s.
   Richards hip endopros-
      thesis s.
   Richards modular hip s.
   Rogozinski screw s.
   Rogozinski spinal fixation s.
   Rossiter S. *(stretching pro-*
      gram)
   Sabolich socket s.
   Scorpio total knee s.
   S-D-sorb E-Z Tac s.
   Segmented Orthopaedic S.
      (S.O.S.)
   Simal cervical stabiliza-
      tion s.
   SITEtrac spinal surgery s.
   skeletal s.
   Socon spinal s.
   Sonic Accelerated Fracture
      Healing S. (SAFHS)
   Sorbie-Questor total el-
      bow s.

system *(continued)*
>   Souter Strathclyde total elbow s.
>   Stableloc II external fixator s.
>   Statak anchor s.
>   StiM s.
>   SurgiLav Plus Hydro débridement s.
>   Synergy s.
>   Synergy neurostimulation s.
>   Synergy titanium posterior spinal s.
>   Synthes CerviFix s.
>   Synthes dorsal distal radius plate s.
>   Synthes Schuhli implant s.
>   Synthes USS (universal spinal s.)
>   T s.
>   Telescopic Plate Spacer (TPS) spinal s.
>   total hip s.
>   total knee s.
>   TransFix ACL s.
>   TriFix spinal instrumentation s.
>   True/Fit femoral intramedullary rod s.
>   True/Flex intramedullary rod s.
>   True/Lok external fixator s.
>   triad s.
>   Ulson fixator s.
>   Ultima hip replacement s.
>   Ultimax distal femoral intramedullary rod s.

system *(continued)*
>   Ultra-Drive bone cement removal s.
>   Ultra-X external fixation s.
>   Universal spine s.
>   Versalok low back fixation s.
>   Versalok low-back fusion s.
>   Versa-Trac lumbar retractor s.
>   Versys hip s.
>   Vertetrac ambulatory traction s.
>   Vilex cannulated screw s.
>   Wagner revision hip s.
>   WalkAide s.
>   WATSMART stereography s.
>   Wiltse pedicle screw fixation s.
>   Wrightlock s.
>   Wrightlock posterior fixation s.
>   Xact ACL graft-fixation s.
>   Xia hook/spinal s.
>   Zickel fracture classification s.
>   Zimmer anatomic hip prosthesis s.
>   Zone Specific II meniscal repair s.
>   ZPLATE-ATL anterior spinal fixation s.

systema
>   s. skeletale

systremma

T
T buttress plate
T-handled awl
T score
T system

tabatière anatomique

tabetic foot

table
Berstein cast t.
hydromassage t.
tilt t.

Tachdjian pin

Tacoma sacral plate

tail
occult t.

tailor
t's ankle
t's bunionectomy

Takahashi forceps

Takayasu
T. arteritis
T. disease
T. syndrome

talalgia

talar
t. axis–first metatarsal
base angle (TAMBA)
t. neck

tali (*plural of* talus)

taliped

talipedic

talipes
t. calcaneocavus
t. calcaneovalgus
t. calcaneovarus
t. calcaneus
t. cavovalgus
t. cavovarus
t. cavus
congenital t. equinovarus

talipes *(continued)*
t. equinovalgus
t. equinovarus
t. equinus
t. planovalgus
t. valgus
t. varus

talipomanus

talocalcaneal
t. fusion

talocalcanean

talocrural
t. fusion

talofibular

talonavicular

taloscaphoid

talotibial

talus *pl.* tali

Tamarack flexure joint

TAMBA
talar axis–first metatarsal
base angle

tank
Hubbard t.

Taperloc femoral component

tapir
bouche de t.

tapotement

TARA
total articular replacement
arthroplasty

tarsal

tarsalgia

tarsalia

tarsalis

tarsectomy

tarsectopia

tarsoclasis

tarsomegaly

tarsometatarsal

tarsophalangeal

tarsoptosis

tarsotarsal

tarsotibial

tarsus
- bony t.
- t. osseus

Taylor
- T. apparatus
- T. back brace
- T. splint

T buttress plate

TCA
- transcondylar axis

TCFO placement wand

T-C pin cutter

Teale
- T. amputation
- T. operation

tear
- anterior horn meniscal t.
- bucket-handle t. of meniscus
- meniscal lateral t.
- meniscal radial t.
- meniscal transverse t.
- oblique meniscal t.
- rotator cuff t.

Teare arm splint

technique
- accessory movement t.
- active release t. (ART)
- adduction traction t.
- Alanson amputation t.
- Alexander t.
- Allgower suture t.
- Amspacher-Messenbaugh t.

technique *(continued)*
- Amstutz resurfacing t.
- Anderson screw placement t.
- anterior iliofemoral t.
- Armistead t.
- Aronson-Prager t.
- Asnis t.
- Bailey-Badgley t.
- Bauer-Tondra-Trusler t.
- Beall-Webel-Bailey t.
- Bell-Tawse open reduction t.
- biframed distraction t.
- Bohlman cervical fusion t.
- Bohlman triple wire t.
- Borggreve-Hall t.
- Brackett-Osgood-Putti-Abbott t.
- Brooks-Seddon transfer t.
- Buncke t.
- Bunnell atraumatic t.
- Bunnell tendon transfer t.
- Burkhalter transfer t.
- Caldwell-Durham flatfoot t.
- Capello t.
- Carnesale t.
- Cave-Rowe shoulder dislocation t.
- Chaves-Rapp muscle transfer t.
- Childress ankle fixation t.
- Chow t.
- Cox flexion-distraction t.
- Crawford-Marxen-Osterfeld t.
- Debeyre-Patte-Elmelik rotator cuff t.
- DePalma modified patellar t.
- Deyerle femoral fracture t.
- DuVries t. for overlapping toe
- Eftekhar broken femoral stem t.
- Eggers tendon transfer t.
- Ellison lateral knee t.
- Essex-Lopresti calcaneal fracture t.

technique *(continued)*
- Evans ankle reconstruction t.
- extremity mobilization t.
- facet excision t.
- Fowles dislocation t.
- Gallie wiring t.
- Ganley t.
- Garceau tendon t.
- Hardinge t.
- Hassmann-Brunn-Neer elbow t.
- Hauser patellar realignment t.
- Jones-Brackett t.
- Kapel elbow dislocation t.
- Kaufmann t.
- Kellogg-Speed fusion t.
- Kumar spica cast t.
- Lambrinudi triple arthrodesis
- Lapidus hammertoe t.
- Leadbetter t.
- McFarland t.
- McKeever-Buck elbow t.
- Moe scoliosis t.
- Matti-Russe t.
- Neviaser acromioclavicular t.
- Ober tendon t.
- Orr t.
- Palmer-Widen shoulder t.
- pants-over-vest t.
- Parrish-Mann hammertoe t.
- Perry-Nickel t.
- Perry-Robinson cervical t.
- Ralston-Thompson pseudarthrosis t.
- Schnute wedge resection t.
- Scuderi t.
- Slocum fusion t.
- Sofield femoral deficiency t.
- spinal fusion t.
- spinal mobilization t.
- Stiles-Bunnell t.
- Stimson anterior shoulder reduction t.
- transfer t.
- Trueta t.

technique *(continued)*
- unlocking spiral t.
- volar plate arthroplasty t. for fracture-dislocation
- Wagoner cervical t.
- Watson t.
- Watson-Cheyne t.
- Weaver-Dunn acromioclavicular t.
- Weber-Brunner-Freuler-Buizy t.
- Weckesser t.
- Westin-Soto-Hall patellar t.
- Whitesides-Kelly cervical t.
- Windson-Insall-Vince grafting t.
- Winograd t. for ingrown nail
- Wirth-Jager tendon t.
- Zariczny ligament t.

technology
- Coblation t.

Teevan law

Teflon cannula

Tegaderm dressing

Tegtmeir elevator

Telescopic Plate Spacer (TPS) spinal system

telophragma

template
- acetabular cup t.

temporomandibular joint (TMJ)

tenaculum
- t. tendinum

tenalgia

tendines

tendinitis
- Achilles t.
- biceps t.
- calcific t.
- de Quervain t.
- digital flexor t.
- infrapatellar t.

tendinitis *(continued)*
    t. ossificans traumatica
    patellar t.
    peroneal t.
    rotator cuff t.
    t. stenosans
    stenosing t.
    ulnar wrist extensor t.
    wrist extensor t.
    wrist flexor t.

tendinoplasty

tendinosuture

tendinous

tendo
    t. Achillis
    t. calcaneus
    t. conjunctivus
    White-Kraynick t. calcaneus

tendolysis

tendomucin

tendon
    accessory communica-
      ting t.
    Achilles t. (AT)
    anterior patellar t.
    biceps brachii t.
    biceps femoris t.
    calcaneal t.
    common t.
    conjoined t.
    conjoint t.
    digital extensor t.
    digital flexor t.
    digiti quinti proprius t.
    EHL t.
    elbow extensor t.
    extensor hallucis longus
      (EHL) t.
    extensor quinti t.
    flexor profundus t.
    hamstring t.
    t. of Hector
    heel t.
    inferior patellar t.
    t. lengthening operation
    lumbrical t.

tendon *(continued)*
    membranaceous t.
    midpatellar t.
    palmaris longus t.
    patelloquadriceps t.
    peroneus longus t.
    peroneus tertius t.
    plantaris t.
    popliteal t.
    pulled t.
    riders' t.
    sartorius t.
    t. stripper
    t. transfer

tendonitis

tendopathy
    plantar t.

tendoplasty

tendosynovitis

tendovaginal

tendovaginitis

tenectomy

tenodesis
    Andrews iliotibial band t.
    Andrews lateral t.
    anterolateral femorotibial
      ligament t.
    calcaneal t.
    t. effect
    Eggers t.
    Ellison iliotibial band t.
    Evans t.
    extensor t.
    femorotibial ligament t.
    Fowler t.
    hallucis brevis t.
    iliotibial band t.
    Müller anterolateral fem-
      orotibial ligament t.
    Perry-O'Brien-Hodgson trip-
      le t.
    semitendinosus t.
    Watson-Jones ankle t.
    Westin-Hall t.

tenodynia

tenolysis

tenomyoplasty

tenomyotomy

tenonectomy

tenonitis

tenonostosis

tenontagra

tenontitis
    t. prolifera calcarea

tenontodynia

tenontography

tenontolemmitis

tenontology

tenontomyoplasty

tenontomyotomy

tenontophyma

tenontoplasty

tenontothecitis

tenophyte

tenoplastic

tenoplasty

tenorrhaphy

tenositis

tenostosis

tenosuture

tenosynitis

tenosynovectomy
    flexor t.

tenosynovitis
    t. acuta purulenta
    adhesive t.
    t. crepitans
    de Quervain stenosing t.
    gonococcic t.
    gonorrheal t.

tenosynovitis *(continued)*
    t. granulosa
    t. hypertrophica
    nodular t.
    t. serosa chronica
    t. stenosans
    stenosing t.
    tuberculous t.
    villonodular t.
    villous t.

tenotomy
    Achilles t.
    extensor t.
    flexor t.
    Fowler central slip t.
    percutaneous t.
    semiopen sliding t.
    Veleanu-Rosianu-Ionescu
        adductor t.

tenovaginitis

tension
    muscular t.

tensor

Tenzel elevator

TEPP repair

Teq-Trode electrode

test
    abduction t.
    abduction contracture t.
    Access Ostase blood t.
    Achilles squeeze t.
    acromioclavicular shear t.
    active drawer t.
    active Lachman t.
    active pivot shift t.
    Adams forward-bending t.
    Adams position t.
    Adams scoliosis t.
    adduction contracture t.
    Adson t.
    Adson maneuver t.
    agility hop t.
    alar ligament stress t.
    Allen t.
    Allis t.

test *(continued)*
    Anderson medial-lateral grind t.
    Andrews anterior instability t.
    anterior drawer t.
    anterior instability t.
    anterior slide t.
    Apley t.
    Apley compression t.
    Apley distraction t.
    Apley scratch t.
    apprehension t.
    approximation t.
    Aspinwall transverse ligament t.
    augmentation t.
    axial compression t.
    axial load t.
    axial manual traction t.
    Ayres tactile discrimination t.
    Babinski t.
    ballottement t.
    Barlow t.
    Barre t.
    Bekhterev (Bechterew) t.
    Berg balance t.
    biceps t.
    biceps jerk reflex t.
    bicycle of van Gelderen t.
    bilateral straight leg raising t.
    Bousquet external hypermobility t.
    bowstring t.
    box and block t.
    Boyes t.
    brachial plexus compression t.
    brachial plexus tension t.
    Bragard t.
    Brudzinski t.
    Brudzinski-Kernig t.
    Buerger t.
    Bunnell-Littler t.
    Burns t.
    carpal compression t.
    cervical compaction t.

test *(continued)*
    Childress duck waddle t.
    Chvostek t.
    Daniel quadriceps neutral angle t.
    De Anquin t.
    de Kleyn t.
    Dellon moving two-point discrimination t.
    distraction t.
    drop arm t.
    Duchenne t.
    Dugas t.
    Dupuytren t.
    elbow jerk reflex t.
    Ely t.
    Erichsen t.
    eversion stress t.
    external rotation-abduction stress t. (EAST)
    fabere t.
    fadir t.
    Fairbanks apprehension t.
    Feagin shoulder dislocation t.
    femoral nerve traction t.
    finger-to-nose t.
    Finkelstein t.
    Finkelstein t. for synovitis
    Finochietto-Bunnell t.
    flexion-extension valgus t.
    foraminal compression t.
    forearm supination t.
    Fournier t.
    Gaenslen t.
    Galeazzi t.
    gravity drawer t.
    grimace t.
    grind t.
    Hamilton t.
    Homans t.
    Hughston-Losee jerk t.
    impingement t.
    Jackson compression t.
    jerk t.
    Lachman t.
    Lasègue t.
    lateral pivot shift t.
    leg length t.

test *(continued)*
 LEAP monofilament t.
 Lewin-Gaenslen t.
 lift-off t.
 lunotriquetrial ballottement t.
 McMurray t.
 Milgram t.
 Mills t.
 Moberg pickup t.
 Morton t.
 Noyes flexion rotation
  drawer t.
 Nafziger t.
 Ober t.
 opposition t.
 paired *t*-t.
 patellar apprehension t.
 patellar retraction t.
 patellar tap t.
 Patrick t.
 Patrick fabere t.
 pinch t.
 pivot shift t.
 posterior apprehension t.
 posterior drawer t.
 reverse Lasègue t.
 reverse Phalen t.
 rheumatoid arthritis t.
 Romberg t.
 ruler t.
 scapular approximation t.
 Slocum t.
 Slocum anterior rotary
  drawer t.
 Slocum lateral pivot-shift t.
 slump t.
 Spurling t.
 square-shaped wrist t.
 stress t.
 Steinmann t.
 supraspinatus t.
 t-t.
 talar tilt t.
 thenar weakness t.
 Thomas t.
 thumbnail t.
 torque t.
 trapeze t.

test *(continued)*
 Trendelenburg t.
 Voshell t.
 Wallenberg t.
 Watson t.
 Wright-Adson t.
 Yeager t.
 Yergason t. of shoulder
  subluxation

testing
 active motion t. (AMT)
 dynametric t.
 isometric strength t.
 shear t.

tetanic

tetaniform

tetanigenous

tetanization

tetanize

tetanode

tetanoid

tetanus
 physiological t.

tetany
 duration t.
 latent t.

Teufel cervical brace

Teurlings wrist brace

TFC
 threaded fusion cage
  Ray TFC

T-foam pad

T-handled awl

Tharies femoral component

theca
 digital t.

thecitis

thecostegnosis

thenal

thenar
    t. weakness test

theory
    sliding filament t.

Theradapt

Thera-Med cold pack

therapist
    physical t.

therapy
    corrective t.
    diathermic t.
    fomentation t.
    heat t.
    physical t.
    short wave t.
    solar t.
    spinal manipulative t.

Thermaphore heat pack

thermatology

thermomassage

thermopenetration

thermophore

Thermoskin brace

thermosystaltic

thermosystaltism

thermotherapy

thermotonometer

Thiele syndrome

Thiemann
    T. disease
    T. syndrome

Thiersch wire

thigh
    cricket t.

Thomas
    T. cervical collar brace
    T. collar
    T. collar cervical orthosis

Thomas (continued)
    T. Kodel sling
    T. sign
    T. splint
    T. test
    T. walking caliper

Thompson
    T. prosthesis
    T. sign
    T. telescoping V osteotomy

thoracalgia

thoracic
    t. facet
    t. facet fusion

thoracispinal

thoracocyllosis

thoracocyrtosis

thoracodynia

thoracolumbar

thoracomyodynia

thorax
    barrel-shaped t.
    pyriform t.

Thornton nail plate

THR
    total hip replacement

thrombophlebitis
    femoroiliac t.

thrombosis
    deep venous t. (DVT)

thrust
    paraspinal t.
    spinal t.

thrypsis

thumb
    bifid t.
    t.-in-palm deformity
    tennis t.

Ti-Bac acetabular component

tibia
    infantile t. vara (ITV)
    saber t.
    saber-shaped t.
    t. valga
    t. vara

tibiad

tibial

tibiale
    t. externum
    t. posticum

tibialgia

tibialis

tibiocalcanean

tibiofemoral

tibiofibular

tibionavicular

tibioperoneal

tibioscaphoid

tibiotarsal

tic
    rotatory t.

Ticonium splint

Tietze disease

Tillaux fracture

tilt
    sacral t.

time
    apex t.

Tinel sign

Tinetti gait assessment

tip
    t. of sacral bone
    Woodruff t.

Tisseel cement

tissue
    bony t.

tissue *(continued)*
    bursal t.
    cancellous t.
    compact t.
    granulation t.
    hypertrophic granulation t.
    myeloid t.
    necrotic t.
    neural t.
    osseous t.
    osteogenic t.
    osteoid t.
    skeletal t.

Tivanium cancellous bone
  screw

TKR
    total knee replacement

TLSO
    thoracolumbosacral ortho-
      sis
        TLSO brace

TMA
    transmalleolar axis
        TMA-thigh angle
    true metatarsus adductova-
      rus
    true metatarsus adductus

TMJ
    temporomandibular joint

toe
    claw t.
    fifth t.
    first t.
    fourth t.
    great t.
    hammer t.
    little t.
    mallet t.
    Morton t.
    overlapping t.
    pigeon t.
    t. plate
    t. plate extension
    second t.
    third t.
    upgoing t.

Tomasini brace

tomography
    helical compound t.
    hypocycloidal ankle t.
    single photon emisssion
        computed t. (SPECT)

Tom Smith arthritis

tone
    t.-reducing ankle-foot or-
        thosis (TRAFO)

tongs
    Gardner-Wells t.
    skull t.

tonic

tonus

tool
    Surgical Anatomy Visualiza-
        tion and Navigation T's
        (SAVANT)

tooth
    t. of axis
    t. of epistropheus

tophaceous

tophus *pl.* tophi
    gouty t.

Torg knee reconstruction

Toronto
    T. Legg-Perthes orthosis
    T. splint

TORP
    total ossicular replacement

torque
    rotatory t.
    t. test

torsionometer

torticollar

torticollis
    congenital t.
    dermatogenic t.

torticollis *(continued)*
    fixed t.
    intermittent t.
    mental t.
    myogenic t.
    neurogenic t.
    spasmodic t.
    spurious t.
    symptomatic t.

torus
    t. fracture

total
    t. articular replacement
    t. articular replacement ar-
        throplasty (TARA)
    t. elbow arthroplasty
    t. elbow replacement
    t. hip arthroplasty
    t. hip replacement (THR)
    t. joint arthroplasty
    t. joint replacement
    t. knee arthroplasty
    t. knee replacement (TKR)
    t. shoulder arthroplasty
    t. shoulder replacement
    t. wrist arthroplasty
    t. wrist replacement

Touraine-Solente-Golé syn-
    drome

Tourni-Cot exsanguinating tour-
    niquet

tourniquet
    Accuflate t.
    Esmarch t.
    Tourni-Cot exsanguina-
        ting t.

Townley
    T. femur caliper
    T. tibial plateau plate

Townsend brace

toxin
    fatigue t.

T-plasty modification of Bankart
    shoulder operation

TPP hip endoprosthesis

TPS
  Telescopic Plate Spacer

trabecula *pl.* trabeculae
  trabeculae of bone

trachelocyllosis

trachelocyrtosis

trachelodynia

trachelokyphosis

Tracker knee brace

tracking
  patellar t.

tract
  iliotibial t.
  Maissiat t.

traction
  AOA cervical halo t.
  Apley t.
  Bendixen-Kirschner t.
  Böhler tong t.
  Borchgrevin t.
  Bryant t.
  cervical t.
  cervical halter t.
  elastic t.
  Georgiade visor cervical t.
  halo-pelvic t.
  Handy Buck t.
  Logan t.
  lumbar t.
  Neufeld t.
  pelvic hyperextension t.
  Russell t.
  skeletal t.
  skin t.
  Steinmann t.
  Vinke tong t.
  Weber-Vasey t.-absorption
  Wells t.

tractus
  t. iliotibialis
  t. iliotibialis Maissiati

TRAFO
  tone-reducing ankle-foot or-
    thosis

tragopodia

training
  gait t.

transcalent

transcervical fracture

transcondylar
  t. axis
  t. fracture

transcondyloid

transducer
  rotatory-variable-differen-
    tial t.

transfemoral

transfer
  Barr anterior t.
  Brooker-James tendon t.
  Brooks-Jones tendon t.
  Brooks-Seddon pectoralis
    major tendon t.
  Bunnell tendon t.
  Eggers tendon t.
  extensor digitorum t.
  fibular t.
  His-Haas muscle t.
  Huber t. of abductor digiti
    quinti
  Manktelow pectoralis ma-
    jor t.
  Ober anterior t.
  patellar tendon t.
  opponens t.
  semitendinosus tendon t.
  tendon t.

TransFix ACL system

transhamate fracture

transhumeral

translocation
  ulnar t.

transmalleolar
  t. axis (TMA)

transmetatarsal

transmitter
  chest-band t.

transplant
  Bosworth femoroischial t.
  d'Aubigné patellar t.
  patellar t.
  Slocum pes anserinus t.

transplantar

transplantation
  femoroischial t.
  tendon t.

transradial

transsacral

transtibial

transtriquetral fracture

transverse
  t. fracture

transversectomy

transversocostal

transversotomy

trapeziometacarpal

trapezium
  t. fracture

trapezoid
  t. bone
  t. bone of Henle
  t. bone of Lyser

trapping
  Conrad-Bugg t.

trauma
  hyperflexion t.

TraumaJet

Trautmann chisel

treatment
  bone cyst t.

treatment *(continued)*
  compression rod t.
  Frenkel t.
  Keesay t.
  Klapp creeping t.
  Lerich t.
  neurodevelopmental t.
  Orr t.
  salicyl t.
  Trueta t.

trench hand

Trendelenburg
  T. gait
  T. limp
  T. sign
  T. symptom
  T. test

trephine
  bone t.
  Castroviejo t.
  Phemister biopsy t.

Trethowan metatarsal osteotomy

Trevor disease

Triad
  T. pin
  T. prosthesis

triad
  t. knee repair
  t. of skeletal muscle
  Waddell t.

triangle
  Alsberg t.
  aponeurotic t.
  cervical t.
  clavipectoral t.
  Codman t.
  deltopectoral t.
  t. of elbow
  infraclavicular t.
  Kanavel t.
  Langenbeck t.
  Petit t.
  popliteal t. of femur
  sacral t.

triangle *(continued)*
 t. sling
 von Weber t.
 Ward t.

Tri-angle shoulder abduction
 brace

tribology

triceps
 t. surae

trichterbrust

tricipital

trick knee

Tricon-M component

tricorrectional bunionectomy

TriFix spinal instrumentation
 system

trigastric

TriggerWheel wand

trigonum
 t. clavipectorale
 t. deltopectorale
 os t.

Trillat osteotomy

trimmer
 calcar t. with Zimmer-Hud-
 son shank

triphalangeal

triphalangia

triphalangism

Tripier amputation

tripod foot

tripsis

triquetral fracture

triquetrolunate dislocation

triquetrous

triquetrum

trochanter
 greater t.
 lesser t.
 t. major
 t. minor
 rudimentary t.
 small t.
 t. tertius

trochanterian

trochanteric

trochanterplasty

trochantin

trochantinian

trochiter

trochiterian

trochlea
 t. fibularis calcanei
 t. humeri
 t. of humerus
 t. muscularis
 peroneal t. of calcaneus
 t. peronealis calcanei
 t. phalangis manus
 t. phalangis pedis
 t. tali

trochoides

Tronzo elevator

tropism
 facet t.

tropometer

trough
 bone t.
 synaptic t.

True/Fit femoral intramedullary
 rod system

True/Flex intramedullary rod
 system

True/Lok external fixator system

Trueta
>   T. method
>   T. technique
>   T. treatment

Trümmerfeld line

truncate

T score (bone density measurement)

T-shaped AO plate

TSRH
>   Texas Scottish Rite Hospital
>>   TSRH double-rod construct
>>   TSRH fixation
>>   Galveston fixation with TSRH crosslink
>>   TSRH implant
>>   TSRH instrumentation
>>   TSRH plate
>>   TSRH rod fixation
>>   TSRH pedicle screw

Tsudi laminoplasty

T system

t-test

tuber
>   t. angle
>   t. calcanei
>   iliopubic t.
>   t. ischiadicum
>   t. ischiale
>   t. radii
>   t. of radius
>   sciatic t.

tubercle
>   adductor t. of femur
>   t. of anterior scalene muscle
>   t. of atlas, anterior
>   t. of atlas, posterior
>   brachial t. of humerus
>   calcaneal t.
>   carotid t.

tubercle *(continued)*
>   cervical t's
>   t. of cervical vertebrae, anterior
>   t. of cervical vertebrae, posterior
>   Chassaignac t.
>   Chaput t.
>   conoid t.
>   deltoid t.
>   dorsal t. of radius
>   t. of fibula, posterior
>   greater t. of calcaneus
>   t. of greater multangular bone
>   t. of humerus
>   t. of humerus, anterior, of Meckel
>   t. of humerus, anterior, of Weber
>   t. of humerus, external
>   t. of humerus, greater
>   t. of humerus, internal
>   t. of humerus, lesser
>   t. of humerus, posterior
>   t. of Humphrey, inferior
>   t. of Humphrey, superior
>   iliac t.
>   iliopectineal t.
>   iliopubic t.
>   infraglenoid t.
>   intercondylar t.
>   intercondylar t., lateral
>   intercondylar t., medial
>   lateral t. of posterior process of talus
>   lesser t. of calcaneus
>   Lisfranc t.
>   Lister t.
>   mammillary t.
>   medial t. of posterior process of talus
>   muscular t. of atlas
>   t. of navicular bone
>   nuchal t.
>   obturator t., anterior
>   obturator t., posterior
>   plantar t.
>   pubic t. of pubic bone

tubercle *(continued)*
  quadrate t. of femur
  t. of rib
  scalene t.
  t. of scaphoid bone
  superior t. of Henle
  supraglenoid t.
  t. of tibia
  transverse t. of fourth tar-
    sal bone
  t. of trapezium
  t. of ulna
  t's of vertebra
  Wagstaffe t.

tuberculosis
  spinal t.
  t. of spine

tuberculum
  t. adductorium femoris
  t. anterius atlantis
  t. anterius vertebrae cervi-
    calis
  t. arthriticum
  t. calcanei
  t. caroticum
  t. conoideum
  t. costae
  t. dolorosum
  t. dorsale radii
  t. iliacum
  t. infraglenoidale
  t. intercondylare laterale
  t. intercondylare mediale
  t. intercondyloideum
  t. intercondyloideum later-
    ale
  t. intercondyloideum medi-
    ale
  t. laterale processus pos-
    terioris tali
  t. majus humeri
  t. mediale processus pos-
    terioris tali
  t. minus humeri
  t. musculi scaleni anterioris
  t. obturatorium anterius
  t. obturatorium posterius

tuberculum *(continued)*
  t. ossis multanguli majoris
  t. ossis navicularis
  t. ossis scaphoidei
  t. ossis trapezii
  t. posterius atlantis
  t. posterius vertebrae cer-
    vicalis
  t. pubicum ossis pubis
  t. quadratum femoris
  t. scaleni [Lisfranci]
  t. supraglenoidale

tuber angle

tuber-joint angle

tuberositas
  t. coracoidea
  t. costae II
  t. costalis claviculae
  t. deltoidea humeri
  t. femoris externa
  t. femoris interna
  t. glutea femoris
  t. iliaca
  t. infraglenoidalis
  t. ligamenti coracoclavicu-
    laris
  t. musculi serrati anterioris
  t. ossis cuboidei
  t. ossis metatarsalis primi
  t. ossis metatarsalis quinti
  t. ossis navicularis
  t. ossis sacri
  t. patellaris
  t. phalangis distalis manus
  t. phalangis distalis pedis
  t. pronatoria
  t. radii
  t. sacralis
  t. supraglenoidalis scapu-
    lae
  t. tibiae
  t. tibiae externa
  t. tibiae interna
  t. ulnae
  t. unguicularis manus
  t. unguicularis pedis

tuberosity
t. for anterior serratus
muscle
bicipital t.
t. of calcaneus
t. of clavicle
coracoid t.
costal t. of clavicle
t. of cuboid bone
deltoid t. of humerus
distal t. of fingers
distal t. of toes
t. of femur, external
t. of femur, internal
t. of femur, lateral
t. of femur, medial
t. of fifth metatarsal
t. of first carpal bone
t. of first metatarsal
t. of fourth tarsal bone
gluteal t. of femur
greater t. of humerus
t. of greater multangular
bone
t's of humerus
iliac t.
infraglenoid t.
ischial t.
t. of ischium
lesser t. of humerus
t. of navicular bone
patellar t.
pronator t.
t. of pubic bone
radial t.
t. of radius
sacral t.
t. of scaphoid bone
scapular t. of Henle
t. of second rib
t. for serratus anterior
muscle
supraglenoid t.
t. of tibia
t. of tibia, external
t. of tibia, internal
t. of trapezium
t. of ulna

tuberosity (continued)
ungual t.
unguicular t.

Tubigrip dressing

tubule
T t's
transverse t.

tuft
finger t.
t. fracture
synovial t's

Tuke saw

Tuli gel-heel cup

tumor
brown t.
Codman t.
Ewing t.
giant cell t. of bone
giant cell t. of tendon
sheath
ivorylike t.
march t.
white t.

tunnel
carpal t.
cubital t.
femoral t.
flexor t.
osseous t.
radial t.
subsartorial t.
tarsal t.

Tuohy needle

Tupoplast

Tupper arthroplasty

Turco
T. release
T. repair of talipes equino-
varus
T.-Spinella tendo calcaneus
repair

turnbuckle
t. ankle brace

turnbuckle *(continued)*
    t. distractor

Turner syndrome

Turyn sign

Tutofix pin

twister
    Axel wire t.
    Mitek wire t.

twitch
    fast t.
    slow t.

twitching
    fascicular t.
    fibrillar t.

Tyrell hook

uarthritis

UCB
  unilateral calcaneal brace

UCBL
  University of California–
    Berkeley Laboratory
      UCBL foot plate

Uematsu shoulder arthrodesis

ulcer
  gouty u.
  ischemic foot u.
  stasis u.
  supramalleolar venous u.
  trophic u.

ulceration
  neuropathic forefoot u.

Ullmann line

ulna

ulnar
  u. anlage
  u. bursa
  u. cubital tunnel syndrome
  u. drift deformity
  u. hemiresection interposi-
    tion arthroplasty
  u. humeral angle
  u. nerve entrapment syn-
    drome
  u. nerve release
  u. neuropathy
  u. rasp
  u. translocation
  u. wrist extensor tendinitis

ulnare
  ligamentum collateral u.
  ligamentum collaterale car-
    pi u.

ulnaris
  extensor carpi u.
  flexor carpi u.

ulnarward

ulnen

ulnocarpal
  u. abutment syndrome
  u. arthrodesis
  u. impingement
  u. ligament

ulnohumeral joint

ulnolunate
  u. articulation
  u. ligament

ulnoradial

ulnotriquetral
  u. articulation
  u. ligament

Ulrich
  U. bone-holding forceps
  U. drill guide

Ulson fixator system

Ultima
  U. calcar stem
  U. hip replacement system

Ultimax
  U. distal femoral intramed-
    ullary rod system

ultimisternal

Ultrabrace brace

Ultra-Drive bone cement removal system

Ultraflex dynamic joint

UltraSure DTU-one

Ultra-X external fixation system

uncarthrosis

uncemented femoral compo-
  nent

unciforme

uncinal

uncinate
  u. hypertrophy
  u. process

uncinate *(continued)*
u. process fracture

uncinatum

uncovertebral
u. arthrosis
u. joint
u. spur

uncus
u. corporis vertebrae cervicalis
u. of hamate bone

undertoe

undisplaced fracture

ungual tuberosity

uniarticular

unicameral bone cyst

unicompartmental
u. knee arthroplasty
u. knee prosthesis

unicondylar
u. fracture
u. prosthesis

Uniflex
U. calibrated step drill
U. humeral nail

Unilab Surgibone

unilateral calcaneal brace (UCB)

union
bone u.
callous bone u.
delayed fracture u.
faulty u.
osteonal bone u.
Osteotone stimulator for bone u.
primary bone u.
radioulnar u., middle
secondary bone u.
slow u.
vicious u.

uniportal arthroscopic microdiskectomy

unit
BioMed TENS u.
Z-Stim 100 u.

Unitek steel crown

uniterminal

univalve cast

Universal
U. acromioclavicular splint
U. bone plate
U. distal radius fracture classification
U. drill point
U. femoral head prosthesis
U. gutter splint
U. hip prosthesis
U. instrumentation
U. modular femoral hip component extractor
PCA (porous-coated anatomic) U. total knee instrument system
U. plantar fasciitis orthosis
U. proximal femur
U. radial components
U. spine classification
U. spine system
U. two-speed hand drill
U. wire clamp

Uni-Versatil sling

unlocking spiral technique

Unna
U. boot
U. boot cast
U. paste
U. paste boot

U-osteotomy

upbiting
u. basket forceps
u. rongeur

upcut rongeur

upgoing toe

V

V blade plate
V nail plate

V1 halo ring

V40 forged femoral head

V-A alignment rod

vacant glenoid sign

vagina

v. communis musculorum flexorum
v. communis tendinum musculorum fibularium
v. communis tendinum musculorum peroneorum
v. femoris
v. fibrosa
vaginae fibrosae digitorum manus
vaginae fibrosae digitorum pedis
v. fibrosa tendinis
v. mucosa
v. mucosa tendinis
v. plantaris tendinis musculi fibularis longi
v. plantaris tendinis musculi peronei longi
v. synovialis
v. synovialis communis musculorum flexorum
vaginae synoviales digitorum manus
vaginae synoviales digitorum pedis
v. synovialis intertubercularis
v. synovialis musculorum fibularium communis
v. synovialis musculi obliqui superioris
v. synovialis musculorum peroneorum communis
v. synovialis tendinis
vaginae synoviales tendinum digitorum manus

vagina *(continued)*

vaginae synoviales tendinum digitorum pedis
v. synovialis tendinis musculi flexoris carpi radialis
v. synovialis tendinis musculi flexoris hallucis longi
v. synovialis tendinis musculi tibialis posterioris
v. tendinis
vaginae tendinum digitorum manus
vaginae tendinum digitorum pedis
v. tendinum musculorum abductoris longi et extensoris pollicis brevis
v. tendinum musculorum extensorum carpi radialium
v. tendinis musculi extensoris carpi ulnaris
v. tendinum musculorum extensoris digitorum communis et extensoris indicis
v. tendinum musculorum extensoris digitorum et extensoris indicis
v. tendinis musculi extensoris digiti minmimi
vaginae tendinum musculi extensoris digitorum longi pedis
v. tendinis musculi extensoris hallucis longi
v. tendinis musculi extensoris pollicis longi
v. tendinis musculi flexoris carpi radialis
vaginae tendinum musculi flexoris digitorum longi pedis
v. tendinis musculi flexoris hallucis longi
v. tendinis musculi flexoris pollicis longi
v. tendinis musculi obliqui superioris

vagina *(continued)*
    v. tendinis musculi tibialis
      anterioris
    v. tendinis musculi tibialis
      posterioris

vaginal
    v. hand ligament

Vainio arthroplasty

Valentine splint

Valeo back support

valga
    coxa v.
    tibia v.

valgum
    genu v.

valgus
    calcaneal v.
    convex pes v.
    hallux v.
    v. stress test
    talipes convex pes v.

Valls hip prosthesis

Valsalva maneuver

value
    mean v.

Van Arsdale triangular splint

Van Beek nerve approximator

van Buchem syndrome

van der Hoeve syndrome

Vanghetti limb prosthesis

van Ness
    van N. rotation
    van N. rotationplasty

Van Rosen splint

Vanzetti sign

vapor
    Mitek v.

vara
    coxa v.

vara *(continued)*
    infantile tibia v. (ITV)
    tibia v.

variangle clip applier

variation
    coefficient of v.
    postural v.

varicosity

Vari-Duct hip and knee orthosis

Varikopf hip prosthesis

Varney
    V. acromioclavicular brace
    V. pin

varum
    genu v.

varus
    calcaneal v.
    cubitus v.
    dynamic hallux v.
    forefoot v.
    hallux v.
    v. malunion
    metatarsus v. (MTV)
    metatarsus primus v.
      (MPV)
    v. rotational osteotomy
      (VRO)

varus-valgus
    v.-v. instability
    v.-v. stress of the elbow

vasculitis
    rheumatoid v.

vasculopathy

vasopneumatic intermittent
  compression

vastus
    v. lateralis (VL)
    v. medialis
    v. medialis advancement
      (VMA)
    v. medialis obliquus

VATER
vertebral defects, imperforate anus, tracheoesophageal fistula, radial and renal dysplasia
VATER syndrome

VAX-D
vertebral axial decompression

V blade plate

VCSPS
variable circumference suprapatellar socket

V-Echinocandin (VEC)

Velcro immobilizer

Veleanu-Rosianu-Ionescu adductor tenotomy

velocity
motor nerve conduction v.

Velpeau
V. cast
V. deformity
V. dressing
V. immobilizer
V. shoulder immobilizer
V. sling

velum *pl.* vela

Venable
V. plate
V. screw
V.-Stuck fracture pin
V.-Stuck nail

Venodyne boot

Venosan support hose

venter
v. ilii
v. scapulae

Verbrugge
V. bone clamp
V. bone-holding forceps

Verdan osteoplastic thumb reconstruction

Vermont spinal fixator

Verneuil disease

Vernier
V. caliper
V. caliper gauge

Versa-Fx femoral fixation

Versalok
V. low back fixation system
V. low-back fusion system

VersaTor tissue cutter

Versa-Trac lumbar retractor system

Verse disease

Versys hip system

vertebra *pl.* vertebrae
apical v.
arcus vertebrae
basilar v.
biconcave v.
butterfly v.
cleft v.
codfish v.
lumbar v.
lumbosacral v.
malposed v.
odontoid v.
olisthetic v.
v. plana fracture
v. prominens reflex
transitional v.
wedge-shaped v.
wedging of olisthetic v.

vertebral
v. ankylosis
v. axial decompression (VAX-D)
v. derangement
v. osteosynthesis
v. ring apophysis

vertebral *(continued)*
v. subluxation

vertebralis
arcus v.

vertebrectomy
Bohlman anterior cervical v.
cervical spondylotic vertebralis

vertebrobasilar

vertebrogenic interference

Vertetrac ambulatory traction system

VertiGraft

Vertstreken closed medullary nailing

vesalianum
os v.

Vesalius
ligament of V.

Vesely-Street splint

vessel
haversian v.

V40 forged femoral head

V1 halo ring

vibratory massage

Victorian brace

Vidal-Adrey modified Hoffman external fixation apparatus

view
Adams v.
axial calcaneal v.
Böhler calcaneal v.
Hermodsson tangential v.

Vilex cannulated screw system

Villadot prosthesis

villondoular synovitis

villus
v. synovitis

vinculum *pl.* vincula
v. breve digitorum manus
v. longum digitorum manus
vincula tendinum digitorum manus
vincula tendinum digitorum pedis
vincula of tendons of fingers
vincula of tendons of toes

Vinertia implant metal prosthesis

Vinke tong traction

Virathene jacket

Visclas orthosis

vise
AlloGrip bone v.

viscosupplementation

Vitallium
V. cup arthroplasty
V. humeral replacement prosthesis
V. implant
V. implant metal
V. plate
V. screw
V. Küntscher nail

Vitalock
V. cluster acetabular component
V. talon locking-cup hip prosthesis

VITOSS scaffold

Vitox femoral head

VL
vastus lateralis

Vladimiroff
V. operation
V.-Mikulicz amputation

VLC compression screw

VMA
    vastus medialis advancement

V-medullary nail

V nail plate

Vogue arm sling

volar
    v. angulation deformity
    v. compartment syndrome
    v. condyle
    v. epineurolysis
    v. plate arthroplasty
    v. semilunar wrist dislocation
    v. synovectomy

volare
    ligamentum carpi v.

volarward approach

Volkmann
    V. bone curet
    V. canal
    V. claw hand
    V. contracture
    V. deformity
    V. disease
    V. fracture
    V. ischemia
    V. ischemic paralysis
    V. rake retractor
    V. splint
    V. subluxation
    V. syndrome

Volkov
    V.-Oganesian external fixation
    V.-Oganesian external fixation apparatus
    V.-Oganesian-Povarov hinged distraction device

Voltaren

Volz
    V. total wrist arthroplasty
    V. wrist

vomer

von Bekhterev reflex

von Gies joint

von Lackum transection shift jacket

von Langenbeck periosteal elevator

von Recklinghausen disease

von Rosen
    von R. abduction splint
    von R. split hip orthosis

voriconazole

Voshell
    V. bursa
    V. sign
    V. test

Vostal classification of radial fracture

V-osteotomy

VOS wrench

VRO
    varus rotational osteotomy

Vrolik disease

VSC
    vertebral subluxation complex

VSF
    Vermont spinal fixator

V-shaped osteotomy

VSP
    variable screw placement
        VSP plate
        VSP plate instrumentation

wad
  flexor w.

Waddell
  W. sign
  W. triad

Wadsworth
  W. elbow approach
  W. unconstrained elbow
    prosthesis

Wagdy double-Y osteotomy

Wagner
  W. acetabular reamer
  W. approach
  W. classification
  W. external fixation appa-
    ratus
  W. line
  W. modification of Syme
    amputation
  W. profundus advancement
  W. retractor
  W. revision hip system
  W. trochanteric advance-
    ment
  W. two-stage Syme amputa-
    tion
  W.-Schanz screw
  W.-Schanz screw apparatus

Wagoner
  W. cervical technique
  W. posterior approach

Wagstaffe
  W. fracture
  W. tubercle

Wainwright plate

Waldenström disease

WalkAide
  W. system

Walldius Vitallium mechanical
  knee prosthesis

Wallenberg
  W. procedure

Wallenberg (continued)
  W. syndrome
  W. test

Walther
  W. fracture
  W. oblique ligament

Walton
  W. meniscal clamp
  W.-Liston forceps
  W.-Ruskin forceps

Wanchik neutral position splint

wand
  ArthroCare w.
  TCFO placement w.
  TriggerWheel w.

Wangensteen needle

Ward
  W. triangle
  W.-Tomasin-Vander Griend
    fixation

Warner-Farber ankle fixation

Warren-Mack rotating drill

Warren White Achilles tendon
  lengthening

Warsaw hip prosthesis

Wartenberg
  W. disease
  W. sign

Wasserstein fixation device

Watanabe
  W. classification of discoid
    meniscus
  W. pin
  W. retractor

Watco
  W. brace
  W. knee immobilizer

Waterman osteotomy

Water-Pik irrigation

Watkins fusion

WATSMART stereography system

Watson
W. scaphotrapeziotrapezoidal fusion
W. technique
W. test
W.-Cheyne technique
W.-Cheyne-Burghard procedure
W.-Jones ankle tenodesis
W.-Jones approach
W.-Jones arthrodesis
W.-Jones bone gouge
W.-Jones classification of tibial tubercle avulsion fracture
W.-Jones fracture repair
W.-Jones nail
W.-Jones reconstruction
W.-Jones spinal fracture classification

Waugh
W. knee prosthesis
W. total ankle replacement prosthesis

wave
A w.
axon w.
contraction w.
double flexion w.
excitation w.
F w.
H w.
M w.
positive sharp w.
stimulus w.

waveform
biphasic w. (*low voltage*)
bipolar IF w.
monophasic w. (*high voltage*)
quadpolar IF w.

Weaver-Dunn acromioclavicular technique

Webb
W. bolt nail
W. fixation
W.-Andreesen condylar bolt

Weber
W. classification
W. hip implant
W. humeral osteotomy
W. paradox
W. Premalok
W. syndrome
W. zone
W.-Brunner-Freuler open reduction
W.-Brunner-Freuler-Buizy technique
W.-Danis ankle injury classification
W.-Vasey traction-absorption

Webril dressing

webspace incision

Weck
W. knife
W. osteotome

Weckesser technique

Wedeen wire passer

The Wedge

wedge
w.-compression fracture
HTO (high tibial osteotomy) w.
w.-shaped osteotomy

Wegner disease

weightbearing brace

Weil
W. pelvic sling
W. splint

Weiland
W. harvesting
W. iliac crest bone graft

Weinstock desyndactylization

Weise jack screw

Weissmann
  W. bundle
  W. fibers

Weit-Arner retractor

Weitbrecht
  W. cartilage
  W. cord
  W. foramen
  W. ligament
  prismatic ligament of W.
  W. retinaculum

Weitlaner retractor

Welander
  W. distal myopathy
  W. myopathy
  W. syndrome

Weller
  W. cartilage forceps
  W. total hip joint prosthe-
    sis

Wells
  W. pedicle clamp
  W. traction

well-seated prosthesis

Wenger plate

Werdnig
  W.-Hoffmann disease
  W.-Hoffmann spinal muscu-
    lar atrophy

Wertheim splint

Wester meniscal clamp

Western
  "W. boot" in open fracture
  W. Ontario and McMaster
    University Osteoarthritis
    Index

Westfield acromioclavicular immobilizer

West Haven–Yale Multidimen-
  sional Pain Inventory
  (WHYMPI)

Westin
  W.-Hall tenodesis
  W.-Soto-Hall patellar tech-
    nique
  W.-Soto-Hall patellectomy

wheel
  Carborundum grinding w.

White
  W. epiphysiodesis
  W.-Kraynick tendo calca-
    neus

Whitecloud
  W.-LaRocca cervical ar-
    throdesis
  W.-LaRocca fibular strut
    graft

Whitesides-Kelly cervical technique

Whitman
  W. femoral neck recon-
    struction
  W. frame
  W. operation
  W. paralysis
  W.-Thompson procedure

WHO
  wrist-hand orthosis

whorl
  bone w.

whorled pattern

WHYMPI
  West Haven–Yale Multidi-
    mensional Pain Inventory

Wiberg
  W. center edge angle
  W. fracture angle
  W. fracture stapler
  W. periosteal elevator
  W. type II patellar contour

Wichman retractor

Wiet cup forceps

Wilde rongeur forceps

Wilke boot brace

Wilkie syndrome

Wilkinson synovectomy

Willauer-Gibbon periosteal elevator

Williams
W. flexion exercises
W. orthosis
W.-Haddad release

Williger
W. bone curet
W. periosteal elevator

Willis
nerve of W.

willow fracture

Wilson
W. sign
W. splint
W.-Burstein hip internal prosthesis
W.-Johansson-Barrington cone arthrodesis
W.-McKeever arthroplasty

Wiltberger anterior cervical approach

Wiltse
W. angle
W. ankle osteotomy
W. approach
W. bilateral lateral fusion
W. diskectomy
W. pedicle screw fixation system
W. system double-rod construct
W. system spinal rod
W. varus supramalleolar osteotomy

Wiltse *(continued)*
W.-Spencer paraspinal approach

Winberger sign

windowed cast

Windson-Insall-Vince grafting technique

wing
Badgley resection of iliac w.
dorsal w.
w. excision of Littler
iliac w.
lateral w. of sacrum
w. plate

Winkelmann rotationplasty

Winograd
W. matrixectomy
W. nail plate removal
W. partial matrixectomy
W. technique for ingrown nail

Winquist
W. femoral shaft fracture classification
W.-Hansen-Pearson closed femoral diaphyseal shortening

Winslow ligament

wire
bayonet-point w.
Bunnell pull-out w.
calibrated guide w.
cerclage w.
Compere w.
w.-cutting forceps
Dall-Miles cerclage w.
Drummond w.
w.-holding forceps
Ilizarov w.
interfragmentary w.
intraosseous w.
Isola w.

wire *(continued)*
    K-w.
    Kirschner w. (K-wire)
    Luque cerclage w.
    Magnuson w.
    Oppenheimer w.
    w.-pulling forceps
    Schauwecker patellar tension band w.
    sublaminar w.
    Thiersch w.
    trochanteric w.

wire passer
    Batzdorf cervical w. p.
    Wedeen w. p.

wiring
    facet fracture stabilization w.
    facet subluxation stabilization w.
    Luque w.
    oblique facet w.
    Schauwecker patellar w.

Wirth-Jager tendon technique

Wissinger rod

Wister wire/pin cutter

Wixson hip positioner

Wohlfart-Kugelberg-Welander syndrome

Wolf arthroscope

Wolfe
    W.-Böhler mallet
    W.-Kawamoto bone graft

Wolferman drill

Wolff law

Wolin meniscoid lesion

Woodruff
    W. screw
    W. tip

Woofry-Chandler classification of Osgood-Schlatter lesion

wormian bone

Wound-Evac drain

wrap
    neck w.

wrench
    Allen w.
    VOS w.

Wright-Adson test

Wrightlock
    W. posterior fixation system
    W. system

Wrisberg
    W. lesion
    W. ligament
    W. nerve

wrist
    w. brace
    w. disarticulation
    w. dislocation
    w. extensor tendinitis
    w. flexor tendinitis
    w.-hand orthosis (WHO)
    SLAC w.
    tennis w.
    total arthrodesis of the w.
    volar w.
    Volz w.

Wristaleve

wryneck

Wu bunionectomy

Wullstein drill

Würzburg plate

Wylie lumbar bulldog clamp

X
- X clamp
- X plate
- X-shaped plate

Xact ACL graft-fixation system

X clamp

Xenophor femoral prosthesis

Xeroform gauze dressing

xerography

xeroradiography

Xia hook/spinal system

XIP
- x-ray in plaster

xiphoid
- x. bone
- x. process

XiScan
- X. fluoroscope
- X. mini C-arm

XMB tibial reaming guide

Xomed drill

x-ray in plaster (XIP)

X plate

X-shaped plate

XTB knee flexion device

Y

Y
- Y axis
- Y bone plate
- Y cartilage
- Y nail
- Y-shaped plate

Yale brace

Yamada myelotomy knife

Yancey osteotomy

Yankauer periosteal elevator

Yasargil
- Y. elevator
- Y. Leyla retractor arm
- Y. ligature guide
- Y. needle holder

Y axis

Y bone plate

Y cartilage

Yeager test

Yee posterior shoulder approach

Yergason
- Y. sign
- Y. test of shoulder subluxation

Y nail

Yoke transposition procedure

Young
- Y. hinged knee prosthesis
- Y. pelvic fracture classification
- Y. Vitallium hinged prosthesis

Youngswick-Austin procedure

Yount
- Y. fasciotomy
- Y. procedure

Y-shaped plate

Y-T fracture

Yuan screw

Y-V plasty

Z
Z axis
Z band
Z disk
Z pin

Zadik total matrixectomy

Zahn
lines of Z.

Zancolli
Z. reconstruction
Z.-Losso procedure

Zang metatarsal cap

Zariczny ligament technique

Zarins-Rowe procedure

Z axis

Z band

Zeichner implant

Zelicof orthopedic awl

Zenker
Z. degeneration
Z. necrosis

Zenotech biomateral

Z fixation nail

Z-plasty
Cozen-Brockway Z-p.
Z-p. local flap graft

Zickel
Z. fracture classification
system
Z. nailing
Z. rod
Z. subcondylar nail
Z. subtrochanteric fixation
Z. subtrochanteric fracture
operation
Z. subtrochanteric nail
Z. supracondylar fixation
Z. supracondylar fixation
apparatus

Zickel *(continued)*
Z. supracondylar medullary
nail

Zielke
Z. gouge
Z. instrumentation for sco-
liosis spinal fusion
Z. pedicular instrumenta-
tion
Z. rod

Ziemssen motor point

Zimalite
Z. implant metal
Z. implant metal prosthesis

Zimaloy
Z. implant metal
Z. implant metal prosthesis

Zimfoam
Z. pad
Z. pin

Zimmer
Z. airplane splint
Z. anatomic hip prosthesis
system
Z. bone cement
Z. cartilage clamp
Z. Centralign Precoat hip
prosthesis
Z. Cibatome Cement Eater
Z. clavicular cross splint
Z. compression screw
Z. compresssion hip screw
Z. driver-extractor
Z. extractor
Z. femoral canal broach
Z. femoral canal extractor
Z. femoral condyle blade
plate
Z. fracture frame
Z. goniometer
Z. gouge
Z. impaction screw-plate
Z. knee immobilizer
Z. low-viscosity bone ce-
ment

Zimmer *(continued)*
  Z. NexGen LPS knee femo-
    ral component
  Z. oscillating saw
  Z. pin
  Z. reamer brace
  Z. rotary bur
  Z. telescoping nail
  Z. tibial nail cap
  Z.-Hoen forceps

Zimmerlin atrophy

Zinco
  Z. ankle orthosis
  Z. CAM Walker brace

Ziramic femoral head

Zirconia orthopedic prosthetic
  head

Zollinger splint

zona
  z. orbicularis articulationis
    coxae
  z. Weberi

zone
  anelectrotonic z.
  Kambin triangular wor-
    king z.
  orbicular z. of hip joint

zone *(continued)*
  peripolar z.
  polar z.
  triangular working z.
  Weber z.

Zone Specific II meniscal repair
  system

Z pin

Z-plasty
  Z-p. release

ZPLATE-ATL
  ZPLATE-ATL anterior spi-
    nal fixation system

Z-Stim
  Z-S. 100 unit
  Z-S. stimulator

Zucker splint

Zuelzer
  Z. awl
  Z. screw

zygapophyseal

zygapophysis
  z. inferior
  z. superior

zygostyle

Zyranox femoral head

Drugs Used in Orthopedics

Below are the names of generic and ℞ brand name drugs used in orthopedics, as shown in the *Saunders Pharmaceutical Xref Book*. The drugs are categorized by their "indications"—also called "designated use," "approved use," or "therapeutic action"—which group together drugs used for a similar purpose. The indications shown below are broad categories of therapeutic action. Individual drugs may be placed in subcategories or have specifically targeted diseases beyond the scope of this listing. For complete information about the drugs listed below, including each drug's availability, specific indications, forms of administration, and dosages, please consult the current edition of *Saunders Pharmaceutical Word Book*.

Anabolic Steroids [*see: Sex Hormones, Androgenic/Anabolic Steroids*]

Analgesics
Analgesics, Nonsteroidal (NSAIDs)
[*see also: Antiarthritics, Nonsteroidal (NSAIDs)*]
acetaminophen
Aclophen
Alumadrine
Amaphen
Amigesic
Anaprox; Anaprox DS
Anatuss
Anoquan
Apo-Etodolac ⊕
Apo-Ketorolac ⊕
Argesic-SA
Arthropan
Arthrotec
aspirin
aspirin, buffered
Axocet
Axotal
Brexidol 20 ⊕
bromfenac sodium
Bucet
Bupap
Butalbital Compound
carprofen
Cataflam

Analgesics, Nonsteroidal (NSAIDs) (continued)
choline magnesium trisalicylate (choline salicylate + magnesium salicylate)
choline salicylate
diclofenac potassium
diclofenac sodium
Diclotec ⊕
diflunisal
Disalcid
Dolobid
Duract
Easprin
Enable
Endolor
Equagesic
Esgic
Esgic-Plus
etodolac
Femcet
fenoprofen calcium
Fexicam ⊕
Fiorgen PF
Fioricet
Fiorinal
Fiorpap
Fiortal
Flexaphen
Gen-Etodolac ⊕
Hyanalgese-D
Hycomine Compound

Analgesics, Nonsteroidal (NSAIDs)
  (continued)
  Ibu
  Ibu-Tab
  ibuprofen
  Ibuprohm
  Indochron E-R
  Isocet
  Isocom
  Isollyl Improved
  Isopap
  isoxicam
  ketoprofen
  ketorolac tromethamine
  Lanorinal
  Lobac
  Lodine
  Lodine XL
  Magan
  magnesium salicylate
  Magsal
  Margesic
  Marnal
  Marten-Tab
  Marthritic
  Maxicam
  meclofenamate sodium
  Meclomen
  Medigesic
  mefenamic acid
  meloxicam
  Micrainin
  Midchlor
  Midrin
  Migratine
  Mobic
  Mobidin
  Mono-Gesic
  Motrin
  Mus-Lax
  Myapap
  Nalfon
  Naprelan
  Napron X
  Naprosyn
  naproxen
  naproxen sodium
  Norel Plus
  Norgesic; Norgesic Forte

Analgesics, Nonsteroidal (NSAIDs)
  (continued)
  Novo-Difenac-K ⒸⒶⓃ
  Orphengesic; Orphengesic Forte
  Orudis
  Pennsaid
  Phenate
  Phrenilin
  Phrenilin Forte
  piroxicam betadex
  Ponstel
  Prominol
  Repan
  Repan CF
  Rexolate
  Rimadyl
  Robaxisal
  rofecoxib
  Saleto-400; Saleto-600; Saleto-800
  salicylamide
  Salprofen
  salsalate
  Salsitab
  Sedapap
  sodium salicylate (SS)
  sodium thiosalicylate
  Sodol Compound
  Soma Compound
  Soma Compound with Codeine
  Tencet
  Tencon
  tenidap
  Toradol
  Triad
  Triaprin
  Tricosal
  Trilisate
  Tussanil DH
  Tussirex
  Two-Dyne
  Vioxx
  Voltaren
  Voltaren ⒸⒶⓃ
  Voltaren Rapide ⒸⒶⓃ
  ZORprin

Antiarthritics
Antiarthritics, Nonsteroidal (NSAIDs)
[see also: Analgesics, Nonsteroidal (NSAIDs)]
Anaprox; Anaprox DS
Ansaid
Apo-Nabumetone ⒸⒶⓃ
Brexidol 20 ⒸⒶⓃ
Cataflam
Celebrex
celecoxib
Clinoril
Daypro
diclofenac potassium
diclofenac sodium
EC-Naprosyn
etodolac
Feldene
fenoprofen calcium
flurbiprofen
Gen-Etodolac ⒸⒶⓃ
ibuprofen
Indocin
Indocin SR
indomethacin
ketoprofen
Lodine
Lodine XL
meclofenamate sodium
meloxicam
Mobic
Motrin
nabumetone
Nalfon
Naprelan
Naprosyn
naproxen
naproxen sodium
Novo-Difenac-K ⒸⒶⓃ
Orudis
Oruvail
oxaprozin
piroxicam
piroxicam betadex
Relafen
rofecoxib
sulindac
Tolectin 200; Tolectin 600
Tolectin DS

Antiarthritics, Nonsteroidal (NSAIDs) (continued)
tolmetin sodium
Vioxx
Voltaren
Voltaren ⒸⒶⓃ
Voltaren Rapide ⒸⒶⓃ
Voltaren SR ⒸⒶⓃ
Voltaren XR
Antiarthritics, Other
Hyalgan
hyaluronate sodium
hylan G-F 20
Synvisc

Muscle Relaxants
Muscle Relaxants, Skeletal
Anectine
Arduan
atracurium besylate
baclofen (L-baclofen)
Banflex
carisoprodol
chlorphenesin carbamate
chlorzoxazone
cisatracurium besylate
cyclobenzaprine HCl
Dantrium
dantrolene sodium
Diazemuls ⒸⒶⓃ
diazepam
Dizac
doxacurium chloride
Flaxedil
Flexaphen
Flexeril
Flexoject
Flexon
gallamine triethiodide
Lioresal
Maolate
metaxalone
methocarbamol
metocurine iodide
Metubine Iodide
Mivacron
mivacurium chloride
Mus-Lax
Myolin

Muscle Relaxants, Skeletal (continued)

Nimbex
Norcuron
Norflex
Norgesic; Norgesic Forte
Nuromax
orphenadrine citrate
Orphengesic; Orphengesic Forte
pancuronium bromide
Paraflex
Parafon Forte DSC
Pavulon
pipecuronium bromide
Quelicin
rapacuronium bromide
Raplon
Remular-S
Robaxin
Robaxisal
rocuronium bromide
Skelaxin
Sodol Compound
Soma
Soma Compound
Soma Compound with Codeine
succinylcholine chloride
Sucostrin
Tracrium
tubocurarine chloride
Valium
Valium Roche Oral ⊛
Valrelease
vecuronium bromide
Zemuron
Zetran

Osteoarthritis [see: Antiarthritics; Analgesics, Nonsteroidal]

Sex Hormones
Sex Hormones, Androgenic/Anabolic Steroids

Anadrol-50
Andro L.A. 200
Androderm
AndroGel
Androgel-DHT
Android-10; Android-25
Androlone-D 200

Sex Hormones, Androgenic/Anabolic Steroids (continued)

Andropository-200
Androtest-SL
Deca-Durabolin
Delatestryl
depAndro 100; depAndro 200
depAndrogyn
Depo-Testadiol
Depo-Testosterone
Depotest 100; Depotest 200
Depotestogen
dihydrotestosterone (DHT)
Duo-Cyp
Durabolin
Duratest 100; Duratest 200
Duratestrin
Durathate-200
Estratest; Estratest H.S.
Everone 200
fluoxymesterone
Halotestin
Hepandrin
Histerone 100
Hybolin Decanoate-50; Hybolin Decanoate-100
Hybolin Improved
Menogen; Menogen H.S.
methyltestosterone
nandrolone decanoate
nandrolone phenpropionate
Neo-Durabolic
Oreton Methyl
Oxandrin
oxandrolone
oxymetholone
Premarin with Methyltestosterone
stanozolol
Tesamone
Teslac
Test-Estro Cypionates
Testandro
Testoderm TTS
Testoderm; Testoderm with Adhesive
testolactone
Testopel
testosterone
testosterone cypionate
testosterone enanthate
testosterone propionate

Sex Hormones, Androgenic/Anabolic Steroids (continued)
Testosterone Aqueous
Testred
TheraDerm
TheraDerm-MTX
Tostrex

Sex Hormones, Androgenic/Anabolic Steroids (continued)
Valertest No. 1
Virilon
Winstrol
Steroids [see: Sex Hormones, Androgenic/Anabolic Steroids]